EBURY PRESS
THE SATVIC REVOLUTION

Subah and Harshvardhan Saraf are renowned health educators, changemakers and authors.

They both experienced chronic diseases since a young age and overcame them through the Satvic lifestyle. Their own healing journeys had such a great influence on them that they decided to dedicate their lives to sharing this timeless wisdom with the world.

Subah enriched her knowledge by learning under the guidance of various Indian masters, as well as at international institutes such as the Hippocrates Health Institute in Florida, USA. Harshvardhan, in parallel, set up holistic health clinics in Mumbai, bringing together a team of natural health doctors to provide hands-on healing.

In 2019, united by a shared vision, Subah and Harshvardhan came together to lead Satvic Movement. Ever since, they have been sharing this knowledge with people through their online videos, health workshops and books. With millions of people watching their videos and over 10,000 people joining their online workshops each month, Satvic Movement has quickly exploded into a thriving community of thousands of people across India, becoming one of the largest health revolutions in the nation.

ADVANCE PRAISE FOR THE BOOK

'For anyone seeking to rediscover joy and well-being, this book is for you. I appreciate the simplicity and relatability with which the tips are presented. My blessings to Harshvardhan and Subah Saraf for their continued good work'—Dr Hansaji Yogendra, director, The Yoga Institute

'I have known of Subah and Harshvardhan since they started their journey. I love the clarity, intensity and the simplicity of their work. In a world where disease rates are rising rapidly, this book provides a clear-cut path for anyone who wants to take charge of their health. No one should miss this'—Dr Nandita Shah, author of *Reversing Diabetes in 21 Days* and Nari Shakti Puraskar awardee

'Easy diet and lifestyle changes can revolutionize your health, and this practical book will walk you through them step by step'—Dr Neal Barnard, MD, FACC, and president, Physicians Committee for Responsible Medicine

'In a world where wellness intersects with sustainability, this book emerges as a competent guide, offering a clear-cut path towards a happier future for all'—Maneka Gandhi, politician and former member of Parliament

'I'm thrilled to see this book, which has the potential to impact countless lives, come together. I am particularly impressed by the section on sleep, which is an important aspect of integrative medicine. I love how the book focuses on circadian rhythms, along with providing simple steps to improve the quality of deep sleep. I wish them the best for this amazing initiative'—Luke Coutinho, holistic nutritionist specializing in lifestyle medicine

'This book holds the power to transform your and your family's destiny. With purity, humility and simplicity in their personality, Subah and Harshvardhan have nurtured the spirit of selfless "giving" to the world and created magical outcomes'—BK Shivani, renowned spiritual teacher

'*The Satvic Revolution* is a perfect blend of health and spirituality. This book will help millions of human beings take control of their life and happiness'—Gauranga Das, spiritual leader and bestselling author

'If health is wealth, then Satvic Movement is the golden key to the treasure trove. Subah and Harshvardhan have put together an outstanding piece of work. Each chapter sparkles in its sweetness, sharpness and simplicity. Profound knowledge is shared through examples from everyday life, insightful quotes, poems and riddles, using engaging and simple language that even a seven-year-old can understand. *The Satvic Revolution* is a book that needs to be read by one and all. Following its teachings would transform our lives and our world. This transformative, all-encompassing and universal knowledge needs to be in our educational curriculum'—Juhi Chawla, actress

THE
SATVIC
REVOLUTION

7 Life-Changing Habits to Discover Peak Health and Joy

SUBAH SARAF
AND HARSHVARDHAN SARAF

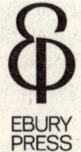

EBURY
PRESS

An imprint of Penguin Random House

EBURY PRESS

Ebury Press is an imprint of the Penguin Random House group of companies
whose addresses can be found at global.penguinrandomhouse.com

Published by Penguin Random House India Pvt. Ltd
4th Floor, Capital Tower 1, MG Road,
Gurugram 122 002, Haryana, India

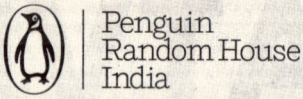

First published in Ebury Press by Penguin Random House India 2024

ISBN 9780143460381

Typeset in Adobe Caslon Pro by Manipal Technologies Limited, Manipal
Printed at Replika Press Pvt. Ltd, India

www.penguin.co.in

*For our community, the heart and soul of this revolution;
for the Satvic team, without whom this book would never
have come to life; and for our families, who have made
countless sacrifices, many of which we will never even know*

Contents

Introduction

The Untold Story of How It All Began

It was the fourth grade, and there I sat at my school desk, diligently taking my maths test. I was a studious girl with my spectacles covering half my face and my hair always tied in a tight ponytail. Growing up in the scorching summers of Delhi, our school didn't have the luxury of air conditioners, so I always had a slightly red face, perpetually sweaty from the heat.

As I focused on my exam, surrounded by pin-drop silence in the classroom, I glanced at my maths teacher sitting in front of me, her face hidden behind a giant newspaper. To my surprise, she suddenly peeked out and locked eyes with me. With a gesture, she signalled for me to come to her at the front of the classroom. My heart skipped a beat.

Pausing my maths exam, I started walking towards her, feeling a mix of curiosity and nervousness. I hadn't cheated, so why was she calling me? As I approached her table, she placed the newspaper in front of me and pointed at an article with the headline 'OBESITY EPIDEMIC on the Rise'. Initially, I didn't understand the connection. I was unsure of why she was sharing this information with me. However, her disappointment became evident as she leaned closer, whispering into my ear, 'You should lose some weight.'

Her words pierced through me. It felt like everyone in the classroom had heard her. My heart sank in embarrassment. I couldn't deny the truth—I was indeed the roundest kid in class, but no one had said it so openly before. I simply returned to my seat, holding back my tears, and hastily finished the rest of the maths exam. As soon as I was done, I gathered my books and backpack, and rushed to my van that carried me and fifteen other children home every afternoon.

That day, I chose to sit in the back seat of the van. I just wanted to be alone. But to my dismay, two older kids joined me. Once the van filled up, it launched into motion. I stared out of the window, my hands clenched tightly in my lap.

Then, suddenly, I felt a sharp kick on my leg. It was one of the boys sitting beside me. I didn't react, hoping it was a mistake.

However, my silence only seemed to fuel them more and another kick followed. Unable to control my emotions,

I screamed at them, asking why they were kicking me. They simply said, 'Because you are so fat!' Their kicks continued until I reached home.

Tired of holding back my tears, I rushed into the bathroom, locked the door and looked at my legs which were covered with the marks made by their shoes. Tears streamed down my face uncontrollably, as I kept wondering why nobody liked me.

I felt embarrassed even talking about this with anyone. I was so shy that I couldn't even discuss it with my parents, and so, I kept it to myself.

Soon after, my mum noticed that my weight was increasing, and inspired me to start exercising. She even created a whole exercise regime for me, and one of the routines I distinctly remember was climbing up and down the stairs of our home ten times. But despite all the effort, nothing seemed to work, and that's when she decided to consult a doctor.

It was during this visit that I was diagnosed with PCOD (polycystic ovarian disease) also called PCOS (polycystic ovarian syndrome), a condition that is typically diagnosed in adolescents and adult women but can, in rare cases, manifest in younger girls. The doctor explained that my body was producing excessive amounts of certain hormones, contributing to my weight gain.

He prescribed a pill, advising me to take it regularly. The idea of the pill brought me a sense of relief, thinking that I had found a solution to my weight problem. But little did I know, this was just the beginning of a tough journey.

Every few months, I was to return to the doctor for a regular check-up, and so I did. I was sitting in the doctor's office with my most recent blood work in his hand, and he told me that I had now developed another disease: hypothyroidism! As a young girl, I thought, 'I have been faithfully following the prescribed medication, so why is it that my health actually got worse?' But before I could make any sense of this, to address the new disease, I was handed another pill to be taken every day.

Despite my compliance, my weight remained stubbornly unchanged. And as the years went by, one by one, I started having more health problems. I developed acne on my face, my hair started falling at an alarming rate, and my menstrual cycles became irregular and delayed. The pills multiplied as well, with a total of four different ones to be taken each day, each representing a unique colour and purpose.

After four years of repeated visits to doctors and trying different treatments to no avail, I genuinely believed that this was how my life was going to be, that I would have to live with these problems for the rest of my life. I often felt that I was less than my peers, and gradually, I began to lose my confidence. I just felt helpless, constantly doubting my abilities in every area of life. I became painfully shy and introverted, as if I had lost a crucial part of myself along the way.

The Turning Point

I was in 11th grade, preparing for my exams, when one morning, my father rushed into my room in a state of excitement, and said, 'Subah, you and I are going to a Nature Cure camp for four days!'

'Nature Cure? Great . . . another false hope,' I thought to myself. Sceptical, I made every excuse to get out of it. However, he persisted, assuring me that this four-day health camp, led by an experienced master, held the answers to all my health problems. Reluctantly, I agreed to go.

The camp took place in a small village between Mumbai and Pune, in a modest two-storey centre. When we arrived, there was a lecture happening in a small hall on the second floor. It was led by a simple old man dressed in a white kurta. He was the master facilitating this camp. Since we were a bit late, we quietly took seats at the back of the hall.

As I looked around, everyone who had come for the camp was at least two or three times my age. I felt like an alien among them. About an hour into the lecture, I found myself yawning every few minutes. I couldn't wait for it to end. On the surface, I put on a smile, but inside, I wanted to run away from that place, back to the comfort of my home.

That night, I was so disappointed with my father for bringing me to this camp that I remember not even talking to him before going to sleep.

On the second day, there was another lecture, and I was prepared to spend the next few hours yawning again. This time, however, something the master said caught my attention. 'Behind every disease lies a cause that no drug can reach,' he proclaimed, sitting with his back erect on a small stage while speaking into a microphone. When I heard his words, something shook deep within me. It felt like for the first time, someone was telling me the truth. But at the same time, another voice inside me crept up and said, 'This is all too good to be true . . . It's not actually going to work.'

He continued, '**When your food is wrong, medicine is of no use, and when your food is right, medicine is of no need.**' He didn't use big, fancy words. He spoke in simple Hindi, in a way that even a child could easily understand.

While I strongly connected with his message, days at the camp were extremely challenging for me. Gone were the large mugs of coffee, biscuits and sandwiches I was accustomed to at home. Instead, we were offered juices and fruit bowls. My usual 10 a.m. wake-up time was replaced with 6 a.m. yoga sessions. As for the four pills I took every day, I was asked to discontinue them for the duration of the camp.

The lectures by the master lasted between four and six hours each day. He made it clear: medicine isn't real healthcare, but food is. He taught us to eat more from the earth and less from packets. He revealed that the best healer isn't found in a pill bottle but is already sitting deep within us. He showed us how most diseases begin in our gut. He even shared that we cannot have optimal health as long as we have major problems in our relationships with other people.

Deep within, I was beginning to sense a profound truth in his words. By the fourth day, I felt I had gained more practical wisdom in those few days of the camp than I had in all my eleven years of modern schooling.

Towards the end of the camp, something extraordinary happened. Just before breakfast, I stepped on the weighing scale and was surprised to see that I had lost 2 kilos. For most people, this might not seem like a big deal, but for someone like me, who had tried numerous pills, exercises and advice to shed weight, it was a massive victory. As a seventeen-year-old, it felt like my ticket to looking good and being accepted by my friends. That 2-kilo weight loss became the single biggest factor that convinced me to give this new lifestyle a chance. Little did I know that this would completely change the course of my existence.

The Twist I Never Anticipated

After returning home, I diligently put into practice the habits taught at the camp. It wasn't easy at first, but I stuck with it. I changed how I lived, from what I ate to how I started my mornings. Three months later, I took a deep breath and went in for my blood tests. When the results came, I was astonished.

- My TSH (thyroid-stimulating hormone), which had always hovered around 10–15 despite the medication, was now just 3—within the normal range!
- The PCOD, which had been a constant struggle, had healed. Earlier, I used to go six months without

getting my menstrual cycle; now I started getting them regularly without fail.

- My skin had cleared up, acne was reduced, and I no longer needed any of those ointments and creams. Even my endless hair fall finally stopped.

- And most importantly, I finally reached my optimal weight! As a result, I felt more active and started waking up each day with much more energy and excitement.

The improvements in my life went far beyond just the physical. It was as if the remote control of my health and my life, which had always felt out of reach, was now back in my own hands. I truly felt like a new Subah was born.

After my healing experience, I found myself questioning a lot of things. I wondered why there were long lines outside hospitals, yet only a handful of people at that health camp. I wondered why, if this knowledge was indeed so powerful, it wasn't reaching the masses. I wondered why, if this knowledge had existed for so many years, nobody knew about it.

I didn't have answers to these questions. However, what I heard was a small voice inside my heart which told me that it was my duty to share this knowledge with as many people as I could.

But the question was—how could I? I still had my traditional schooling to complete. How could I pursue this radical new path ahead of me while continuing my conventional education? And more importantly, where would I even start?

When I revealed this inner voice to my father, he reassured me that if this was really what I felt my life's calling was, I should pursue it, determined and unafraid. He urged me to quit my traditional education and fully commit to the new path that lay ahead. He spent countless hours crafting my new curriculum, deciding which subjects I needed to study.

That's when I immersed myself in the science of natural health, diving into books by various masters and scholars. For two years, I locked myself in a room, rarely stepping out. I lost touch with my friends but found new ones in the authors whose books filled my days. Later, I travelled to renowned health institutes across the globe, from Florida to Los Angeles, becoming a certified health educator. (For those curious about who these mentors are or which institutes I visited, a detailed list of all sources is included in the acknowledgments section at the end of this book.)

Though, throughout this period, my greatest guide and mentor remained my father. He taught me how to think, work and dream. He revealed a vision that extended way beyond my own limited perception, infusing me with the belief and spirit of this revolution.

As the years passed and my confidence grew, I felt ready to share the knowledge I had received. That's when I began creating online videos and hosting offline events in Delhi and Mumbai. On one occasion, I had the opportunity to host a workshop in Mumbai for a group of 120 people. It was during this time that another miracle followed in my journey.

How I Met Harshvardhan

The venue that I was hosting the workshop at was a beautiful health centre led by a young man named Harshvardhan.

When I met him, I was simply awestruck. He, too, had experienced the cycle of endless doctor visits, a lengthy list of medications, and no lasting results. The only difference was that, in his case, he suffered from sinusitis, asthma and psoriasis throughout his childhood. After ten years of searching for a solution, he also came across the concept of using food and lifestyle to not only reverse but also prevent disease. Within just a month of adopting these changes, he was able to breathe comfortably at night without nasal sprays, he no longer needed creams to suppress his psoriasis patches, and he regained his confidence in life.

When the two of us met each other and discussed our stories, we were surprised to find one thing in common: reversing our diseases was the *smallest* thing we gained from following our new habits. Actually, we gained our lives back. We regained our potential to dream, to grow and to truly live life. We both individually felt a fire inside us to spread this message of natural health to the world. And so, we decided to come together as one force and lead the Satvic Movement: **a mission dedicated to spreading authentic and timeless health knowledge to the world in an accessible and practical manner.**

For those of you who are not aware of the term 'Satvic', it is one of the three virtues laid out in our ancient Indian philosophies. It originates from the Sanskrit term 'Satva' and represents the mode of goodness inherent in each of us. It symbolizes purity, wisdom, compassion, clarity and joy. Adopting this way of life, or these habits, doesn't just improve our physical health—it awakens the Satva within us. Thus, the term 'Satvic Movement' perfectly captures the essence of this mission.

The Revolution Begins

It all started simply by sharing our knowledge through online videos. Little did we know that in just a few short years, Satvic Movement would rise to become one of India's largest and fastest growing health and wellness movements. Today, it's not just hundreds or thousands, but millions of people who are a part of this movement. As of 2024, over 4,00,000 individuals have learnt about the Satvic way of life through our online workshops, while the movement's digital community has expanded to more than 9 million followers.

At its core, this revolution is fuelled by people who want to lead a conscious life, not just in terms of what they put on their plate, but also in the lifestyle choices they make, the thoughts they cultivate, the relationships they create, even extending to the career choices they make. What excites us the most about this revolution is that it starts small—with each individual making a change in their own life, but its impact ripples far and wide, creating a revolution in society at large.

Why We Wrote this Book

The moment Penguin Random House India approached us in 2023 with the opportunity to write a book, we knew we wanted to share the seven life-changing habits that have transformed our lives and have the power to transform yours too.

The knowledge you'll find in this book is a culmination of both mine and Harshvardhan's life learnings, gathered from the wisdom imparted by our masters, teachers and institutes across the globe. Our role in all of this has simply been to distil this valuable knowledge into an accessible seven-habits framework. We have tried our level best to make each chapter easy to understand, interesting to read and practical to follow, even for those living a busy, fast-paced lifestyle.

While the both of us have written this book together, for the sake of simplicity and consistency, I (Subah) will be the one narrating the chapters.

Why the Seven Habits

We have come to the realization that habits are everything in life. Essentially, a habit is a routine or practice performed so often that, over time, it becomes second nature, happening almost instinctively, even without our conscious thought.

In our view, what you do repeatedly shapes who you are and what you achieve. Put simply, successful habits make up a successful life.

I am your constant companion.
I am your greatest helper or heaviest burden.
I will push you onward or drag you down to failure.
I am completely at your command.

Half the things you do, you might as well turn over to me
and I will be able to do them—quickly and correctly.

I am easily managed—you must be firm with me.
Show me exactly how you want something done
and after a few lessons, I will do it automatically.

I am the servant of all great individuals
and, alas, of all failures as well.
Those who are great, I have made great.
Those who are failures, I have made failures.

I am not a machine though,
I work with all the precision of a machine
plus the intelligence of a human.

You may run me for profit or run me for ruin
It makes no difference to me.

Take me, train me, be firm with me,
and I will place the world at your feet.

Be easy with me and I will destroy you.
Who am I?

Answer: Habit

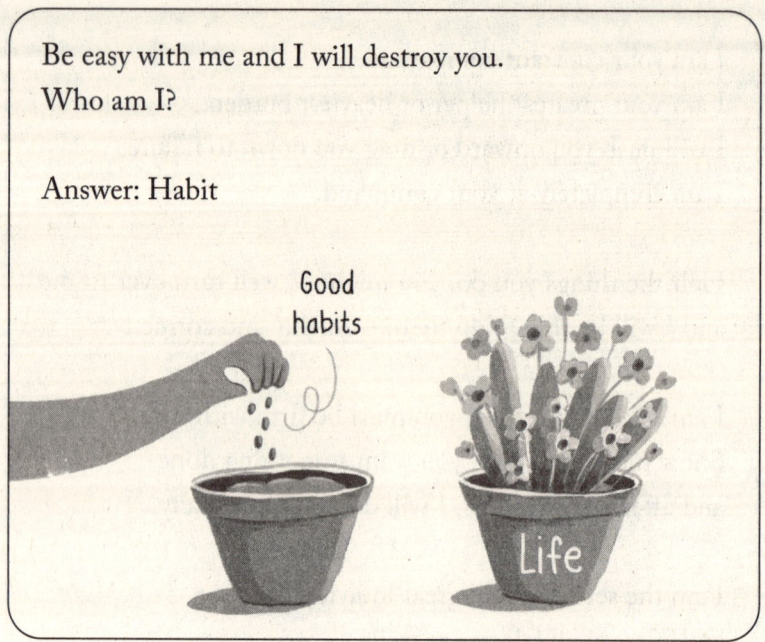

What you just read is a profound poem by an unknown author. To us, it perfectly encapsulates the idea of how powerful a habit can truly be in our lives. Throughout our journeys, whether it was to reverse our health problems, become physically stronger, live a life of optimal health, become writers or run Satvic Movement at a young age, we had to rely on strong habits. Specifically, there are seven habits that have been crucial in our journeys, and we're excited to share them with you in this book.

Before you start learning about each habit, there are three important things you need to know about them:

1. The Seven Habits Work on Raising Your Level of Health

When we share the seven habits during our seminars, people often ask us, 'Will these help with my diabetes?' or 'Will they help me with my hypertension?' This is an important question that we want to clarify.

Most chronic diseases that we suffer from today are nothing but a symptom of a fall in one's health level. To put it very simply, disease = fall in your level of health. Now, when you raise the body's health level, there is automatically no room left for disease.

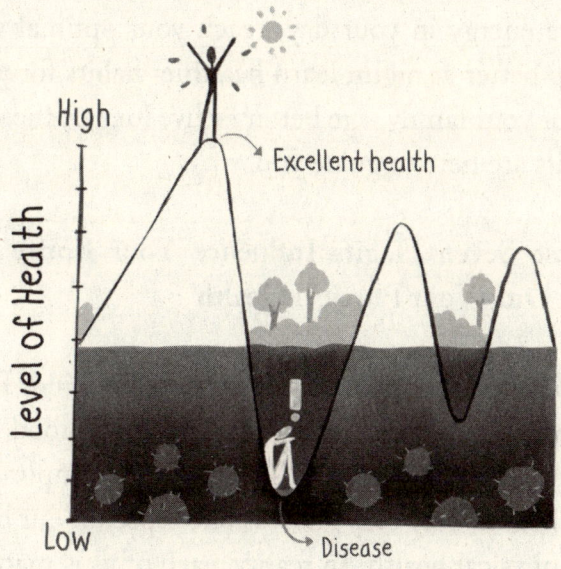

So, dear reader, please remember that our goal through the seven habits is not to treat any particular disease, but to simply elevate your level of health.

When your health level rises, most chronic lifestyle diseases automatically disappear.

The seven habits you're about to learn are equally beneficial for someone who wants to overcome health challenges as well as someone who is already healthy and wants to achieve the next level of mastery in their well-being. So, whether you're looking to heal an existing health problem or you simply want to gain more energy in your day, reach your optimal weight, sleep better at night, learn healthier habits for yourself or for your family, age better or live longer, these seven habits are here to guide you.

2. **These Seven Habits Influence Your Entire Being, Not Only Your Physical Health**

When we think of health, what comes to mind? Perhaps a person in a gym or a plate of healthy food. While nutrition and exercise are undoubtedly important for our health, they only address one aspect of our being— our physical health. In reality, each of us is made up of multiple dimensions, including:

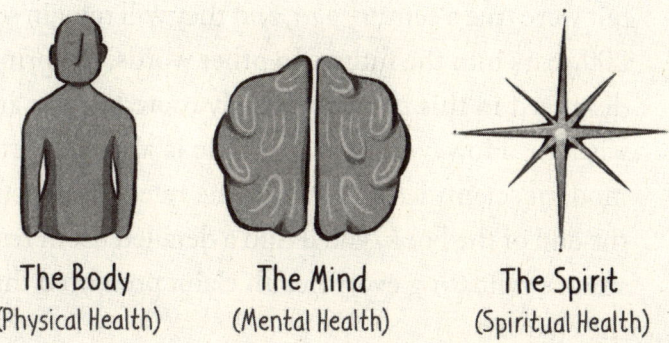

The Body
(Physical Health)

The Mind
(Mental Health)

The Spirit
(Spiritual Health)

Modern-day health wisdom often focuses excessively on the physical dimension, neglecting the other dimensions. However, the truth is that health is not just about the absence of disease or about being physically fit. Health is so much more! Real health comes when your physical, mental and spiritual health are all well-nourished and thriving.

While the first four habits in this book focus primarily on physical health, as you advance through the chapters, the habits will begin to address deeper aspects of your being—from your relationships with others to your purpose in life and even your spiritual health—allowing you to grow across all areas of your well-being.

3. **Each Habit Is Rooted in Timeless Wisdom But Is Backed by Modern Science**

It's important to know that these habits are based on timeless principles, which hold true not just for today, but were true a century ago, and they will remain so even 200 years into the future. In other words, the principles discussed in this book are deeply rooted in our ancient wisdom. However, each principle is also supported by modern scientific research. In the references section at the end of the book, you'll find a detailed list of research studies validating every health claim presented through the chapters.

In the next chapter, you will have the opportunity to take a twelve-step health test, which will help you understand your current health status and serve as a launching pad towards a life filled with vitality, purpose, joy and peak health!

1

The Twelve-Step Health Test

It was the winter of 2012. I still vividly remember sitting in the chilly corridor of one of Delhi's most renowned hospitals, with my mum by my side. The hospital had a striking theme: from the walls to the staff's uniforms, everything was green. Beside us stood a big water cooler. As we sat and waited, every few minutes a nurse would come by, reminding me, 'You need to drink more water!' I had my third glass of water in my hand and still needed to drink about two more. As soon as I felt an intense urge to pee, I was led to a small, dimly lit ultrasound room. Lying there, a nurse moved a device over my abdomen, examining my internal organs.

The ultrasound was almost always coupled with a blood test. We would take the elevator down to a small room. My mum would wait outside while a nurse tightly tied a band around my arm to draw blood. I dreaded needles (I still do), but these tests, which had to happen every few months, were an unavoidable part of the treatment routine. A few days later, my mum and I would go to the doctor with the test reports in our hands, and in most cases, it would result in an increase in the dosage of my medicine.

Fast forward ten years, shortly after Harshvardhan and I got married, a master in the field of natural health visited our home. He was in his seventies and renowned worldwide for his expertise in this field. I vividly recall the three of us—Harshvardhan, the master and myself—seated on our living room floor, deeply engrossed in conversation. While he was sharing his wisdom with us, he happened to talk about how in the past, before modern medical science was invented, our ancestors measured the quality of their health.

He said, 'There are eight signs that any healthy person would meet. These signs are as relevant today as they were 200 years ago.' His words struck a chord with me. As he was sharing, I *had* to stop him. I felt the need to capture what he was saying. I quickly took out my phone, and, with his permission, started the voice recorder, requesting him to repeat. He then began to chant this Sanskrit shloka from a traditional Nature Cure text:

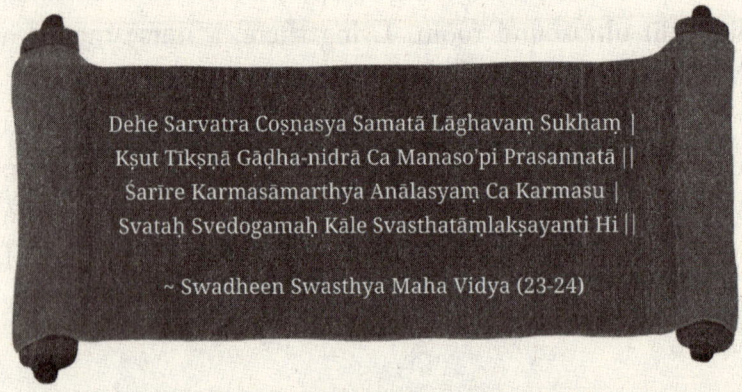

Dehe Sarvatra Coṣṇasya Samatā Lāghavaṃ Sukham |
Kṣut Tīkṣṇā Gāḍha-nidrā Ca Manaso'pi Prasannatā ||
Śarīre Karmasāmarthya Anālasyaṃ Ca Karmasu |
Svataḥ Svedogamaḥ Kāle Svasthatāmlakṣayanti Hi ||

~ Swadheen Swasthya Maha Vidya (23-24)

Translation:

Equal distribution of heat in the body,
a sense of lightness and comfort,
experiencing sharp hunger,
deep and unbroken sleep,
a sense of peace in the mind,
the ability to do work with ease,
no sign of laziness,
and timely defecation,
these are indeed the signs of good health.

The master explained each of these signs to us in depth and taught us how to use them to gain a clear understanding of what's happening inside our bodies.

This was an eye-opener for us; the idea that we can conduct a self-assessment of our health so easily, from the comfort of our homes, without a single needle, machine or rupee, was very new.

Looking back, I couldn't help but think how, growing up, I had become a slave to medical tests to get the slightest hint of what was going on inside my body. I was so reliant on external diagnostics, so dependent on machines and lab results, that I lost the intuitive understanding of my own body.

On the other hand, the simple signs that the master outlined were incredibly empowering. In an instant, one could evaluate one's own health and get a real picture of the body's internal state.

Over the next four years, Harshvardhan and I consistently assessed ourselves using these health parameters to understand how we were doing. Along the way, we realized the need to simplify some of the original parameters and add a few more, particularly focused on subtler levels of our health, to make the test even more complete.

In this chapter, we're excited to introduce you to the twelve-parameter health test, which is inspired by the same shloka mentioned earlier.

Before we proceed, it is important to note that medical tests or blood tests are not wrong or unnecessary. Not at all. In fact, they serve a vital purpose, and even we get them done at least once every year. The health test shared below serves a very different purpose and should not be considered a substitute to medical tests.

With that said, are you ready to take the test and discover your current health score? Let's get started.

The Twelve-Step Health Test

As you read each statement, please circle the number that best describes your response (0=Never, 2=Sometimes, 4=Always). Mark your responses based on your experiences in the last two weeks. Also, be honest with yourself. This test is for you to become aware of your current health status, and not for anyone else to see.

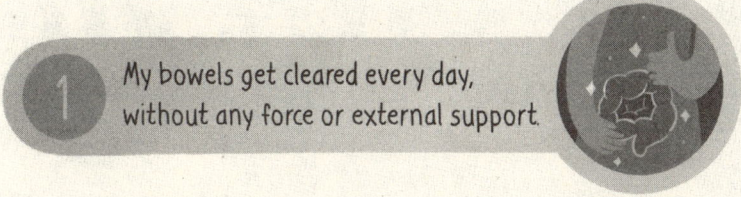

1 My bowels get cleared every day, without any force or external support.

If your bowels get cleared easily at least once every day during your bathroom visit, without the need for laxatives or excessive water intake, choose 'Always' (4).

If not, choose 'Never' or 'Sometimes' based on your experience.

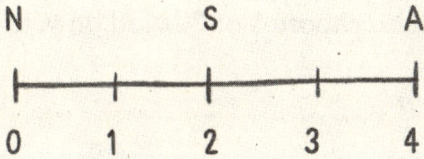

Why is this important? Well, if you're not clearing your bowels every day, it means that the waste that was supposed to exit your body is staying and collecting inside. Accumulation of waste inside the intestines is a major root cause of many chronic lifestyle diseases.

In fact, more than 2000 years ago, Hippocrates—commonly called 'the father of modern medicine'—even said, 'All disease begins in the gut.'

~

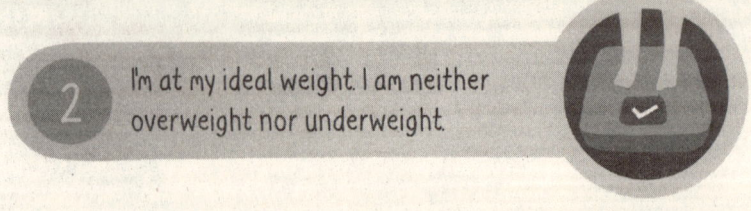

2   I'm at my ideal weight. I am neither overweight nor underweight.

If you're satisfied and happy with your weight, choose 'Always' (4).

If you're a little away from your ideal weight (as per you), choose 2.

If you're far away from your ideal weight (as per you), choose 0.

You can also choose 1 or 3 based on your situation.

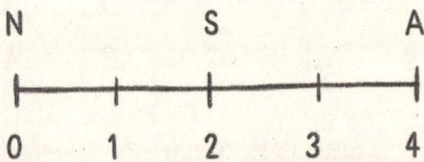

Being at your ideal weight isn't just about looking good; it's a reflection of the internal state of your body. If you find yourself underweight, it might mean that your body is struggling to absorb essential nutrients from the food you're eating. On the other hand, if you find yourself obese or overweight, it could indicate that your digestive and elimination systems aren't functioning as efficiently as they should.

Regardless of where you stand today, there's no need to worry. By implementing the habits you're going to learn about in this book, your body will naturally come to its optimal weight.

~

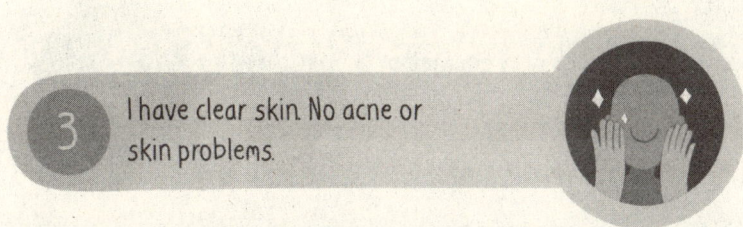

If you always have clear skin with no acne, pimples or skin problems, choose 'Always' (4).

If not, choose 'Never' or 'Sometimes' based on your experience.

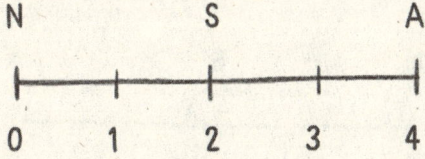

You might be wondering, 'What's the connection between my skin and my health?' Well, your skin is one of your largest detox channels. If there are waste and toxins accumulated inside your body, it will attempt to throw them out through your skin. In essence, **your skin is like a mirror, showing the reflection of your body's internal state.**

When your gut is clean, clear skin naturally follows. How to achieve this?

We will discuss it in the next chapter.

~

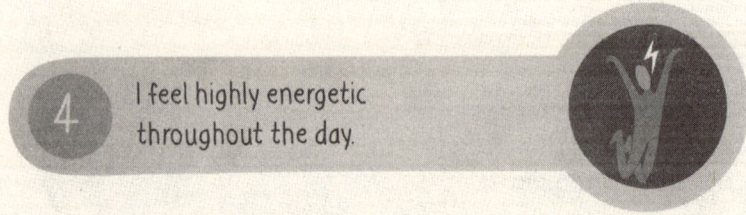

If you feel energetic and excited to do your daily tasks without feeling tired, choose 'Always' (4).

However, if you find yourself yawning frequently during the day, struggling to stay awake after waking up, or feeling tired, lazy or lethargic, then choose a lower score that reflects your energy levels accurately.

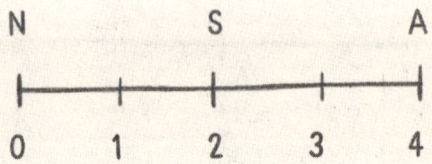

In reality, nature has given us so much energy that we have the potential to work from morning until night without feeling tired, without needing a nap in between, and without relying on energy drinks or stimulants.

~

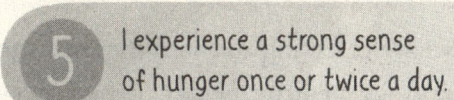 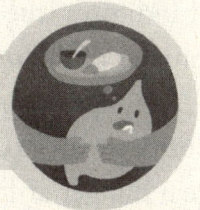

5 I experience a strong sense of hunger once or twice a day.

If you experience true hunger (a rumbling sensation in your stomach) once or more than once a day, give yourself a score of 4.

However, if you always feel full, heavy and rarely experience genuine hunger, choose a lower score based on your current situation.

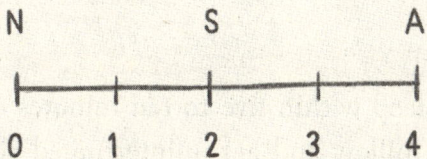

N   S   A

0   1   2   3   4

Hunger can be categorized into two types: **hunger of the stomach** and **hunger of the mind**. Hunger of the mind is the kind that craves something spicy, salty or sweet every few hours. It's that feeling of wanting to eat again, even if you've already eaten a satisfying meal.

On the other hand, real hunger, also known as hunger of the stomach, remains consistent regardless of the food available. Here's a simple way to differentiate between genuine hunger and the mind's cravings: If you were to place a bowl of plain chopped cucumber in front of you, would you genuinely feel like eating it? If the answer is yes, it indicates true hunger of the stomach. If not, it indicates hunger of the mind.

In this parameter, we are referring to the hunger of the stomach, not of the mind. A healthy person experiences real hunger at least once a day. It's a sign that digestion is working well and the previous meal was properly digested.

~

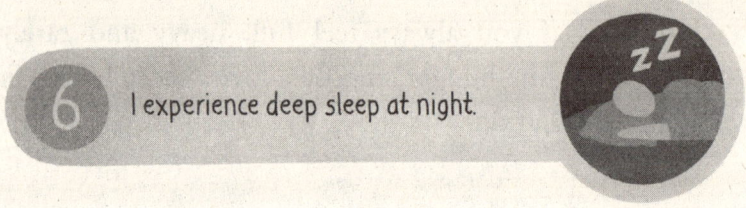

If you fall asleep within five to ten minutes of your head touching the pillow and get uninterrupted sleep at night without waking up in the middle, choose 'Always' (4).

If you struggle to fall asleep or frequently wake up in the middle of the night, choose a lower score based on the frequency.

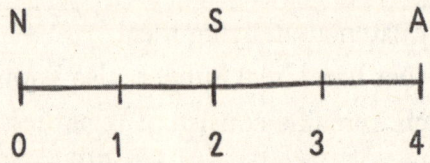

It is during deep sleep when the maximum healing of the body takes place, and hence it is an important sign of health.

Your sleep quality also directly reflects the state of your mind. A highly chaotic mind will struggle to enter a state of relaxation. In habit three, we will delve into the topic of sleep, and even discuss how to create a night routine that will help uplift the quality of your sleep.

~

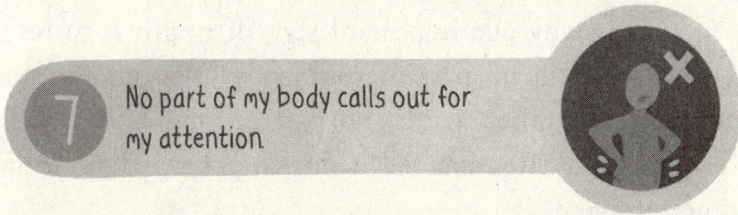

If you do not experience any chronic pains in your body and if you're able to move effortlessly without experiencing any discomfort in your joints or other parts, choose 'Always' (4).

However, if you experience any kind of pain in your body, such as in your shoulders, back, neck or joints, or even constant headaches, then give yourself a lower score.

P.S. We are not referring to the soreness that comes after a workout or menstrual cramps. Instead, we're referring to persistent and recurring pain in the body that is felt on a more regular basis.

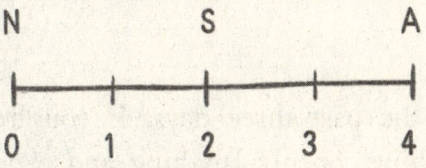

We observe that many people complain about pain—whether it is in the lower back, neck and shoulders, or the head. They even normalize pain in their lives, believing that they have to spend the rest of their lives with it. However, chronic pain in any part is not normal. It's your body's way of whispering to you that something is not right within, and if you listen to your body whisper, you won't have to hear it scream.

This is why one important sign of health is to be in a state wherein no part of your body calls out for your attention. In other words, no part of your body should demand your attention, be it due to aches, pains or any other problem.

Now, let's shift our focus to assessing some more subtle aspects related to your mental and emotional dimensions. As you proceed, you might find that these parameters aren't as black and white. But, don't overthink it. Just do your best to mark your responses.

~

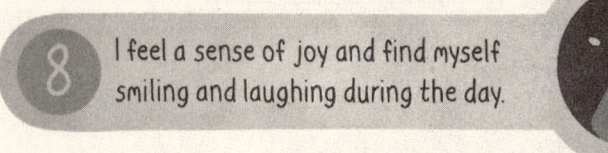 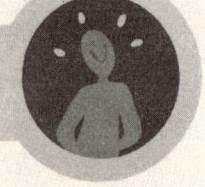

8 I feel a sense of joy and find myself smiling and laughing during the day.

Reflect on the past three days. If you frequently find yourself smiling, openly laughing and experiencing joy, choose 'Always' (4).

However, if you often feel uptight, rarely smiling or laughing, and not being able to embrace the simple joys of life, give yourself a lower score based on your current state.

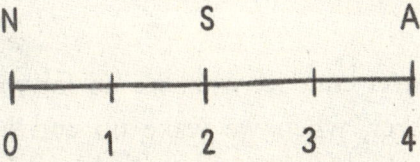

One aspect that impacts how joyful you feel is your relationship with others. When your relationships are well nourished, when you don't hold grudges or ill feelings for anyone, inner joy becomes easily attainable. We'll go deeper into this in habit five of this book, understanding how to nourish our relationships and experience more joy in our lives.

~

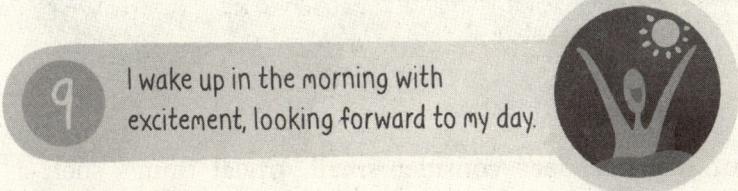

9 I wake up in the morning with excitement, looking forward to my day.

If you feel eager to start your day when you get out of bed in the morning, genuinely enjoying the work you do, choose 'Always' (4).

However, if you find yourself lacking motivation when you rise in the morning, disliking your work or constantly waiting for the weekend, choose a lower score.

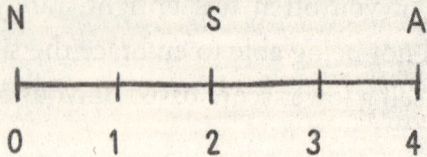

Most of us never connect what we do for work with our health. However, when we wake up and have nothing to look forward to in our day, or dread going to work, it takes a toll on our mind's health, which greatly affects our physical health. In habit six, we'll delve deeper into how to live a life aligned with your purpose, so you actually wake up every morning with a sense of excitement!

~

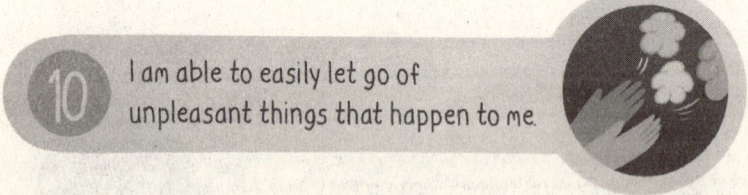

10 I am able to easily let go of unpleasant things that happen to me.

For instance, let's consider small, trivial things such as someone making a remark you don't like, a loved one preparing a dish that doesn't suit your taste, or a friend forgetting an important occasion like your birthday or anniversary. Similarly, when someone fails to meet your expectations or if you find yourself in a disagreement with a partner or a loved one, how do you feel about it after two or three days? In such situations, do you find it easy to let go without getting caught in a cycle of constant overthinking and going in circles?

If you can easily let go and move on from these incidents, choose 'Always' (4).

If you struggle to let go and tend to dwell on issues and overthink, choose a lower score.

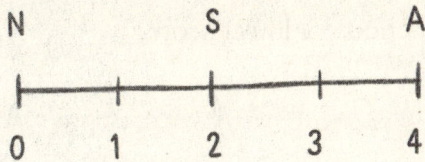

Not being able to let go of situations, overthinking or dwelling on past events leads to chronic stress. As you may already know, prolonged stress elevates levels of stress hormones like cortisol in your body, which is linked with problems such as heart disease, high blood pressure and weakened immune function.

~

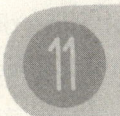 **11** My mind is stable, and it's not easy for someone to make me angry or annoyed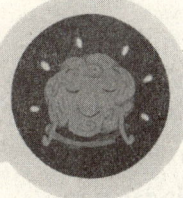

Reflect on your recent experiences. When was the last time you lost your temper, or said something to someone which you regretted later? How often do you manage to remain calm, even when someone does something which is not as per your expectations? Are you quick to lose your temper and give them a mouthful?

If you consistently remain calm and composed even in challenging situations, choose 'Always' (4).

If you are quick to lose control of yourself and tend to react quickly, choose a lower score.

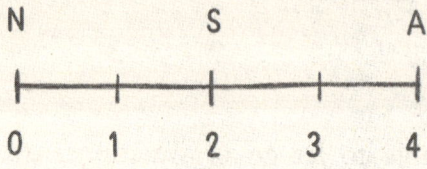

N   S   A

0   1   2   3   4

~

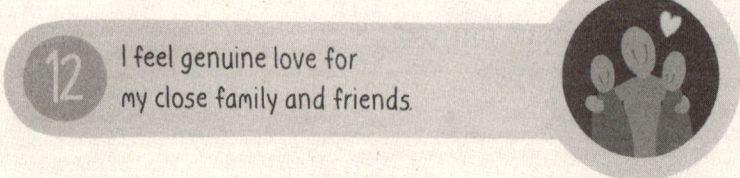

12   I feel genuine love for
     my close family and friends.

Whether it's your spouse, children, parents, siblings or close friends, ask yourself: Do you feel true, genuine love in your heart? Or is it merely superficial, with no depth or sincerity?

To determine if your love is genuine, consider the following indicators. Do you find yourself talking negatively about them behind their back? Are you even slightly jealous when they achieve great success? Do you respect their individuality, opinions and choices, even if they differ from your own?

Mark your score accordingly, keeping in mind that it can be challenging to reach a 4 in this parameter.

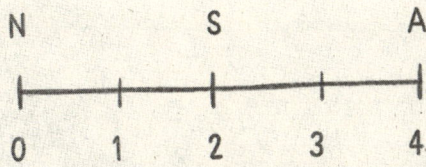

~

It's Time to Score Yourself

Now that you've gone through the test, please add up your total score and measure yourself with the following key:

40–48: Peak Health

Congratulations! A score in this range indicates that your current approach to life is working exceptionally well for you.

25–39: Average Health

A score falling in this range suggests that there is room for improvement. Fortunately, following the seven habits outlined in this book can make a significant difference in your life.

0–24: Poor Health

A score falling in this range suggests that you may be facing underlying health issues and experiencing low overall well-being. We understand how it feels to receive a score in this range because we have been here before. However, please know that following the right habits can show you amazing results in a short period of time.

Now that you know what your score means, let's move ahead.

As we journey together through this book, there is one term that will come up again and again. The term is 'peak health'. You might wonder what it really means. To clarify, we've encapsulated its essence in the figure below.

In your PEAK HEALTH, you experience:

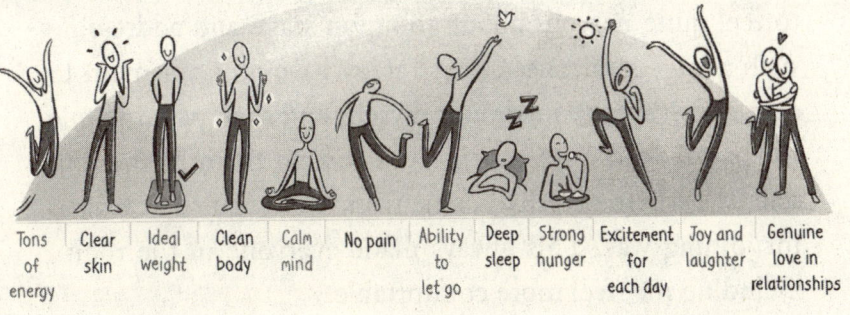

| Tons of energy | Clear skin | Ideal weight | Clean body | Calm mind | No pain | Ability to let go | Deep sleep | Strong hunger | Excitement for each day | Joy and laughter | Genuine love in relationships |

No matter where you are today on your health journey, regardless of the score you've received, we encourage you to retake the test three weeks after reading this book and applying the habits. You might be surprised by what you see.

We say this because every now and then, Harshvardhan and I come across people whose stories blow our minds. These are real experiences that remind us of how rapidly the human body can change, transitioning from a state of poor health to peak health in just a matter of a few months. Among the many stories that have left a mark on us, here is one that stands out vividly in our memory.

The Unexpected Guest at the Seminar

This particular experience takes me back to one of our first few seminars which was held in Mumbai on a Sunday. It was an eight-hour workshop in a spacious hall with approximately 120 participants. As I walked into the room, I saw people of all ages sitting closely packed together, many with notebooks in their hands, patiently waiting for the seminar to begin.

In the early days of starting Satvic Movement, I used to feel quite nervous about going on stage and addressing such a large audience. One strategy I would implement to ease into it was to introduce myself, and then pass the mic to anyone who raised their hand, asking them to share in one line where they had come from and what their reason for joining was. This always made everyone in the room, including me, feel more comfortable.

I distinctly remember one young woman in the group who enthusiastically raised her hand. She was seated on the far left in the middle row, wearing a pink top. With a certain sternness in her voice, she began speaking, 'I'm Seema, and I haven't come here to learn anything. In fact, I already know everything you're going to teach us . . .'

Upon hearing this, I felt a bit confused. Why was she sharing this, especially in front of the other people there, who had come quite eager to learn? Based on my past seminar experiences, I had encountered a few troublemakers, and I was almost certain that she might be one. Worried that her comments could potentially disrupt the flow of the seminar for others, I politely responded, 'Thank you, Seema. Would you like to continue our conversation during lunch?'

However, Seema had other plans. 'I have come here to show everyone what these habits have done for me,' she interrupted, almost disregarding my earlier response, her tone still authoritative.

She continued, 'Six months ago, I couldn't even walk. I had a disease called rheumatoid arthritis, which caused severe inflammation and stiffness in my joints. I had to call my father from the other room just to even walk me to the bathroom. If this seminar had taken place six months ago, I wouldn't even be here.'

As she shared this, the faces of everyone in the audience had turned towards her, and I could sense that they were all a bit perplexed.

She went on, 'I was in the worst health condition of my life. I used to watch my friends live normal lives, but I couldn't do any of that. I felt like I was trapped in my body. I felt that I was a burden on my family members.'

I still wasn't sure why she had chosen to raise her hand and share so much of her personal life at the beginning of an educational seminar. However, as she continued to express her pain, her eyes welled up with tears. I decided not to interrupt her and allowed her to complete.

She went on, 'I came across the Satvic lifestyle through your videos. Watching them completely changed my perspective on health, and I started following the habits you shared.'

Suddenly, a member of the audience, their voice full of anticipation, boldly interrupted, 'And then what happened?'

She continued, 'Well, four months ago, I wasn't able to walk. My whole body screamed with pain whenever I tried. But this morning, I completed thirty surya namaskars before coming here. After just a few months of following these habits, my inflammation began to significantly decrease. From not being able to leave my house, today I feel an unstoppable energy within me. When I tell the doctors about this, they don't believe what happened to me; they simply call me a "living miracle". It's not just my health that I've gotten back, but my whole life. That's why I'm here today—not to learn, but to show all of you the incredible impact of these habits.'

The audience was awestruck, and so was I. The same member who had interrupted her broke into applause, and the rest of the audience joined in.

Hearing her story, I felt re-energized with a heightened sense of responsibility to continue the seminar and my own life's journey with even greater dedication.

In that moment, I simply thanked her for sharing her story, asked her to take a seat, and continued the seminar as planned. However, during the lunch break, I couldn't resist finding her among the crowd and giving her a big hug for being such a warrior.

During our conversation, I asked if she'd like to share her experience with a wider audience, and while Seema initially felt a bit camera shy, she said that she'd like to give it a shot. The next day, I called two of our team members from Delhi to capture her incredible story, which we later uploaded on Satvic Movement's YouTube channel, aiming to inspire thousands more.

Concluding Thoughts

Over the last few years, we have met hundreds of people who've had stories similar to Seema's. Some regained their ability to walk, while others regained their ability to breathe freely once more. Some were able to fit into dresses they thought they'd never wear again, and others broke free from the burdens of chronic ailments that had held them captive. Some were able to experience much deeper sleep at night, and others said that they were able to feel a sense of joy and bliss they hadn't experienced since their childhood days.

Even though the reasons people started to live these habits were different, their end result was the same: they all told us that it's not just their health that improved, but their experience of life that was uplifted.

However, dear reader, we encourage you not to solely rely on our words or theirs. There are countless stories and countless theories in this world, but only your own practice and heart will guide you towards the truth. Experience is a much better teacher than any theory you read. So, embrace the habits taught in this book and experience their impact for yourself. Start with what you find most practical, and the rest will take care of itself.

In the next chapter, we'll dive into the first of the seven habits. It begins with a small change in your evening routine, but its impact on your life is tremendous.

Habit 1

Keep a Clean Body Within

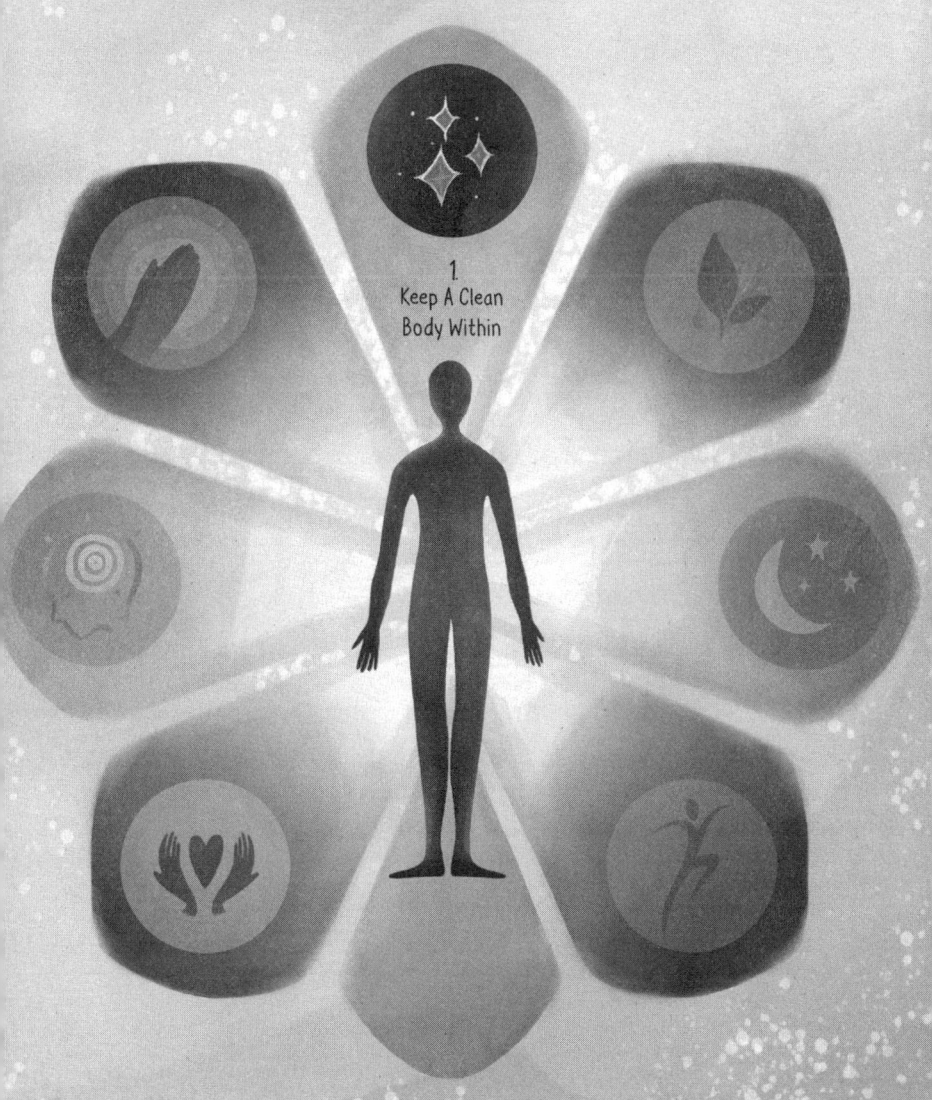

1.
Keep A Clean
Body Within

2

The Surprising Ancient Practice for Inner Cleansing

Visualize a flower vase—a transparent, wide-mouthed, glass vase. Over time, it's become murky and covered in patches of dirt. Now imagine that I hand you this dirty vase and ask you to remove the stains. I also give you a brush, some detergent and a cloth. As you begin cleaning, you pour the detergent on the vase, scrub it vigorously with the brush and use the cloth to wipe it. But, to your surprise, no matter how much you scrub, the vase remains dirty.

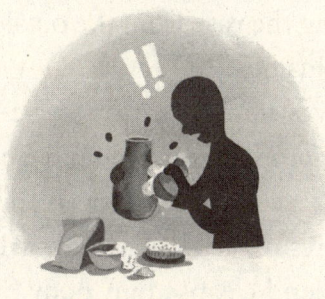

Feeling a bit puzzled, you pause for a moment, catching your breath from the intense scrubbing. That's when it suddenly dawns on you that the dirt making the vase appear unclean is not on the outside, but on the inside! So, you decide to scrub the vase from the inside, and voilà, it becomes sparkling clean.

When we think of a vase, it's quite easy to understand that **internal cleanliness is the key to how it appears from the outside**. But when we consider our own bodies, this concept seems much harder to grasp.

As a result, we spend a lot of time and money in our lives trying to 'look' and 'appear' clean and beautiful from the outside. We buy expensive face washes, creams and serums, hoping for clear skin. We spend vast amounts on make-up products, concealers and spot removers, to cover our blemishes. It's not only skincare—we also invest in deodorants and perfumes to mask the body's odour. However, what we don't realize is that the root of the problem that we often try to mask or cover lies not outside, but on the inside.

These products may temporarily give some results. However, expecting any external quick-fix solution to work, without cleaning our bodies from within, is just as useless as scrubbing the vase from the outside when the dirt is actually on the inside.

For years, I was trapped in this cycle—dependent on medicines, beauty products, creams and face washes to look a certain way. But each time I stopped these routines, the problems would resurface. It was only when I addressed the root cause, when I cleansed my body from within, that my skin, hair and health problems naturally healed, once and for all.

What I learnt later in my life was that for peak health, the primary prerequisite is an internally clean body. As long as the body is cluttered with accumulated waste and toxins, one cannot be in their peak health.

Therefore, I welcome you to the first of our seven habits: 'Keep a Clean Body Within'. Many aspects of our health—digestion, skin quality, energy levels, mood, clarity of thought—are directly tied to how clean our bodies are from the inside. While this might sound vague right now, as you read on, you'll have absolute clarity.

Here's what you can expect to learn from this chapter:

- What makes our bodies dirty in the first place?
- Who is the best cleaner in the world? Is he/she sitting in a clinic, hospital, chemist shop or somewhere entirely unexpected?
- A powerful practice is to give your body a chance to cleanse. This is something I saw my grandfather doing when I was a little girl, but didn't realize how valuable it was until much later.

With our foundation set, let's dive into our first topic.

What Makes Your Body Dirty from Within?

How do toxins even form within our bodies? Does this just happen automatically? Or, is there something we consciously do that gives rise to these toxins?

In order to understand this, we need to take a closer look at our digestive system. We need to first know what happens to our food after we swallow it. Every time we take a bite, that food begins an incredible process inside our body. As it passes through our stomach and intestines, it is broken down into small particles, and all the good stuff is extracted from it—the vitamins, minerals and energy we need. The components that our body can't utilize are converted into waste material, which is gently expelled from the body.

Now, let's think about those highly processed foods that we sometimes (or often) indulge in—like fried samosas, crispy pakoras, cheesy pizzas, loaded burgers, greasy cookies, sugar-loaded colas. Or think about those instances when we overeat, burdening our digestive system with far more food than it can handle. In such situations, do you think that the food can be broken down as easily? Sadly, the answer is no.

When this happens, our stomach is like, 'Whoa, what's this? How do I even handle all of this?' It struggles to digest the excessive amount of food, or the heavy, denatured and greasy food. Hence, some of it is left undigested, lingering in our digestive tract.

Over time, as we keep indulging in our unnatural eating habits, this undigested food forms a thick layer on the walls of our intestines. As time passes, the undigested matter gets older and older and converts into what we call 'toxins'.

This toxic overload might initially manifest as small problems—lethargy, bloating, weight gain, bad breath, a constant sense of tiredness, acne or even brain fog. But if we ignore the symptoms for several years, these toxins, or this accumulated waste matter, can also lead to chronic lifestyle diseases such as diabetes, thyroid imbalance, hypertension, skin problems, digestive issues, etc.

In summary: incorrect eating habits result in undigested food within our bodies. Undigested food, over time, is converted into toxins. It's the collection of these toxins that eventually leads to many of the health problems that we, as a society, face today.

Ayurveda, the ancient system of medicine, provides a detailed explanation of this concept of toxins. In the *Aṣṭāṅga Hṛdaya*, one of the primary classical Ayurvedic texts, these 'toxins' are referred to as '*āma*'. Āma is described as the improperly digested essence of food that resides in the *āmāśaya*, or stomach. It is a toxic, sticky, cloudy, foul-smelling substance that can spread from the gastrointestinal tract to other parts of the body.

'Every tissue is fed by the blood, which is supplied by the digestive system. When the digestive system is unclean and inefficient, our blood is thickened with toxic poisons, and our body is open to disease.'

—Dr Bernard Jensen
Renowned doctor and health advocate

Aṣṭāṅga Hṛdaya Sutra Sthana 13/23–24:

Srotorodha balabhramsa gaurav anila mü dhatäh
Älasya apakti nishtheeva malasanga äruci klamähl
lingam malanâm samanâm nirâmânäm viparyayah

Translation:

The symptoms of āma in the body are given as follows:

1. *Srotorodha*—Obstruction of the channels and pores
2. *Balabhramsha*—Loss of strength
3. *Gaurav*—Feeling of heaviness of the body
4. *Anila Mü Dhatäh*—Disruption of internal movements
5. *Älasya*—Laziness and lethargy
6. *Apakti*—Loss of digestive power
7. *Nishtheeva*—Cough or phlegm in the throat or lungs
8. *Malasanga*—Constipation
9. *Äruci*—Lack of enthusiasm or disinterest
10. *Klamähl*—Exhaustion

Ayurveda goes on to explain how the **majority of diseases stem from an accumulation of āma**. In fact, āma is said to be responsible for 90 per cent of all diseases.

Personally, this was the first learning I received from my master that blew me away. All these years, I questioned, 'Why am I sick?', 'Why am I getting these health problems?', and nobody seemed to know the answer.

'It's just happening to everybody these days,' they said. But that answer never satisfied me. It was many years later that I learnt how the accumulation of waste in the body is one major cause of many chronic health challenges. For me, this was a huge revelation.

So far, we've learnt that improper eating habits are one of the biggest causes of undigested food residue in our system. However, is this the only cause? Well, no. Many factors in our modern-day lifestyles add to this toxin build-up, whether it's the pollution in our air, the pesticides in our crops, or the stressful lifestyle of modern cities. In other words, we, as a generation, are more exposed to toxins today than ever before. And that's also why we, as a generation, need constant detoxification today more than ever before.

To guide you on this journey of internal cleansing, let us move to the next part of this chapter. So far, you've understood how our bodies start to accumulate internal impurities. Now it's time to learn about the force which will help to cleanse them, re-establishing health within the system. I want to introduce you to an extraordinarily powerful cleaner and healer—possibly even the best one in the world!

Who Is the World's Best Healer?

Who do you think this is?

Is he or she sitting in some fancy clinic?

No.

Is the answer locked away in some magic drug?

No.

Do you have to spend a lot of money to access it?

No.

In reality, the extraordinary force that heals you is present somewhere you may never look.

The best healer is sitting within you.

Mark it down, underline it, circle it.

Don't go looking for the healer outside, because it's already present within you.

And there's proof for this!

When you break a bone, plaster is placed on your arm to keep it in place and give it rest. In a few days, what happens? The bone automatically joins itself back together. It's not like there's some medicine in the plaster. The plaster is simply a support system that allows the right ends of the joint to meet and be in a rested state. So, what is that power that joins the broken bone? It's your healing power.

This healing power is an enormous, magnificent force of nature, which lies within each one of us. At Satvic Movement, we call this healing power our 'praanshakti'.

'Praanshakti' is basically the energy which manages the entire body without our conscious thought. It's the energy that runs our respiratory, circulatory, nervous and other vital systems. It's constantly scanning its environment, destroying diseased cells and fighting for survival.

When was the last time you reminded your heart to beat, your lungs to expand and contract, or your digestive system to secrete the right digestive juices? These and a myriad of other processes happen involuntarily, without us having to do anything. The inner intelligence that manages these processes is what we are calling the 'praanshakti'.

The conceptual basis of 'praanshakti' is not unique to our natural healing sciences. In fact, it is recognized across several modern and ancient cultures. In Traditional Chinese medicine and Taoism, praanshakti is referred to as 'qi' (chi). The ancient Greeks recognized it as 'pneuma'. To the ancient Egyptians, it was 'Ka'. In science, it's referred to as 'homeostasis', and in modern medicine, it's often called the 'Life Force'.

> 'Natural forces within us are the true healers of disease.'
> —Hippocrates
> The Father of Modern Medicine

Whatever be the name, if this praanshakti, this healing power, can rejoin such a massive broken bone, can it not cleanse our body from within? Can it not remove the accumulated waste? Can it not heal us? Of course it can!

Once the healing power (praanshakti) starts working, it has the capability to fix pretty much everything, no matter where the problem is located, no matter how long it's been there.

Praanshakti

She is someone who never goes on leave.
Always by your side, never will she deceive.

She loves you like your own mother.
To protect you is her only intention, no other.

From the moment you were born, till your last breath.
She will be with you till your very death.

About her, most of us don't know much.
She's a silent worker, always there with her healing touch.

In different cultures, she's given different names.
The yogis call her Prana, while the Egyptians call her Ka.
    The Chinese call her Chi.
And at Satvic Movement, we call her our very own
    Praanshakti.

She heals, she cleans, she protects and she digests.
She's the life force sitting inside you. She's truly the best.

If you break a bone, what does the doctor do?
He puts it in plaster so you can no longer move.

But in this plaster, there is no special pill.
All it does is to keep your bone still.

So what's this power that joins such a big broken bone?
Does it come from somewhere outside, or is it your
very own?

And what about those times when you get a cut on your
skin?
Even with no Band-Aid, it heals from within.

So what's this power that fixes things unknown?
Does it come from somewhere outside, or is it your
very own?

It's none other than your very own praanshakti.
Truly magnificent, she deserves all our *bhakti*.*

She's your internal doctor, the world's best cleaner.
But in our lives so far, we've not really seen her.

Now, the natural question that comes is that if this
praanshakti is truly so strong,
Why have we had toxins inside us for so long?

Even though she's powerful, there's something about her
you must understand.
In one thing at a time she can put her hand.

---

* 'Bhakti' stands for love and devotion.

Either she can digest and break down the food you send
     her way,
or she can clean and remove the toxins away.

She cannot do two things at a time, whether you like it
     or not.
She can either digest or clean the rot.

Can you guess what percentage of your praanshakti
     digestion takes up?
70 to 80 per cent. You read that, right? Yup.

Now, you may be wondering, this poem has been going
     for quite some time,
but dearest reader, did you like the rhyme?

Now, to understand praanshakti's workings a little better,
let us take an example.

The Busy Road with a Pothole in the Middle

Imagine a busy road connecting Mumbai to Delhi. There
are cars, scooters, buses and even big trucks travelling along
it every day. On one busy weekend, due to heavy rainfall
and a poor drainage system, a large pothole has developed
in the middle of the road. Now, let's assume that you're in
charge of repairing this pothole. What's the first thing you
would need to do?

The answer is obvious: you'll need to stop the traffic. As long as cars continue to drive on this road, there's no way you can repair the pothole.

Well, the same holds true for the body. Consider your body as the road. If there's a 'pothole' that has developed (any issue needing attention), can it be fixed with constant 'traffic' coming in all day and night? No. What's the first thing you would need to do in order to initiate the repair? You'll have to stop the cars.

What are these 'cars', in the context of our body? They are the never-ending supply of food that we keep sending inside. They're the wake-up chai with biscuits, the breakfast paranthas, the mid-morning snacks, the plateful of roti and sabzi, those afternoon cookies, the evening namkeen and the post-dinner munchies. Even before one meal has a chance to get fully digested, we already send in the next.

Now, if there's constant traffic of food entering the body continuously, what's happening inside all the time? Twenty-four hours a day, seven days a week? Digestion,

digestion and digestion. As a result, your praanshakti gets very little time to clean, to repair, to heal and to maintain health within the system. We keep eating all day, and our praanshakti keeps digesting all day. It keeps working, never getting a break.

But here's an important question: If we want our praanshakti to engage in internal cleansing, in repairing damaged cells, in healing any ailments, in maintaining the general upkeep within our system, shouldn't we set aside a little time every day free from digestion? Shouldn't we allow some time every day when it can uninterruptedly focus on these other important tasks?

Well, to experience peak health, this is absolutely crucial. From time to time, we need to give our praanshakti a break from digestion, so that it can clean, heal, repair, fix and purify our bodies from within.

In the next section, we will delve into exactly how this can be achieved. But before that, it's important to understand that there isn't a 'single' right way to accomplish this. Each healing modality has its own unique approach to purification of the body. If you explore Ayurveda, there's *panchakarma*. Yoga offers *shat kriyas*, and in Chinese medicine, there's acupuncture. These practices are valuable. However, they typically require you to visit a centre or clinic, or to be under the guidance of a professional.

Yet, there is one method which is propagated by each of these disciplines—whether it's Ayurveda or yoga. It involves a transformative shift in lifestyle, and can be adopted by anyone, without leaving the home or incurring any additional expenses. Let's discover what it is.

A Simple, Yet Powerful Practice for Daily Cleansing

I grew up in a Jain family. Jainism is a spiritual path originating in ancient India that follows the principles of non-violence, compassion and the pursuit of spiritual purity. I lived in a joint family with my parents, four *taiji*s (aunts) and four *tauji*s (uncles), their children, my grandmother and grandfather. At one point, there were twenty-one of us living in one home!

Though I didn't understand most of the concepts of Jainism back then, I used to observe all the elders in the house practising certain rituals.

One of their rituals was to eat their dinner before sunset (which was around 6 p.m.) and only have their next meal after sunrise the next day. My grandparents were especially particular about this. After coming back from school, when I used to be having my snack at 5 p.m., they used to be getting ready to eat their dinner. To be honest, I found this quite odd. I always wondered how they didn't feel hungry at night.

Whenever I used to ask them why they ate their dinner so early, they simply said, 'Because we've always done it this way. Our elders did it, so we do it.' As you can imagine, I never felt inspired to try it myself.

Fast forward to years later, I went to a health institute in Florida. There, I noticed something similar happening. This institute was essentially a healing and education centre where people would typically come and spend two to three weeks. By following the guidelines shared, people were able to reverse even serious health problems. While I was there, I observed that there was one key practice followed by the institute every single day. This was the practice of having an early dinner. Every day dinner was served by 6 p.m. and cleared away by 7.30 p.m.

For me, this was a revelation! I realized that **what** you eat is as important as **when you eat it**. That's when I also realized that what my grandparents had been doing as an age-old practice all this while was actually grounded in deep wisdom.

From then onwards, I inculcated the habit of eating early dinners in my own life, and saw massive improvements in my energy levels and overall health.

While eating the last meal by 6 p.m. is ideally recommended, feedback from many members in our Satvic community (those who diligently follow this lifestyle) and my own observations made me realize that this time isn't practical for most. Hence, we suggest 7 p.m. as a more feasible option. Eat your dinner by 7 p.m. every evening. You might think that this is too minor a shift to have an impact, but remember:

Health ≠ making massive changes.
Health = small, simple changes, done consistently.

Now, you may be wondering, 'But what is the connection between cleansing my body and having an early dinner?'

Come, let us understand.

How Your Digestive Fire Is Connected to the Sun

Any food you consume enters the stomach. Within the stomach resides a digestive fire. In the *Charaka Samhita*, one of the foundational Ayurvedic texts, this digestive fire is termed *'jatharagni'*. *Jathar* translates to stomach, and *agni* translates to fire. This jatharagni is responsible for breaking down food in the stomach and is crucial for effective digestion.

Now, do you think that the intensity of this digestive fire remains constant throughout the day? No. As per Ayurvedic texts, its intensity varies. When the sun is at its peak, our digestive fire is believed to be at its strongest. This is why it is often recommended to eat the heaviest meal of the day during this period. As the sun goes down, our digestive fire tends to wane, and by night-time it's at its weakest.

This is why dining late at night or eating a very heavy dinner, regardless of how nutritious the meal is, can lead to improper and incomplete digestion. As we saw earlier, if our food isn't digested well, it isn't eliminated well either. This undigested food residue stays in the body, fermenting over time, leading to a build-up of waste.

Don't get me wrong—it's not like if you eat a late-night dinner once or twice, there will be accumulated waste the next day. It's only when we regularly eat late, night after night, that impurities begin to develop within the body.

How a Simple Switch in Dinner Timing Impacts Health

Let's consider a scenario where you have dinner at 10 p.m. and then eat breakfast at 9 a.m. Assume that it takes about nine hours for your stomach to completely digest the meal. This means that digestion continues until 7 a.m., with your praanshakti occupied with actively digesting food for most of the night.

In such a case, how many cleaning hours would you get in a night?

Only two.

Such limited time is insufficient for any deep cleaning work, or proper elimination of toxins from the body.

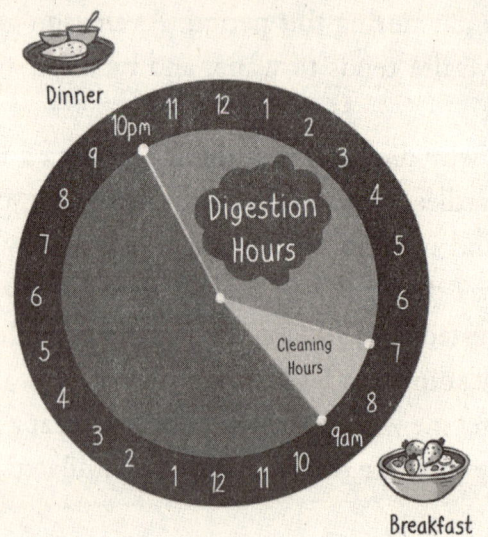

Now, let's see what happens when we eat an early dinner. By having an early dinner, let's say around 7 p.m., digestion happens faster because our digestive fire is stronger in the early evening. If it took nine hours to digest a meal before, it would now take roughly eight hours. So, if you had dinner at 7 p.m., it would get digested by around 3 a.m. the next morning. **This means that eating early leaves you with six hours of cleaning time, which is roughly three times more compared to late eating!**

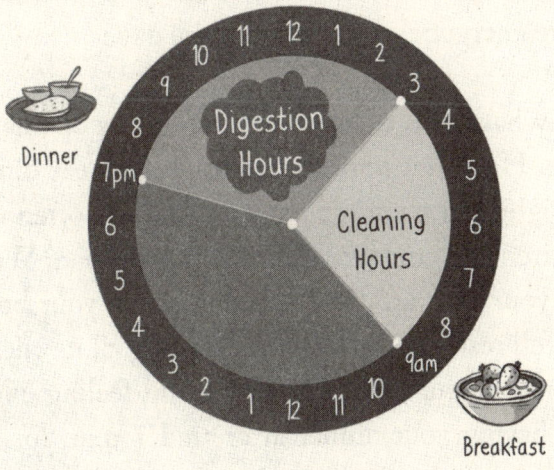

Remember, these numbers are estimates. They vary greatly depending on your age, your lifestyle and your activity level. But here's the beautiful part: by simply shifting your dinner a couple of hours earlier, you're gifting your body with many more healing and cleansing hours every night! Day after day, night after night, this small change adds up to something truly extraordinary:

- Your praanshakti finally gets the time it needs to engage in deep cleaning, something it couldn't do before.
- Your organs—the stomach, pancreas, liver and intestines—get a few hours to rest every day, which in turn increases their efficiency.
- Excess fat around your belly and body begins to melt away.
- Your sleep becomes much deeper.
- The morning grogginess that you may experience becomes a thing of the past, and you wake up much more energetic, ready to seize the day.

You may have also experienced the effects of this in your own life. Have you noticed that when you eat dinner late in the night and sleep soon afterwards, you often wake up feeling tired and groggy? Why does this happen? Well, even though your eyes are closed during sleep, your body isn't getting full rest. It's too busy channelling all its energy into digestion and thus, you don't wake up feeling energized. But try having your dinner at around 7 p.m. for a week. You'll be amazed at how much more energy you wake up with the next morning.

For this very reason, at our Satvic headquarters, which serves as the workspace from where the Satvic Movement team operates, dinner is served at 6 p.m. in the evening.

Today, even research studies are reaffirming what our age-old traditions have always said. Circadian rhythms, our body's natural built-in clock that regulates the sleep–wake cycle, play an important role in how our body functions. These rhythms, driven largely by our exposure to sunlight, suggest that our metabolism and digestive ability are more active during daylight hours.

In a recent study published in 2022, scientists looked at data from nine rigorous clinical trials involving 485 adults. They found that people who consumed most of their calories earlier in the day lost more weight than people who did the opposite. They also had greater improvements in their blood sugar, cholesterol levels and insulin sensitivity, a marker of diabetes risk.

In essence, whether we look at the time-tested teachings of Ayurveda or Jainism or cutting-edge scientific studies, the message is clear: eating dinner early isn't just a tradition—it's foundational to our well-being.

Making this Practical: Overcoming Everyday Challenges

When we discuss the practice of early eating with our Satvic community members, they all recognize its value. They agree that it's great for them. However, the question always arises: 'How do we realistically follow this given our busy daily routines?' This is an important concern, and in this section, we want to address a few potential obstacles that could come your way.

How can I possibly manage to have an early dinner if I return late from work?

- If you return late from work, **consider the possibility of adjusting your routine so you come back from work earlier,** preferably by 6 p.m. Maybe you can request for flexibility to start your day a bit earlier and finish earlier as well. This may sound too idealistic, but we believe that some of you reading this may actually be able to make it happen.

- If the above-mentioned solution is impossible for you, then the next best option is to eat a light, easy-to-digest dinner at the earliest possible time. To ensure the meal is light, avoid having an excess of grains and pulses in it. Eating a light dinner allows your body to digest it more quickly, providing ample time in the night for cleansing, repair, and healing.

If I eat my dinner by 7 p.m., I will feel hungry in the night and won't be able to sleep. How can I deal with this?

- It's natural to feel hungry in the night when you first start this routine. **Give your body some time to adjust.** Consider how many years you've been accustomed to eating late at night—perhaps twenty, thirty or even forty years! It's not realistic to expect the body to suddenly adapt to a new early dinner routine. However, within one week of consistently following this practice, you will likely no longer experience hunger pangs at night.

- During the transition phase, which could last for about a week, here are a **few options of foods you can consume when you feel hungry at night:**

  o   Warm herbal tea using fresh or dried herbs
  o   Any light fruit
  o   A few soaked nuts
  o   A light soup made with seasonal vegetables

What can I do if my family/partner eats late at night? It's challenging for me to have an early dinner alone.

Both Harshvardhan and I have personally experienced the same challenge. Here's what we suggest:

- **Have an open conversation with your family or partner** about the benefits of having an early dinner. Share with them the knowledge you've gained and explain why it could be beneficial for everyone. If they agree, you can start the ritual together and hold each other accountable.

- However, if they are unable to adjust their routines to have an early dinner or if they don't agree, don't worry. **Be the first person in the family to start this practice** and stay committed to it.

For example, when Harshvardhan and I spent time in Kolkata with his mum and grandma, they were used to eating a late dinner. However, we had our dinner prepared early and ensured that we ate it by 7 p.m. Initially, we were alone at the table for the first two days. But on the third day, when our granny saw us eating early, she decided to join us. When everyone was eating early, Mum couldn't resist. She also joined us, and early dinners became a new ritual in the house. Now, they're the ones who are ready at the dining table by 7 p.m., eagerly calling us to join them.

In other words, as you consistently live the practice, you become a beacon of light to others around you. Remember, you have to **inspire, not enforce.** Lead by example, and others will be automatically inspired to follow.

We hope the questions and answers above have shed some light on how to transform what you've read from a theory in a book into an actionable practice in your everyday life. Initially, setting up systems in your home for this change might be challenging, but gradually, as you keep doing it, you'll observe that early eating will become a new rhythm for your body; it'll become second nature. As Robin Sharma rightly said, in his book *The 5 AM Club*, 'Any change is hard at first, messy in the middle, and gorgeous in the end.'

Now that you've learnt everything you need to know about the principle of 7 p.m. dinners, we would like to share with you one additional principle, if you're looking to maximize your cleanse. This bonus suggestion is for those of you who want to go the extra mile.

A Bonus Suggestion to Maximize Your Cleanse

If you want to go one step further in your journey, start your day with a glass of cleansing juice each morning.

One of the most effective options is the juice of a vegetable called 'ash gourd'. I began the practice of drinking this juice during my own healing journey and have continued it ever since.

If you're unfamiliar with ash gourd, it's a vegetable with a pale green or ash-grey exterior and white, spongy flesh inside. In Sanskrit, it's called *kushmaand*, which translates to 'tiny egg of energy'. It's commonly available with most vegetable vendors. They might recognize it by its local names, such as '*Safed Petha*' or '*Kumhara*'.

What's the benefit of this juice? Well, drinking a glass of ash gourd juice in the morning on an empty stomach immensely helps the praanshakti in its cleansing work. Think of ash gourd juice like a magnet, drawing waste particles from within your body. As the juice exits your system, it takes out those waste particles along with it.

Ideally, after consuming ash gourd juice, you should wait for one to one and a half hours before eating anything. As for its taste, it's quite neutral, similar to cucumber juice.

In the references at the end of this book, you will find two research studies detailing the clinical significance of drinking ash gourd juice.

If you want to learn how to prepare the juice, we have created a detailed video that demonstrates the preparation method. You will find the link at the end of this chapter.

A word of caution here: while ash gourd juice is suitable for most people, some, especially those with cold or sinusitis symptoms, may find that it exacerbates their condition. If, after three to five days, you feel that ash gourd juice doesn't suit you, please listen to your body and stop its consumption.

If you cannot find ash gourd juice, an excellent alternative would be any fresh green juice, coconut water, or celery juice.

Concluding Thoughts about This Practice

As you walk on this path, there's one thing we'd like to emphasize: **don't become a hardliner or extremist.** For instance, even we are not able to follow the practice of eating a 7 p.m. dinner 100 per cent of the time. We strive to follow it for five to six out of seven days of the week. If we are visiting our families, and if they have lovingly prepared dinner for us, whether it's 8 p.m. or 9 p.m., we'll enjoy it with love in our hearts. We understand that we are making an exception, and it's not the norm. We know fully well that from the next day, we must come back to our practice of eating early.

In your life too, there may be occasions when you have an event to attend or when you're travelling. Treat those days as exceptions. Understand the essence of the habit and try your best to live it *most* of the time, if not *all* the time. In case you fail, try again. It takes time to change habits that you've been following for decades.

The ultimate essence of habit one, 'Keep a Clean Body Within', comes down to this: this human body is Mother Nature's precious gift to us. Soon, we will return it to Her. In the time we have, it's our duty to keep it clean, bustling with energy and health—the way She has designed it to be.

In the next chapter, we will move on to habit two, where we'll take a deep dive into understanding the topic of food. You'll learn certain truths about your food that you will wish you had learnt in school or college—truths that the media and food companies are hiding from us. You will gain another powerful tool to help you achieve peak health and understand how it lies right at the end of your fork.

To access the ash gourd juice preparation video, scan the QR code or visit satvicmovement.org/book/ashgourd

Habit 2

Eat Living, Wholesome and Plant-Based

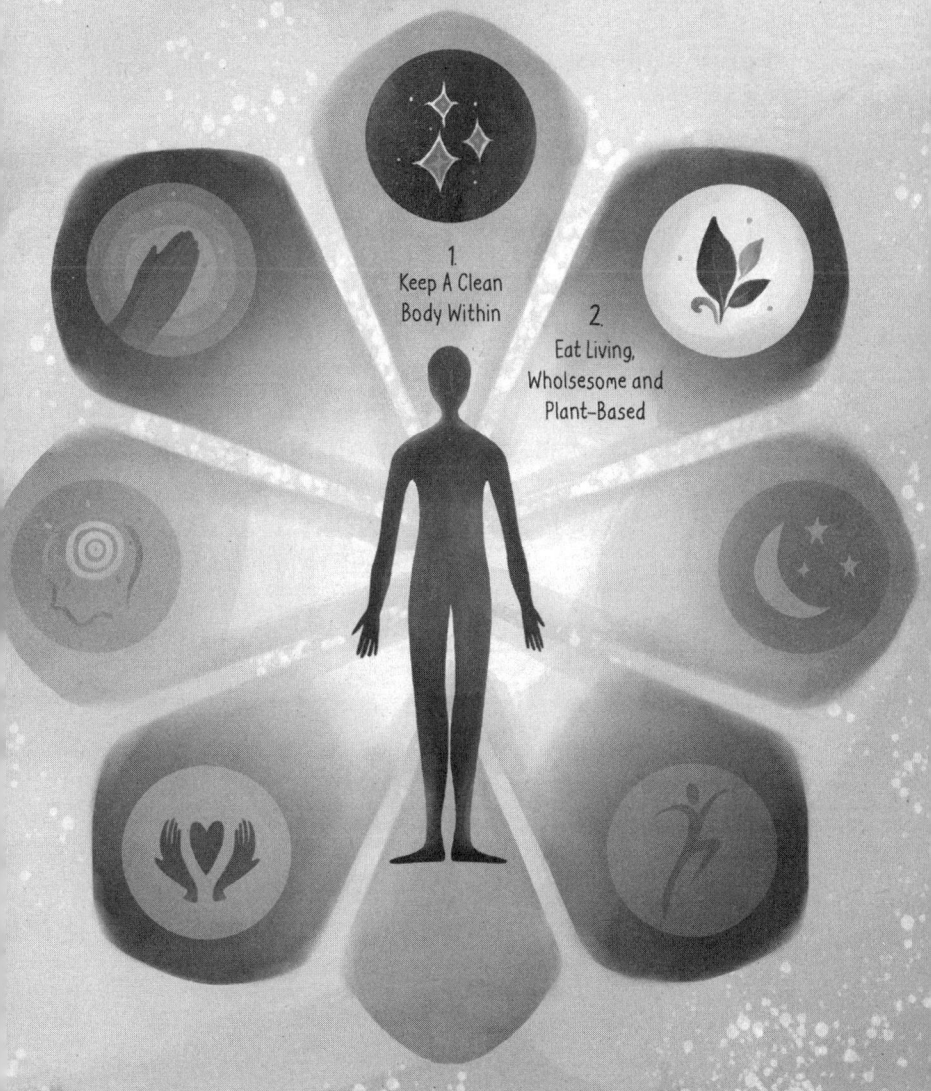

1.
Keep A Clean
Body Within

2.
Eat Living,
Wholsesome and
Plant-Based

3

Truths That Packaged Food Companies Hope You Never Find Out

What is the one ritual that you perform every single day, without fail? It's as fundamental as breathing and as routine as the ticking of a clock. It's a ritual you perform from the cradle to the grave. Whether at home or travelling, whether alone or with friends, it's a ritual you don't miss. Every few hours, as the day unfolds, you find yourself drawn to it.

What is it?

Well, the ritual we're talking about is EATING FOOD.

Now, think about this: How many hours during your school or college years were devoted to teaching you about food? Specifically, which foods nourish you best and why?

Not many. Most of us go through our formal education with only a superficial understanding of food and nutrition. It's a bit surprising when you think about it: something we engage in every few hours, our primary source of energy, and yet, it's rarely given its due attention in our educational systems growing up.

Hence, today our food choices are strongly influenced by:

1) What we see our parents or families eating (many of whom struggle with health challenges themselves)
2) The media (TV, newspapers or billboard advertisements by big food companies, which care very little about our health, and much more about their own profits)
3) The 'special offers' section of food delivery apps (perhaps this one is most recent)

In reality, most of us have never really questioned, 'What's the best food for our bodies to thrive? To stay healthy and strong till the end of our lives?'

In this habit, we're going to find answers to these questions and further explore the topic of food.

As the habit's title—'Eat Living, Wholesome and Plant-Based'—suggests, the Satvic food philosophy stands on three foundational pillars. In the upcoming chapters, we will delve into each of these pillars, one at a time. This particular chapter is dedicated to our first pillar: living foods.

Before we proceed, I also want you to know that both Harshvardhan and I absolutely love food. We understand that food is more than just a means to fill the stomach.

Food is also about enjoying the flavours and textures of the meal, about bonding with your family when you sit at the dining table together, about communities coming together over a lavish feast during festivals and gatherings. Realizing how food plays such a multifaceted role in our lives, we acknowledge that changing long-standing food habits can be daunting. We've been there. That's why we've designed this chapter to be not only theoretical but also highly practical. While the first half will provide you with deep knowledge, the second half will offer clear action steps to help you implement that knowledge into your life with ease.

Here's what you can expect to learn in this chapter:

- What does living food actually mean?
- The two secret truths about packaged foods that big food companies hope you never find out.
- How to decode ingredient lists in the supermarket to avoid falling into marketing traps.
- Practical swaps you can make in your kitchen today for better health.
- How to overcome cravings and temptations? (Yes, it's possible!)

So sit tight, get comfortable, and let's begin!

What Is Living Food?

What does it mean for food to be living? At its core, living food is that which has the presence of a life force within.

This life force is termed 'prana' in Sanskrit. In many Indian spiritual traditions, prana is recognized as a vital, life-sustaining energy that flows through the universe. Because living food contains this life energy, it also has the power to generate new life.

To understand this concept better, here's an example. Imagine that you take a ripe tomato and bury it in the soil. After a few days, what will happen? If the conditions are right, you will find tiny plants sprouting out of the ground you put the tomato in. Now, let's say you bury a piece of chocolate or some potato chips, or a cookie in the soil. You even water it and provide all the right conditions. Will it ever sprout into new life? No!

Why? Because the tomato, bursting with prana, can give birth to new life, while the processed cookie or chip, devoid of such energy, cannot.

Another example to understand living food is that of a lentil. When allowed to soak and germinate, it transforms into a sprout! This represents the life force within the lentil.

Please remember that these analogies are not a literal representation—not every living food when put in soil will grow into a plant. They are simply examples to help understand the concept of the life force.

In a nutshell, living foods are those which are full of life energy, and are as close to their original form as possible, as given by Mother Nature. These include fruits, vegetables, grains, nuts, seeds and sprouts. Living foods are beautifully packaged in divinely created wrappers called skins and peels.

Here are three interesting markers to know if something is living or not:

Marker #1: Living Food Is Farm-to-Kitchen

If a food item comes straight from the farm to the kitchen, it's most likely living. But if it visits a factory in between for heavy processing, it likely loses its life force.

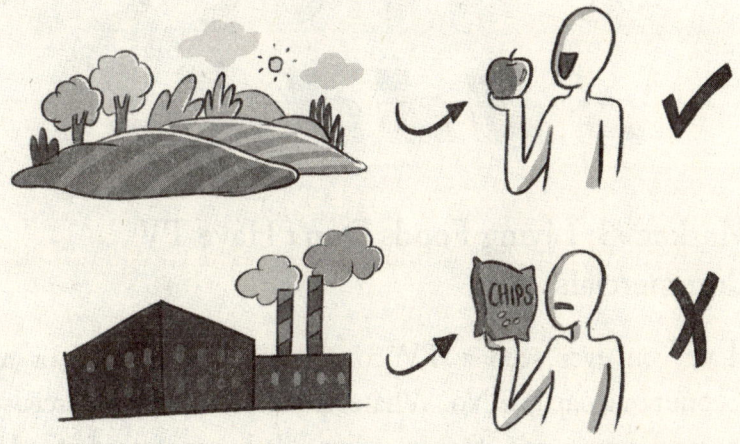

Marker #2: Living Food Rots Fast

It might seem counter-intuitive, but food that decays quickly is actually real food. Why? Because only life attracts life. Bacteria and microorganisms are drawn to those foods that are filled with life force.

Think about it: If you leave a banana or an apple on your kitchen counter, it'll only take a few days before it starts to turn brown. Contrast that with a fast-food burger.

Some anecdotal accounts showed that even after several weeks of being left on the counter, some burgers hardly changed in their appearance or composition! What's inside them that doesn't allow them to rot or decay? We'll learn more about this further in the chapter.

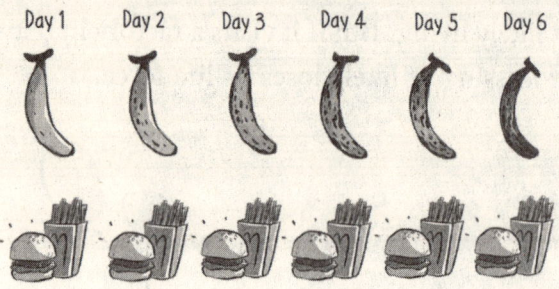

Marker #3: Living Foods Don't Have TV Commercials

Have you ever seen a TV commercial for broccoli or a coconut or a papaya? No. Whatever you see TV commercials or newspaper ads for is most likely processed food, manufactured for the primary purpose of making profit.

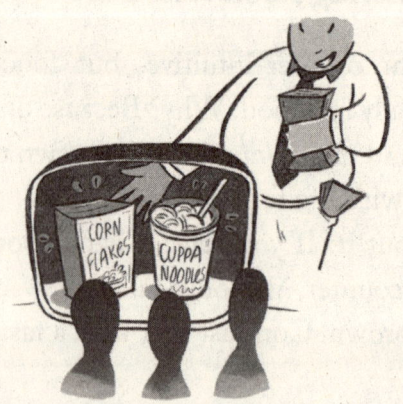

'The key to eating healthy? Avoid anything that has a TV commercial.'

—Anonymous

Now, if these three markers define what living foods are, what do you think lies on the opposite end of the spectrum? What's the category of food that's the polar opposite of living foods?

Well, **the absolute opposite of living foods are highly processed foods**. These are foods that are manufactured or heavily altered in laboratories or factories, and are then:

- Bottled (aerated drinks, store-bought milkshakes, factory-made sauces and dressings, commercial fruit juices)
- Packaged (commercial chips, biscuits and cookies, breakfast cereals, namkeen and masala mixes, instant noodles, packaged jams and spreads, ready-to-eat curries)
- Frozen (ready-to-cook parathas, frozen pizzas, frozen samosas, frozen spring rolls and nuggets, frozen yogurt)
- Tinned (factory-made soups, canned vegetable purees, commercial broths and stocks)

In other words, when a living food goes to a factory, where it is completely altered from its natural state, and then bottled, packaged, frozen or tinned, it is converted into a processed food.

Now, whenever the talk of processed foods arises, I'm sure you stumble upon this question: 'But is it really a problem if we consume them occasionally? If we eat them only sometimes?'

In order to answer this question, we would like to share with you two secret truths about packaged foods that big food manufacturers hope you'll never find out. These are two truths that are never spoken about on the TV or in the newspapers. These are truths that are deliberately kept hidden from the mass population because if we knew, we would take very different actions.

Once you know these truths, you can make a more informed choice as to whether you would like to include these processed foods in your diet frequently, occasionally, sometimes or not at all.

Two Secret Truths that Big Food Companies Hope You Never Find Out

The First Truth: Packaged Food Has More Additives Than We Are Led to Believe

Take a moment and think about the ketchup bottle sitting in your kitchen. Reflect on these questions:

- When do you think the tomatoes inside were picked, crushed, boiled, seasoned and finally bottled?
- After being bottled, how long might it have sat in a warehouse, waiting for distribution?

- Once it reached the retail store, how many days or weeks did it sit on the shelf before you purchased it?

Piecing this together, can you estimate the time between when that ketchup was made and when it reached your table?

If you think the time frame is anywhere between a few weeks and a few months, you're right.

Now, imagine making fresh tomato ketchup at home. You place it in a bottle and leave it out on your kitchen shelf. After five to seven days, what do you expect would happen? It might separate, with the water on top and a thicker pulp at the bottom. You might see mould growing on its surface. It might even start to ferment, tasting sour, the fresh tomato aroma replaced by a pungent, unpleasant smell.

Yet, when you open the commercially packaged tomato ketchup, despite being manufactured months ago, how is it that it pours bright red, doesn't separate, smells like tomatoes, and shows no signs of mould?

Similarly, home-made biscuits last two to three weeks, but how do the biscuits in the store-bought packet stay good for many months or even years?

Well, as you may have guessed, these store-bought products are laden with **preservatives and synthetic chemicals** to keep them looking, tasting and smelling fresh.

I remember, during my childhood days, how every day while returning from school, my friend and I would persuade our van driver to stop at a local store. We would hastily go in and buy a few packets of chips, along with chocolate or jam biscuits for our ride home. I had these packaged treats every single day (not exaggerating). Of course, my mum and my aunts would keep telling me that these are bad for me, but it simply didn't matter because they tasted so good!

It wasn't until years later, after overcoming my health issues and diving into research on these additives, that I fully grasped the impact of what they really do within our bodies. I was genuinely taken aback. Here's a glimpse of what I discovered these processed products contain:

- **Food colours:**
  Did you ever wonder about those vibrantly coloured cereals frequently advertised to children? Or biscuits with unusually dark, orange or pink creams? That burst of colour comes from added food dyes that are designed to make products appear bright and attractive.

- **Chemical preservatives:**
  This is the main reason why these products don't spoil easily. These chemicals stop yeast and fungus growth, in order to make the food look, smell and feel 'fresh' for a long time.

- **Artificial flavours:**
  When genuine flavours are expensive, food manufacturers use lab-produced chemicals to replicate tastes like cherry, blueberry or vanilla. This means

there's a possibility your store-bought strawberry-flavoured yogurt might not contain any real strawberries at all, but rather a synthesized, lab-created imitation of strawberry flavour.

These are just a few of the additives used. There's a long list of other chemicals that are also used, including emulsifiers, gelling agents, thickening agents, etc.

While these preservatives and chemicals are listed in the ingredient list in small font at the back of the product's packaging, what's not mentioned anywhere on the packet is how **multiple studies have indicated these additives have carcinogenic properties (cancer-causing properties).***

If only we could see the harmful effects of these synthetic chemicals immediately, we wouldn't even go near them. However, because the damage these chemicals cause is so incremental (often spread over many years), we tend to turn a blind eye to them. When I read the research on how harmful these chemicals are, especially for children, I couldn't help but question why our food regulation authorities don't do anything about it. How is it that they allow these products to be marketed to our children and sold outside their schools and colleges?

To put it bluntly, **these preservatives and added chemicals may prolong the shelf life of the product, but they actually shorten ours.**

---

* For detailed studies on the health implications of these chemical additives, see this book's reference section.

'Don't ask why healthy food is expensive.
Ask why processed food is so cheap.'

—Anonymous

This reminds me of something that happened at one of my first-ever workshops, which was with a group of children in my aunt's basement. I was sharing the concept of processed foods when a child raised his hand and asked, 'If they are laced with chemicals, if they have no nutrition, and if their life force is taken away, do you mean that these packaged foods are dead foods?' Another one raised his hand and asked, 'How can we expect to gain life by eating something that's dead?'

Their understanding, and the way they articulated it, left me pleasantly surprised. Today, I find the term 'dead foods' quite an accurate descriptor of these products.

All of this said, I also fully understand how tough it is to resist the temptation of these treats. Our taste buds have been conditioned to crave these flavours. Have you ever picked up that packet of chips and then tried to set it aside after a few bites? I've been there, and I know how hard it is. But remember:

It's not your fault.

It is not your fault that you can't stop yourself. It's not your fault that you find yourself reaching for another, and then another.

Because the Second Truth Is That:
Packaged Foods Are Engineered for Addiction

This truth is best illustrated through a personal experience I had during the early years of my journey. It was a cold afternoon, and I was staying at my relatives' home while training to become a plant-based chef. I had decided to stay with them as their home was conveniently close to the academy where I was studying.

One day when I came back home from class, the house was empty and my stomach was rumbling with hunger as I'd had a light lunch. I entered the kitchen, intending to prepare a simple meal. Yet there it was—an open bag of chips, half eaten.

Despite my commitment to clean eating, my growling stomach tempted me. 'Just four or five chips,' I thought. I gave in to the temptation, ate a few pieces, and put the packet away. I felt happy with myself.

But then, I couldn't stop myself. I opened it again and emptied out the whole packet.

I knew it wasn't good for me. I knew it was full of chemical additives. In fact, I was studying health and nutrition day in and day out. Yet, I couldn't stop myself. (I'm sure you've experienced this in your own life—you open a bar of chocolate thinking you'll eat just one piece. But, in no time, the whole bar disappears into nothingness!)

Once I finished that packet of chips, I felt guilty. How could I inspire others to remove these processed foods from their lives when I wasn't able to control myself?

But then, as I was about to discard the empty bag of chips, I read the label: 'No one can eat just one.' That sentence was a revelation, because that's exactly what had happened to me!

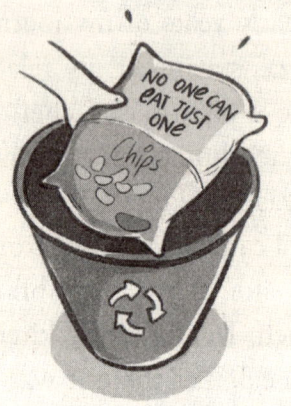

Intrigued, I started researching more, only to make an astonishing discovery. We can't eat just one chip because they're simply not designed that way. Shortly after eating one, we become chemically addicted to it, much like we become addicted to a drug. Initially, I rejected such a provocative claim, deeming it an irresponsible exaggeration. Yet, as I delved deeper, I found hard evidence in the insightful book *Hooked* by Michael Moss.

It exposed the lengths to which food companies go— investing millions in research to perfect an addictive taste, a satisfying crunch, a tantalizing aftertaste—all aimed to get us, the consumers, hooked on their products. Their sole goal? Making us **addicted** to their offerings so that we buy it again and again and again.

To achieve this, they use three ingredients in excessively high doses. Do you know what they are?

Well, the three ingredients are:

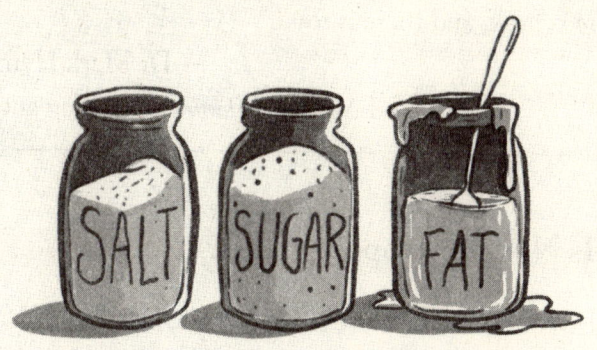

Salt, sugar and fat—these three ingredients, in high doses, hijack our brain's reward system.

Think about it: After the twenty-fifth bite of a cucumber, how do you feel? Full, right? Maybe even bored of eating it.

But after the twenty-fifth bite of a potato chip, how do you feel? You want one more, and then one more, and then one more. Isn't it?

This is because it's loaded with salt, sugar and fat. High amounts of salt, sugar and fat in anything keep you coming back for more and more and more.

While the price tag on a packet of chips may seem cheap, the actual cost is expensive. With each purchase, these companies are handcuffing us, trapping us in a vicious cycle of dependency: buy, consume, crave, repeat. This ruthless cycle continues endlessly until we fall prey to diseases.

To summarize, that was the second truth: packaged foods are engineered for addiction.

'There is no such thing as "junk food".
There is junk, and there is food.'

—Dr Mark Hyman,
MD and *New York Times* bestselling author

Why Is Nobody Stopping This?

If these packaged foods are so addictive, filled with harmful chemical additives and devoid of nutritional value, why are they still so freely available in our markets? Why is no one putting a stop to them? Did these questions cross your mind as you read the two truths in the previous pages?

Well, here is an interesting historical fact to help you understand.

Do you know that back in the 1930s, the tobacco industry marketed cigarettes as completely fine for our health and even beneficial? They even used to publish articles in newspapers saying that doctors also used them, so you should too. Here are some actual articles:

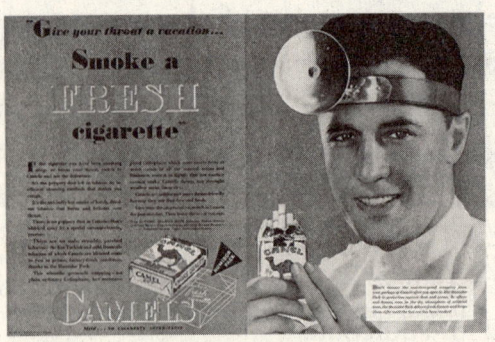
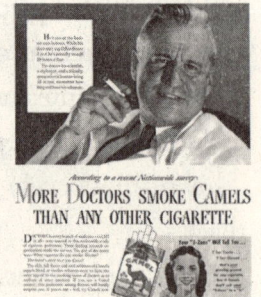

Some articles even claimed that cigarettes would help you stay slim and attractive.

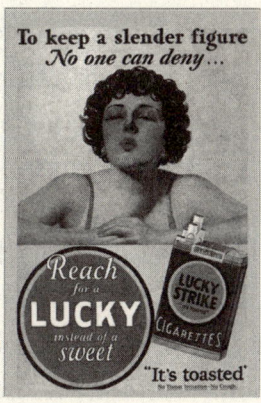

But today, what do we know about cigarettes? That they cause lung cancer, among other health issues. But industries like tobacco and junk food have successfully built billion-dollar empires on the back of deceptive advertising.

Likewise, packaged food today is considered normal and safe. Throughout my life, I believed it was normal to kick off my day with a packet of cookies or to whip up a packet of instant noodles every other day. Have you, too, normalized the consumption of processed, packaged food in your life? Yes, I'm asking **you**.

But ninety years from now, perhaps someone will take a stand and declare that this isn't normal. That these packaged foods that we've come to accept as the norm are destroying our health. That it's not normal to eat this rubbish in the name of 'food'.

But why should we wait for that time?

Why should we wait for the government to fix things?

Why should we wait for institutional changes to improve laws?

Why should we wait ninety years for someone to raise their voice and tell us that the health risks posed by these foods are worse than we imagined? Perhaps by that time, it will be too late. We can take control of our health right now!

You see, once you put this book down, you will have two paths.

Path one: Wait for the system to change. Wait for the government to step in. Wait for yet another research study to confirm that these products are carcinogenic.

Path two: Take full responsibility for what you put into your body each day.

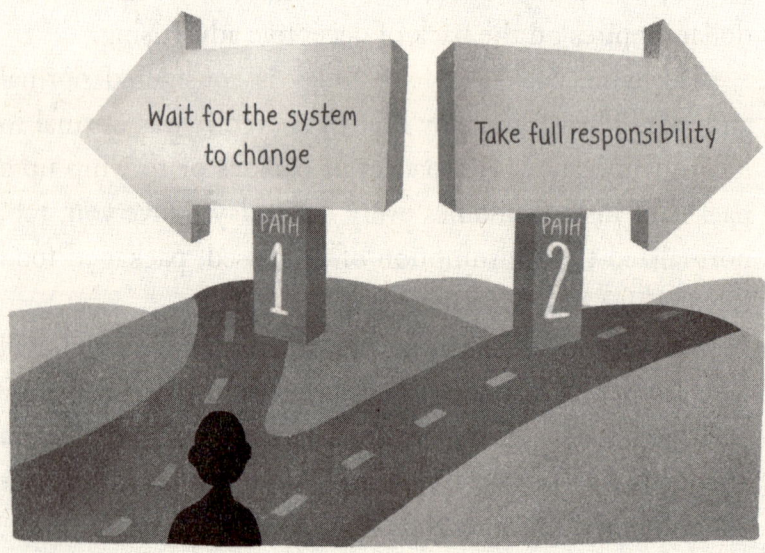

The choice is yours to make. What do you choose, dear reader?

We're aware that the topics we've covered so far have been somewhat grave and heavy. But rest assured, in the upcoming section, we will focus on solutions rather than problems. We aim to equip you with not one or two, but three strategies to resist the manipulative marketing tactics of large corporations and regain control of your health. You may find one, two or all three of these strategies applicable to your situation. Start with what resonates with you and what you find doable.

Three Steps to Not Fall into the Marketing Gimmicks of Food Companies

#1: Choose Foods from the Green and Yellow List

Here's a silver lining—not all packaged foods lining supermarket shelves are bad. The key lies in distinguishing the clean options from the harmful ones. Essentially, every food item falls into one of three categories: red, yellow or green. By simply reading the ingredient list of a product, we can know which category it fits into.

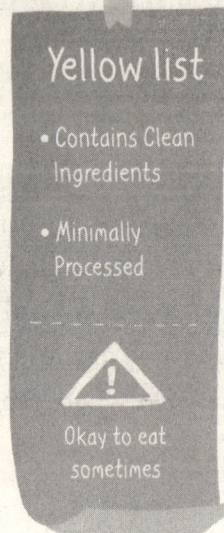
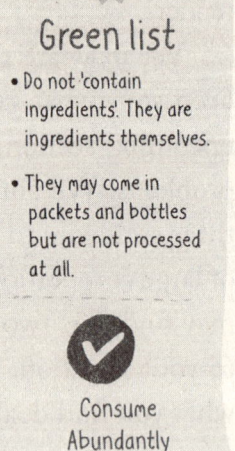

Red list

- Contains Nasty Ingredients
- Highly Processed

Avoid consuming completely

Yellow list

- Contains Clean Ingredients
- Minimally Processed

Okay to eat sometimes

Green list

- Do not 'contain ingredients'. They are ingredients themselves.
- They may come in packets and bottles but are not processed at all.

Consume Abundantly

Thankfully, the law mandates food manufacturers must declare every ingredient used in their product on the ingredient list. Due to this requirement, manufacturers often print the ingredient list, a very important piece of information, in extremely tiny font on the back of the pack.

For instance, a packet of chips with ingredients like this would fall into the red category.

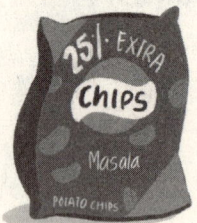

Ingredients

Potato, Vegetable Oil, Corn Starch, Iodised Salt, Maltodextrin, Tomato Powder, Acidity Regulators, Flavouring Substances, Anticaking Agent, Citric Acid.

A nut and date bar with ingredients like this would fall in the yellow list since all the ingredients are clean ingredients. You could easily find them in a regular kitchen. Plus, they don't sound like chemical names. You can easily pronounce them.

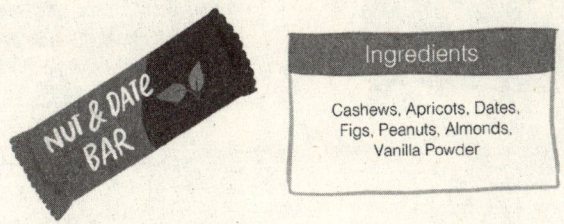

A box of dates or a bag of pumpkin seeds would fall in the green category, because these foods are actually ingredients themselves.

Here are images and ingredient lists of eight packaged products. You have to determine which category each product belongs to and write your answer in the blank. Please turn the page once you've filled your answers.

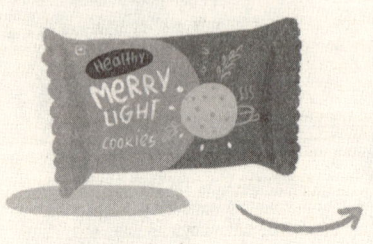

Ingredients

Refined Wheat flour, Edible Vegetable Oil, Malt Extract, INS 504, Butter, Milk Solids, Invert Sugar Syrup, Dough Conditioner, Artificial Flavours

_____

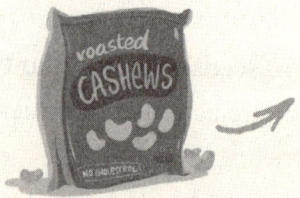

Ingredients

Cashew Nuts, Chili Powder, Salt, Chaat Masala, Jaggery

_____

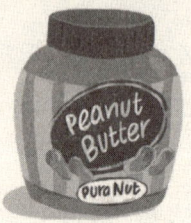

Ingredients

Peanuts and Rock Salt

_____

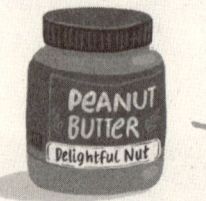

Ingredients

Corn Flour, Sugar, Peanut Butter, Edible Vegetable Oil, Caramel Colour, Stabilizer, Molasses, Iodised Salt

_____

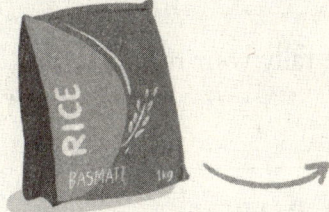

Ingredients

Rice

_____

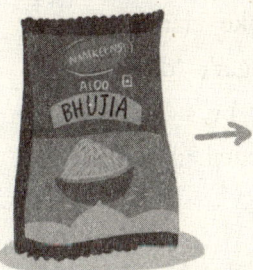

Ingredients

Potato, Refined Palmolein Oil, Bengal Gram Flour (Besan), Tapioca Starch, Red Chilli Powder, Black Salt, Cardamom, Dried Ginger Powder, Bay Leaves, Nutmeg, Acidity Regulator and Nature Identical Flavours

_____

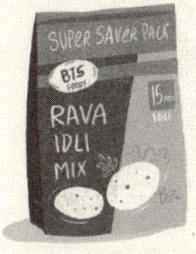

Ingredients

Semolina, Hydrogenated Vegetable Fat, Bengal Gram Dal, Salt, Dehydrated Curry Leaves, Raising Agent, Sodium Bicarbonate (INS 500 ii), Anti Caking Agent Silica (INS 551), Mustard Seeds, Chili

_____

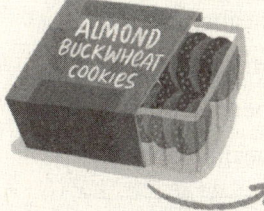

Ingredients

Buckwheat, Sunflower Seeds, Coconut Powder, Raisins, Jaggery, Almonds, Cinnamon Powder, Rice Bran Oil, Vanilla Powder, Salt

_____

If you've completed the quiz, please tally your results with the answers below:

1. **'Healthy' Merry Light Cookies—Red List**
   Despite claiming to be 'healthy', the ingredient list reveals artificial flavours, emulsifiers, and preservatives. Supermarket products frequently make claims like 'healthy', 'natural', 'fat-free', 'low-sugar', 'diabetic-friendly' and 'no-preservatives'. Don't be swayed by the front labels—always check the actual ingredient list.

2. **Roasted and Spiced Cashews—Yellow List**
   This pack of cashews passes the test because its ingredients can easily be found in a typical kitchen.

3. **Peanut Butter by Pura Nut—Yellow List**
   Simple and pure with only peanuts and salt. No additives.

4. **Peanut Butter by DelightfulNut—Red List**
   If some ingredients are hard to pronounce, it's a red flag. Also, food regulation authorities mandate that all ingredients must be declared in decreasing order of the quantity they are used in. This means that the most used ingredient is listed first, and the least used ingredient is listed last. In this jar of peanut butter, cornflour and sugar are listed before peanut butter,

which means that it actually contains more cornflour and sugar than peanut butter!

5. **Packet of Rice—Green List**
   While it's packaged, this rice is just that: rice. It doesn't contain ingredients. Rather, it's an ingredient itself.

6. **Namkeen Bhujia—Red List**
   Though most ingredients seem safe, don't be fooled by the 'Nature identical flavours'. These might sound natural, but in reality, these are chemically synthesized equivalents of natural flavours, not extracted from source materials.

7. **Rava Idli Mix—Red List**
   You may see ingredients starting with **INS or E acronyms.** If an ingredient is represented by a number, not a name, and begins with these acronyms, please understand that it's just a synthetic additive.

8. **Almond Oat Cookies—Yellow List**
   These cookies are made with straightforward, recognizable ingredients commonly found in kitchens.

If you got most of the answers correct, congratulations! You've learnt a new skill: reading ingredient lists. And today, in the 21st century, with the majority of the population heavily relying on packaged foods, we believe this is as important a skill as knowing how to cook or how to code. Now you can also read the labels on the products in your kitchen cabinet and identify which list they belong to.

Our suggestion is to avoid items from the red list altogether, or have them sparingly. If you want to enjoy packaged foods, go for products from the yellow list. Today, there are more and more conscious brands emerging that offer clean packaged foods that belong to the yellow list. The best, though, are foods from the green list, which can be consumed abundantly, either whole or transformed into delicious dishes at home.

Now let's delve into the second strategy to avoid falling prey to the marketing gimmicks of food companies.

#2: Replace, Don't Remove

Many of us (including us!) cannot sustain a lifestyle of restraint and strict control. So instead of removing our favourite foods, if we can learn how to replace them with their cleaner, living food counterparts, we can actually sustain this habit. Replace, don't remove. Switch, don't quit.

To assist you in this process, we have identified substitutions for the top six processed foods that are most popular today. For each item, we have provided two alternatives: a quick option that can be prepared in under five minutes, and a more elaborate option that can be made in fifteen minutes and then stored to be consumed over the following weeks.

Instead of	Do this ✔ (the quickest option– under 5 mins)	Or do this ✔ (If you have time to prepare– under 15 mins)
Savoury snacks (chips, namkeen)	Roasted nuts, Roasted gram, Roasted corn on the cob 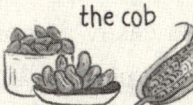	Home-made Chips, Popcorn or Chivda 
Biscuits or cookies 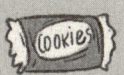	Fresh fruits, Slices of coconut 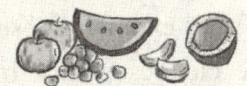	Home-made biscuits and cookies 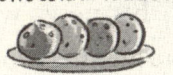 Apple slices dipped in peanut butter
Packaged chocolates 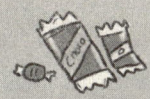	Chocolate smoothie bowl made using cacao 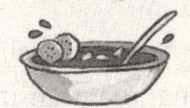	Home-made chocolate coated nuts, Chocolate laddoos 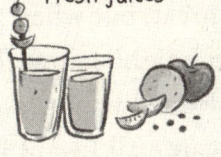
Packaged drinks and sodas	Fresh lime water, Fresh coconut water 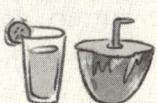	Fresh juices 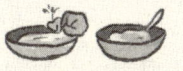
Packaged sauce, ketchup and salad dressings 	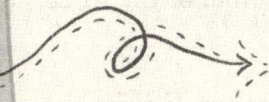	Home-made dips, sauces and chutneys
Commercial ice creams 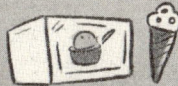	Smooothie bowls made at home using fruits and bananas 	Home-made ice creams 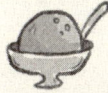

Our Satvic team has created a detailed document sharing recipes for each of these substitutions. You will find the link to these at the end of this chapter.

Now, we know that many of you might be able to make these replacements easily at home, whereas others may find them impractical, perhaps due to a lack of time, a busy schedule or any other reason. Well, we'd like to tell you that today, there are many conscious brands out there committed to making cleaner foods—those that fall in the 'yellow list'. After extensive research, our team has curated a list of the cleanest snack brands that exist in India. We have left the link for this list at the end of this chapter (this compilation is entirely unbiased and not sponsored in any way.)

By now, we hope you are feeling a little bit more confident about making the transition to living foods. However, you might still wonder, 'These substitutes are great, but when a craving strikes, my motivation crumbles. I might know that the buttery cookie in front of me is loaded with preservatives, but at that moment, I just don't care. All I want is to savour it.'

We've all been there. That's why we would like to introduce you to the final of the three steps.

#3: Tweak Your Kitchen Environment

One of our most profound learnings from the book *Atomic Habits* by James Clear was this:

Motivation is overrated.

Environment matters more.

Please note this. Circle it, highlight it and underline it.

If you rely on motivation to quit packaged foods or eat more living foods, you're most likely going to fail. Motivation may work for the next two or three days. But after that, you'll be back at square one, even after reading this long chapter. Because if the item is kept in front of you, controlling yourself requires way too much willpower! Most of us don't have it. Your environment matters much more than how much motivation you have.

Often, you make food choices not based on **what** the foods are, but **where** they are.

If you walk into your kitchen, open the fridge and see a tub of delicious ice cream, what would you do? Chances are that you will get a spoon, scoop some ice cream into a bowl, and convince yourself that it's just one bite! It does not matter how much self-control you have or how much willpower you possess. The layout and design of your space impact your behaviour more than self-discipline or motivation.

So what's the solution? Redesign your environment. **Make packaged foods invisible.** If they are in your home, they can only go three places: your stomach, your family's stomach or out of the house. You need to decide their destination. The choice is yours.

If you're serious about achieving peak health, we suggest removing all highly processed foods (those on the red list) from your kitchen. Whether you discard them or give them away is up to you, but the key is to get them out of sight.

In case you're thinking, 'Oh, but if I do this, my family/partner/flatmate will send me out of the house,' well, we understand. Take the second-best option: reduce their exposure. Create a separate processed-food cabinet. Collect all the processed red-list items from your house. Don't leave anything anywhere. Collect everything in the bedroom, kitchen, everywhere. Place it all in this one dedicated cabinet. Ideally choose a cabinet that's difficult to reach. Label it with a reminder like 'Beware, dead food inside'. Lock the cabinet if possible, and share the key with someone else in your home. This will make it harder for you to access the unhealthy options.

Once you've removed the processed foods from your sight, replace the empty spaces with healthy cues. In other words, make the living foods more visible. Keep a basket of fruits on your kitchen counter and stock up on wholesome snacks. Make it easy to reach for healthy options when hunger strikes.

This approach has truly worked for us. People often ask, 'Do you guys genuinely follow everything you share? Is it possible to live without eating packaged food?' And then we ask ourselves, 'How have we managed so effortlessly without these processed foods?' We realize it's because we don't keep them in our home. When they're out of sight, they're out of mind. There's no temptation. The fact that we don't have to resist them every moment is a huge reason we've been able to sustain this habit.

'You **don't** have to be the **victim of your environment.** You can also be the **architect of it.**'

—James Clear,
author of *Atomic Habits*

In summary, there are three practical ways to reduce your consumption of processed foods:

1. **Read the ingredient list** every time you make a purchase. If a product is on the red list, it's best to put it back on the shelf.
2. Don't merely eliminate your favourite processed foods. If you do, you might find yourself craving them in a few days and giving in to the temptation. Instead, swap them for more nutritious alternatives. **Replace, don't remove.**
3. **Tweak your kitchen environment.** Remove the processed food from your sight. Out of sight, out of mind. Instead, fill your kitchen with healthy reminders of fresh, living foods.

Concluding Thoughts about This Practice

Dear reader, we understand that implementing drastic changes just by reading a chapter can be hard, but we sincerely hope that you start with the steps that you find most practical.

And don't forget: the essence of the first pillar, 'Eat Living', is to enjoy the abundance provided by Mother Nature. She's gifted us so many incredible living foods. Each living food provided by the earth pulses with life-giving energy. Mother Earth fills it with minerals. The water element makes it juicy. The Wind God gives it freshness and cleans it, while the Moon God infuses it with divine medicinal qualities. If we consume dead foods, we ingest death, and if we consume living foods, they fill us with life, which radiates through our energy, eyes and our entire being!

Also remember, when you bring a revolution in your own kitchen by choosing fresh, living foods, you automatically become a catalyst for positive change for society at large. This revolution extends beyond your personal health. It creates a wave of inspiration for your family and loved ones, it supports the farmers who work day and night to grow real, nourishing food, and it promotes a shift in our food industry—from prioritizing profits to prioritizing humanity's health. With every purchase you make, you vote for a different world.

In the next chapter, we will proceed to the second pillar of habit two, which is to eat 'wholesome'. You'll learn about the crazy rat experiment, the common kitchen ingredient that doubles up as the perfect glue, and many more surprises.

To access the snack replacement recipes, scan the QR code or visit satvicmovement.org/book/snack

To access the 'India's Cleanest Snack Brands', scan the QR code or visit satvicmovement.org/book/list

4

The Two Most Sneaky Culprits in Your Kitchen

Growing up, the aroma of toasted sandwiches stuffed with melting cheese, crunchy bhujia, and tangy tomato ketchup is what filled the kitchen every morning. Alongside, a comforting glass of milk or the invigorating scent of fresh coffee marked the start of my day. Lunch was simple—a plateful of basmati rice paired with either dal, rajma or chola. Snacks typically consisted of buttery biscuits, chocolate cookies or generous bowls of my favourite namkeen. Dinner was a humble serving of vegetables (various Indian sabzis) accompanied by soft wheat chapatis and a bowl of curd (dahi).

I loved my meals. They were delicious, satisfying and comforting. And also, my family felt at ease knowing I was mostly eating at home. I genuinely believed that I was maintaining a healthy, balanced diet.

However, it wasn't until I attended a talk by my master in June 2016 that I realized that a shocking 60–70 per cent of what I was consuming was not wholesome. In fact, it was far from it. That's when the dots connected; I realized that many of the chronic health issues I was suffering from were directly caused by this missing quality in my food.

Perhaps you're wondering what 'wholesome' even means. So, before we go further, let's understand its meaning and why it even matters.

What Does 'Wholesome' Even Mean?

At its core, 'wholesome' refers to food in its purest, unaltered and unfragmented form. It is food from which its vital components have not been extracted.

You see, Mother Nature has invested a great deal of time into every food She provides. Whether it's a banana, pumpkin, coconut or even a humble grain of rice, each has been designed with care. Nature ensures that each food possesses a perfect balance of nutrients so it can be easily digested by our human body.

However, when we subtract any vital component from this natural composition, perhaps to extend its shelf life or for our convenience, we unknowingly refine and alter the food's intrinsic value. In doing so, we transform a wholesome food into a **refined** or **fragmented** one.

Consider corn, for instance. We harvest corn on the cob, a food which is in its wholesome state. The roasted version of this is also commonly sold on the streets of India, known as *bhutta* in Hindi. I'm sure you've seen it. While most of us eat it directly, did you know there are different products made out of it?

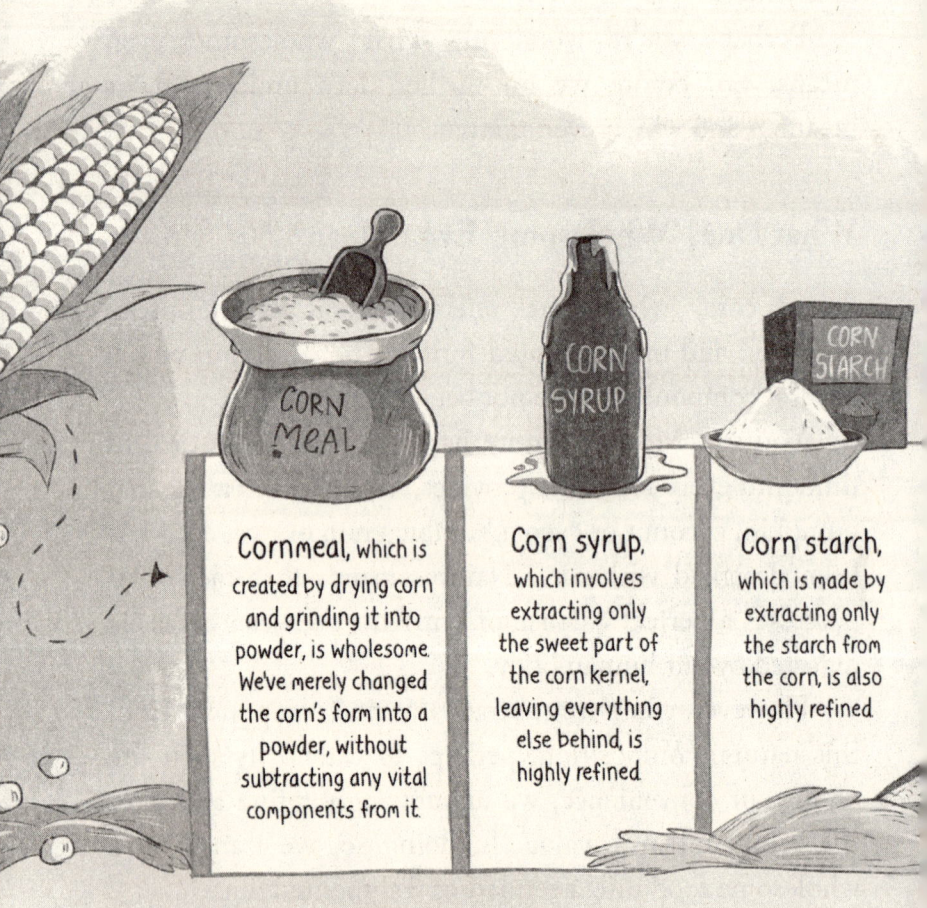

Cornmeal, which is created by drying corn and grinding it into powder, is wholesome. We've merely changed the corn's form into a powder, without subtracting any vital components from it.

Corn syrup, which involves extracting only the sweet part of the corn kernel, leaving everything else behind, is highly refined.

Corn starch, which is made by extracting only the starch from the corn, is also highly refined

Hopefully, that provides a bit more clarity on what 'wholesomeness' means.

Now, what percentage of your own diet do you think is wholesome? Are there any **highly refined foods** that you might be consuming every day?

Well, by the end of this chapter, you'll have clear answers to these questions. Here's what you can expect to learn in this chapter:

- What are the two most refined foods you may be consuming every day?
- Where could they be hidden apart from the obvious places?
- Whether or not it's possible to remove them from your diet.
- If it is, what are wholesome substitutes to these refined foods that could lead to better digestion, a healthier gut and greater energy in your day?

With our foundation established, let's dive right in.

The First Refined Food

From breakfast cereals to coffee mugs,
One taste of me and joy erupts!

My ancestors were the beets and the canes,
And in their legacy, my sweetness reigns.

I hide myself behind innocent names, I won't lie,
What do you think, who am I?

Answer: Sugar

If you walk into your local grocer and request for 'sugar', you'll be handed a packet of pure white crystal-like particles. But, have you ever paused to think—where do these come from? Well, as the rhyme suggested, sugar comes from two major sources: sugar cane (80 per cent of global sugar production) and sugar beets (they're like beetroots, except they're white).

To make sugar,
first this raw material (sugar cane or sugar beet) is harvested,
then crushed,
then extracted into juice,
then clarified,
then boiled,
then evaporated,
then crystallized,
then centrifuged
and then refined.

Finally, we get sweet, sparkling sugar crystals.

But you see, Mother Nature never provided us with these. She provides us with sugar cane, which is filled with life-giving nutrients. However, when that natural food is converted into white sugar, all of those beneficial minerals and vitamins are leached out in the refinement process. Finally, there is only one thing that remains in the white sugar crystals, and that is the sweetness! (Even the colour completely changes—from the natural yellow of sugar cane to the pure white of sugar).

Now chances are, if you're reading this book, you're already aware about the harmful effects of sugar. Many of us grew up hearing our parents warn us about those dreaded cavities or the extra kilos of weight sugar might bring (I know I did). But even with those warnings ringing in our ears, why is it that saying no to those sugary cakes, donuts, chocolates, jalebis and barfis is so difficult? When we know it's bad for us, why is it so hard to avoid? The answer may surprise you. Let's find out.

Why Is It so Hard to Say No to Sugar?

Picture this: you walk into a room, and there's a table in front of you with five items on it. You're asked to identify the most addictive substance among them. Which would you select? Think deeply and place a check mark next to your choice in the image below.

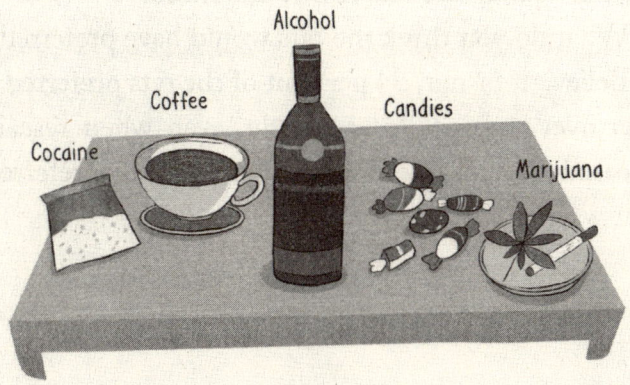

Most people would instinctively choose 'cocaine'. And it's no surprise—it's one of the world's most addictive and harmful drugs, illegal in most countries.

But here's a twist: the right answer isn't 'cocaine'. It's the innocent-looking 'candies'. The reason for this is pretty simple. Candies are laden with refined white sugar, and **sugar is highly addictive, even more addictive than cocaine!** And I don't mean addictive in the way that people talk about delicious foods. I mean addictive, literally, in the same way as drugs. This may sound like an overstatement but as we progress further, it will become clearer.

There was a fascinating study conducted in 2007 by researchers at the University of Bordeaux. In this experiment, forty-three rats were placed in cages with two levers. One lever, when pressed by the rats, gave them an intravenous hit of cocaine, making them feel an instant 'high'. The other lever, when pressed by the rats, gave them a sip of sugar water.

The researchers allowed the rats to do a couple of sample tries, so that the rats could understand each lever's offerings. Then, the real test commenced.

What do you think the rats would have preferred?

Believe it or not, **94 per cent of the rats preferred sugar water over cocaine!** Interestingly, even when researchers increased the cocaine dosage, the rats still preferred the sugar water.

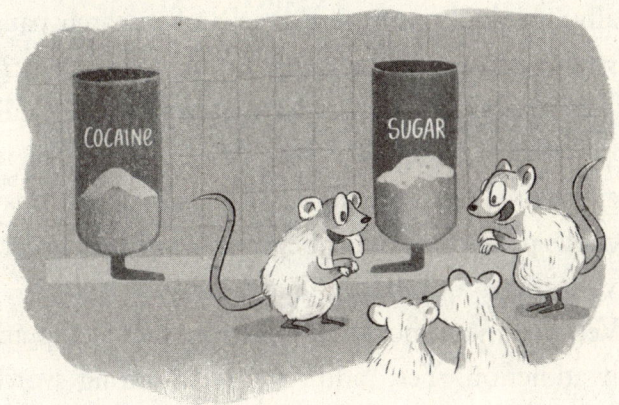

What's the science behind this? When we consume sugar, the amount of dopamine released in the brain increases, just like the response triggered when we take an addictive drug. Over time, with repeated exposure, our brain becomes dependent on sugary foods to get this dopamine rush. What's surprising is that researchers suggest the brain finds the rewards from sugar even 'more rewarding and attractive' than those from cocaine.

'When society finally discovers that refined sugar is just another white powder, along with pure cocaine, it will change its mind and attitude toward refined food addiction.'
—Dr Serge Ahmed,
Scientist with the University of Bordeaux in
France and author of the above-mentioned study

Actually, we don't even need stacks of research papers to understand how addictive sugar is. We can see it in our everyday life. Have you ever experienced how difficult it is to stop after just one sugary treat, like a cookie? You intend to eat just one, but before you know it, you've consumed the whole pack! Soon you begin craving the sweet even after your meals and throughout the day.

Well, you must know that this isn't a mere temptation—it's an addiction. Yes, 'addiction' is a strong word, but research, as well as our personal experience, shows us exactly that.

Beyond its addictive nature, sugar has numerous other downsides. Strong evidence indicates that excess sugar in our diet is stored as fat in our body, causing excessive weight gain. Short-term studies also link high sugar intake to elevated blood sugar levels, diabetes, high triglycerides, increased blood pressure and heart disease. It's no wonder some experts have labelled refined sugar a '**slow white poison**'.

Now, having understood the addictive and harmful nature of sugar, there's no denying that most of us love desserts! It's hard to imagine life without them. The good news is that we don't have to give them up. At our Satvic headquarters, we love preparing desserts. We frequently bake cakes to mark celebrations with our team, prepare Indian mithais like kheer and rabdi for festivals and occasionally indulge in scrumptious desserts to end our meals. The only difference is that we don't use refined white sugar. Instead, we prepare or find treats made from wholesome sweeteners. Yes, there are some excellent alternatives to white sugar. But before sharing the best ones, let's do a short activity.

When you read the word 'sugar' in this chapter, you might be picturing that spoonful you stir into your morning tea or coffee, or the sugar you sprinkle over your breakfast cereal. But you'd be surprised where else refined sugar is sneakily hiding!

A Quick Activity

Here are some popular food products many of us enjoy. Next to each, jot down your best guess: what percentage of it is sugar? Let's see how close you get!

a) A Can of Cold Drink

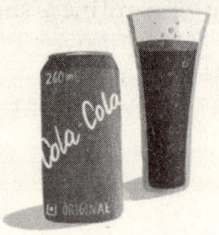

What % of this can do you think is sugar?

_____

b) Children's Cacao Based Drink Powder

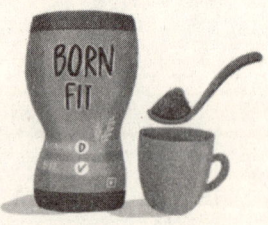

What % of this bottle do you think is sugar?

_____

c) Store-bought Tomato Ketchup

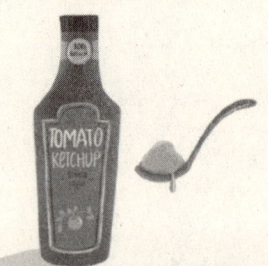

What % of this bottle do you think is sugar?

_____

d) Well-known Wake-up Biscuits

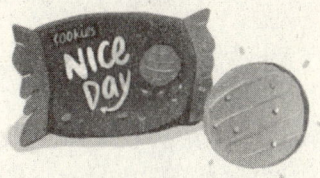

What % of this biscuit
do you think is sugar?

_____

e) Motichoor Laddoo

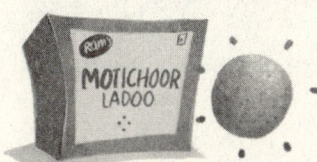

What % of this laddoo
do you think is sugar?

_____

f) Popular Creamy Milk Chocolate

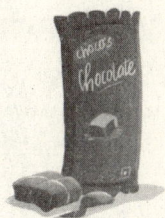

What % of this bar
do you think is sugar?

_____

9) Popular Store-bought Chocolate Spread

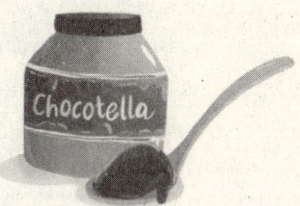

What % of this bottle
do you think is sugar?

_____

Let's check your answers now!

a) A Can of Cold Drink

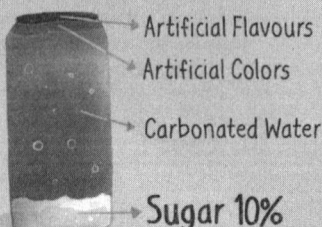

Artificial Flavours
Artificial Colors
Carbonated Water
Sugar 10%

> While 10% sugar may seem little, it actually means that 1 can of cold drink contains 9 teaspoons of sugar!

b) Children's Cacao-Based Drink Powder

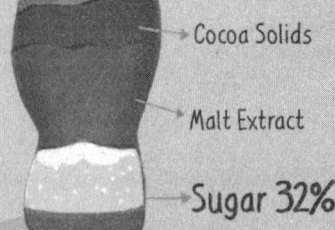

Milk Solids
Cocoa Solids
Malt Extract
Sugar 32%

> Though 32% sugar might seem like a small amount at first glance, it translates to 40 teaspoons of sugar in a 500 gram bottle of this powder.

c) Store-bought Tomato Ketchup

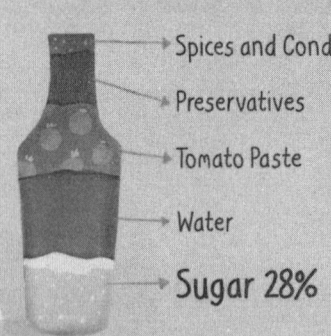

Spices and Condiments
Preservatives
Tomato Paste
Water
Sugar 28%

> Can you believe that the bottle has more sugar than tomato paste?

d) Well-known Wake-up Biscuits

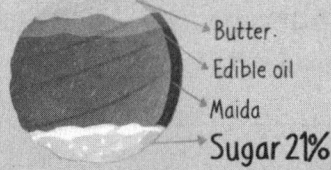

Butter.
Edible oil
Maida
Sugar 21%

Do you realize that almost a quarter of this biscuit is sugar?

e) Motichoor Laddoo

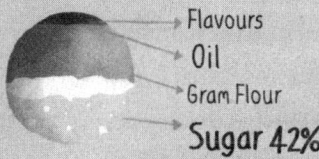

Flavours
Oil
Gram Flour
Sugar 42%

Traditional doesn't always mean wholesome. Almost half of this laddoo is sugar.

f) Popular Creamy Milk Chocolate

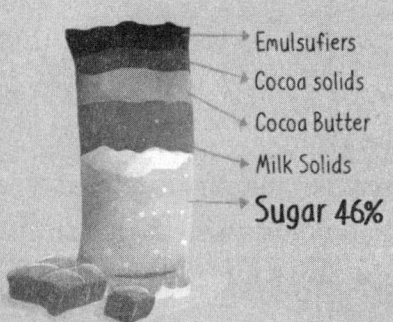

Emulsufiers
Cocoa solids
Cocoa Butter
Milk Solids
Sugar 46%

This bar consists of almost 50% sugar, equivalent to 30 teaspoons of sugar in just one 250 gram bar!

g) Popular Store-bought Chocolate Spread

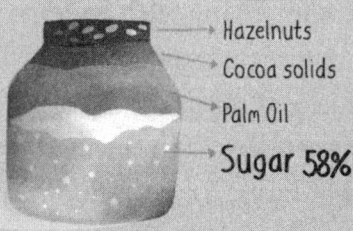

Hazelnuts
Cocoa solids
Palm Oil
Sugar 58%

As you can observe, the jar is essentially half sugar. That's roughly 50 teaspoons of sugar in a 180 gram jar.

The next time you're out grocery shopping, you can try this exercise in real time. Take a moment to read the sugar content listed on the ingredient label. In many cases, you'll find the percentage of sugar directly printed on the packaging.

> **Heads-up:**
>
> Sugar is not always called 'sugar' in ingredient lists. Instead, it's often hidden behind more complicated terms, such as sucrose, dextrose, glucose, maltose, molasses, maltodextrin, sorbitol, xylitol, maltitol or high fructose corn syrup. Don't let these fancy names confuse you—they're essentially the food industry's synonyms for sugar. A handy tip: if an ingredient ends in 'ose', 'syrup' or 'ol', you can be pretty sure it's just another form of refined sugar.

The Alternatives

The most sustainable way to actually eliminate refined sugar from your life is to *replace*, and not *remove*. There are many replacements of refined sugar. Let's categorize them from the worst to the best:

The worst are the highly refined sweeteners. These include brown sugar (essentially white sugar coated with brown molasses), khaand, mishri and commercial honey. Our recommendation would be to remove these entirely from your diet, or at least, reduce their intake as much as possible.

Better are minimally refined sweeteners. This includes jaggery, which is commonly found in India. You can find it in block, syrup or powder form. Aim to purchase chemical-free jaggery from an authentic brand, keeping in mind that the darker the jaggery, the purer it tends to be. While jaggery is less refined than white sugar, it is still a refined food, and hence, you should practise restraint while consuming it.

The best are unrefined sweeteners. These include dates, figs and raisins. And let's not forget fresh fruits like bananas, mangoes, oranges, pineapples, berries, melons and more. These are Nature's candies and are the most wholesome of all.

Satvic desserts are primarily sweetened using dates, jaggery and fresh fruits. This includes everything from cheesecakes, chocolates, pies and cakes to traditional Indian sweets like gulab jamun, halwas, kheers and ladoos.

We've also noticed that earlier, it used to be quite a challenge to find desserts that didn't contain refined sugar. However, today, as awareness is growing, many conscious brands are emerging, offering desserts like chocolates, nut bars, brownies and ladoos prepared using only dates or jaggery as sweeteners. We've included names of a few such brands in the 'India's Cleanest Snack Brands' list shared at the end of previous chapter. The more we demand wholesome food, the more such brands will thrive.

What Happens When You Quit Refined Sugar for Three Weeks?

When you eliminate refined sugar from your life, it's amazing how quickly your body responds. Here's what you might expect after just three weeks:

1. **You'll notice reduced puffiness in your face and belly** (there are two things your body can run on—sugar or fat. When you remove the refined foods with high sugar content, the body will be forced to live off and burn the fat fuel).

2. **Your skin will look better** (because refined sugar increases insulin levels, which causes hormonal imbalances, leading to acne).

3. **You'll experience sustained energy throughout the day** (because blood sugar levels will be normal, not going up and down, you won't feel fatigued easily during the day).

4. **Cravings for unhealthy foods will decrease** (as your brain's dependency on the dopamine spikes triggered by sugar begins to diminish, it'll also reduce your brains' dependence on food for pleasure).

If you feel inspired, give it a try; you might be surprised by what happens.

'A person in good health has a hundred wishes.
A person in bad health only has one wish—to be healthy again.
We take so much for granted.'
—Anonymous

The Second Refined Food

I come from a family of white and smooth,
Early in my youth, my outer skin was removed.

My ancestor is the humble wheat grain,
But, sadly, from me, no nutrition can you gain.

Once I enter your body, I find it hard to leave, no matter
   how much I try,
Take a guess, who do you think am I?

Answer: Refined Wheat, aka Maida

Like with sugar, when you think about maida, many of
you might already know it's not good for you. However,
pause for a moment, think about the last three times you
consumed it, and jot down your answers below.

1 _____
2 _____
3 _____

Where Is Refined Wheat Flour, aka Maida, Hiding?

While recalling the last three times you consumed refined
flour, you might have considered common items like

bhaturas (fried dough) or pizza bases. But did you think of these:

- Samosas
- Momos
- Naans
- Noodles and chow mein
- Breads (both white and brown)
- Pastas

- Cakes
- Biscuits and cookies
- Croissants
- Frankie wraps and rolls
- Buns—for paavs and burgers
- Namkeen (mathri, namak para, etc.)

Most readers who take a moment to reflect on their consumption of refined flour proudly declare, 'Maida? We don't use that at home!' Yet, when they look closer, they're often surprised by how much they're eating without realizing it.

When you pick up something from a bakery or store, almost every item is prepared using maida, unless it's explicitly labelled otherwise. Why? Because it's the cheapest flour available in the market.

Now that you know where maida hides, let's understand how it's made, and what it does once it enters your body (it's going to get slightly technical, but I promise that it's worth understanding).

How's It Made?

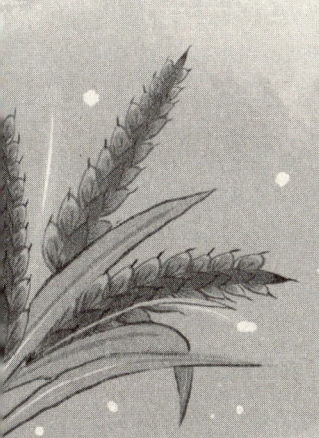

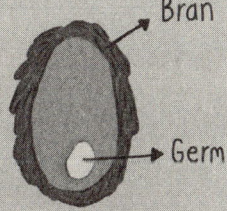

Bran

Germ

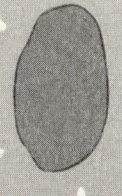

Nature provides us with wheat in this form. Within those golden stalks are small, rounded

wheat kernels.

When you take a closer look at a whole wheat kernel, you'll find it's wrapped in a layer known as the **'bran'.**

This bran is packed with fiber, B vitamins, and essential minerals like iron, copper, and magnesium. The bran is essentially the nutritional powerhouse of the grain.

Now peek inside the wheat kernel, and you discover the 'germ'. Think of this germ as the heart, the essence, or the life giving force of the grain.

However, when wheat is refined, the nutritious bran and germ are thrown away to make the end product softer and to prolong its shelf life.

What's left is the inner white part, which is then ground into flour, which we commonly know as **'maida'.**

What Does It Do within the Body?

Stripped of its nutrition and missing its fibrous bran, maida congests the system. Our digestive system has to work extra hard to push it out of our body, and often, it isn't fully eliminated, resulting in incomplete digestion and thus the creation of toxins inside.

Here's a fun experiment to try (especially for the kids):

The Maida Experiment

Grab two pans. In the first, toss a few tablespoons of maida. In the second, an equal amount of wholewheat flour. Now, add a few tablespoons of water into both and set them up on the stove. Give both a good mix and after about two or three minutes, switch off the flame.

Now, touch and feel the mixtures. Notice how the maida mixture turns into this gooey, super-sticky mess, clinging to your spoon and the bowl? The wholewheat mixture does thicken up, but it doesn't get as sticky.

This sticky consistency of maida (due to the missing fibre) mirrors its behaviour in our digestive tract. Hence, it's no surprise that it's infamously also referred to as the 'glue for the gut'.

Here's an interesting piece of history: In many cultures, especially during the era before commercially available adhesives became widespread, maida was mixed with hot water and used as gum to stick posters on walls!

A study published in the *American Journal of Clinical Nutrition*, involving about 2800 people, found that those who consumed more refined grains ended up with more belly fat and weight gain. In another study, known as *The Nurses' Health Study*, researchers followed over 74,000 women for twelve years. They discovered something striking—the more refined grains these ladies had on their plates, the higher their risk of developing obesity. So, it's not merely an observation from our kitchen experiments; but even long-term research studies show how maida ruins our digestive health.

At this point, it's important to clarify that having maida-based treats once in a while is okay. Our bodies are powerful and can handle these occasional indulgences. However, the challenge emerges when such foods become a regular staple.

So, should we never again consume our beloved cakes, pastries, bhaturas, samosas, pizzas and momos? Well, our intention in this chapter is not to tell you to 'do this' or 'do that'. It's simply to share behind-the-scenes insights about the foods that we eat so frequently. By gaining this knowledge, you empower yourself to make informed decisions. You might choose to eliminate maida completely, or have it occasionally; the choice, ultimately, is yours to make. However, if you're considering alternatives to maida or refined wheat flour, here are some fantastic suggestions.

The Alternatives

The worst are the highly refined flours

This includes all-purpose flour, semolina flour (sooji) and tapioca pearls (sabudana).

Much better are unrefined flours

This includes wholewheat flour, chickpea flour (besan), or millet flours.

A Note about Millets

Millets are ancient grains that are even better for you than wheat. They're not new; our ancestors have been eating them since forever. However, back in the 1960s, when the green revolution came and new farming methods were introduced, wheat and rice became more popular, and millets were forgotten.

Millets are excellent for various reasons. Firstly, they can even grow in less fertile soil, and don't need too much water. This means that farmers don't need to use a lot of chemicals in order to grow them. Plus, they have a much lower glycemic index than wheat. This basically means that they don't cause spikes in your blood sugar levels. They're also packed with many nutrients.

A few common varieties of millets include barnyard millet (sama), sorghum millet (jowar), finger millet (ragi) and pearl millet (bajra). You can use their flours to make chapatis or even enjoy them whole.

At Satvic Movement, we've embraced these swaps with open arms. From tasty wholewheat pizzas and colourful momos, to millet upmas and ragi pancakes, the Satvic menu remains vast and inviting. If you're curious about these recipes, they're available in our food books and also shared on the YouTube channel.

> 'Society eats so much junk food that eating real food is considered dieting.'
>
> —Anonymous

Now that we've covered both the refined foods, below are answers to two of the most common questions asked by our community members.

Practical Answers to Practical Problems

> **What do I do when I go out to eat at restaurants? There's refined items in practically everything on the menu!**
>
> Here are three suggestions:
>
> 1. **Choose Conscious Restaurants**
>   In most cities, there are restaurants or cafes that serve healthier food options. Use keywords like 'healthy restaurant near me' or 'plant-based restaurant near me'

when searching. Additionally, some cuisines, like south Indian for example, naturally tend to offer cleaner food options. Opt for such conscious restaurants when you can.

2. **Choose the Best from the Menu**

   Yes, it's true that most of the menu will be full of items made of refined flour. However, most restaurants will offer at least some relatively clean options: for example, a sprout chaat, or a filling salad, or rice with stir-fry veggies. Use your best judgement and order what aligns best with the principles you want to imbibe.

3. **Don't Become too Rigid**

   Prepare yourself that when you're eating out, you might not be able to meet 100 per cent of the principles you wish to follow. That's when you need to practise flexibility, let go of rigidity, do your best, and if it's not as per the principles, enjoy it nonetheless, knowing you're making an exception.

As the revolution spreads, we envision a world with multiple Satvic restaurants in almost every city, where you can eat food that makes you happy while nourishing each cell of your body. Until that becomes a reality, we hope these suggestions help you whenever you go out to eat.

Dates, jaggery, millets, fruits and living food—isn't this way more expensive? Won't this increase my kitchen budget?

Yes, it may increase your kitchen budget. There's no denying that certain whole foods can be more expensive than their refined counterparts.

But for a moment, we'd like you to put aside your short-term glasses and look at this situation from a pair of long-term glasses. When you truly embrace the recommendations in this book, you'll not only *add* things to your cart, but you'll also *eliminate* many others.

Consider this: How much do you spend every month on bread, biscuits, cookies, noodles, ketchup, spreads, cornflakes and snacks? And when the repercussions of such dietary choices crop up, how much of your earnings go towards medical bills, painkillers, steroids, skin creams, serums, doctor's appointments, hospital visits and various tests and scans?

A fair bit, right?

Now, if you genuinely adopt the habits shared in this book, you'll likely reduce your dependence on many of those things.

So in the immediate future, yes, you might feel the strain of purchasing whole foods. But if you take a step back and look at the bigger picture, it becomes apparent that this approach isn't just an expense—it's an investment.

Think of it as the best health insurance you can offer yourself.

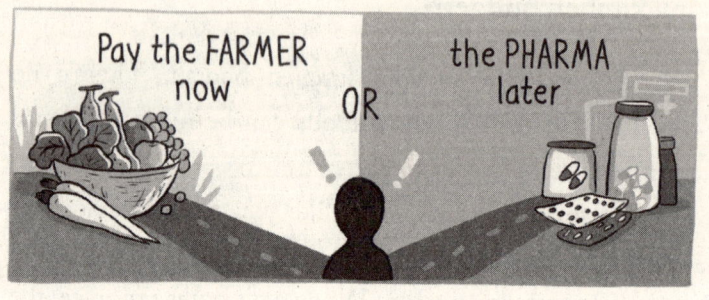

Concluding Thoughts about This Practice

Dear reader, while much can be said about wholesome food, and we could share many more swaps, we have shared with you the two that we believe to be the most powerful and impactful for your health. Make sure you don't let this knowledge remain mere theory confined to the pages of this book. Make it a part of your life.

The journey towards eating living and wholesome foods will not be a cake walk. You will encounter challenges along the way. As you move away from white sugars and refined flours, you'll notice just how deeply these fragmented foods have penetrated our food system, from our traditional dishes to the sweets in the markets, to the menus in restaurants. In your journey, you'll face temptations, and sometimes, others may even ridicule you for not indulging in the same habits as them.

But remember, when you follow this change, you are becoming a part of something much greater: a Satvic Revolution. You are taking a stand against the wrongdoings that are happening in our food system today, and a step closer to Mother Nature.

As you walk this path, don't forget that the food industry will continue to entice and tempt you. For all those times, remember: **people are fed by the food industry that pays no attention to health, and then have to get treated by the health industry, which pays no attention to food.**

By embracing living and wholesome foods, you're breaking free from this cycle and taking your health back into your own hands, setting yourself up for a lifetime of peak health and joy.

In the next chapter, we will move on to the third topic within this habit, which is 'plant-based'. We'll discover the five places in the world with the highest rate of people living beyond the age of 100 and reveal a lesser-known secret behind their longevity. We'll also talk about the pig that played video games and the transformative change that some of the world's top sportsmen are making to reach their peak performance, all while answering one of the most controversial questions that has ever existed in humanity: 'Animals: To Eat or Not to Eat?'

5

Animals: To Eat or Not to Eat?

Growing up, Sunday was my favourite day of the week. It was the only day when my parents, my brother and I would be relatively free. My parents didn't have to go to the office, and we didn't have school. On almost every Sunday, we would go out for dinner; having Sunday dinner at restaurants was sort of a tradition.

My mum often let me pick the restaurant. I remember one particular Sunday when I chose a Chinese spot. I loved Chinese food, especially manchurian. We reached the restaurant and I placed our order for some manchow soup and honey chilli potatoes to begin with. I was excitedly awaiting our food when, just a few minutes after, I observed my parents having a quiet discussion. Suddenly, they said that they wanted all of us to leave the restaurant immediately.

I was taken aback. 'But why?' I asked. 'We have just arrived.' Their answer confused me even more: they didn't want to eat at a restaurant that also served meat. From the smell of the meat to watching waiters carry it around, it was unsettling for them (to provide some context, I grew up in a strict vegetarian family, where meat and fish had never entered our home).

So, they paid for our untouched starters, and we quietly made an exit. This whole episode was quite confusing for me. I was only fifteen, and found myself internally rebelling: 'Isn't this a bit much? What's wrong with eating at a restaurant that serves meat? Why be so extreme?' My mind was flooded with questions, yet, I bottled them up inside.

There were other situations, too, where I found myself questioning my vegetarian upbringing. In my science class at school, when our teacher introduced us to the food pyramid, I learnt that protein, which is important for strength, is primarily found in animal foods. 'But how will I get this nutrient without eating meat?' I often thought. In the school canteen, I watched my friends relish their rumali roti with butter chicken, licking their fingers. 'Should I give it a try? Am I missing out?' I often thought. Over time, I began to feel that my family's strong vegetarian principles were too traditional, too religious or perhaps too radical. I felt embarrassed to tell my meat-loving friends that I came from a vegetarian family, fearing that they would view me as too purist, backward and uncool.

All this while, I grew up with the notion that I was a part of the minority. I believed that most people abroad eagerly consumed and loved meat. However, as time went by, I grew up, ventured out and travelled to different parts of the world. Through my journeys, I had a surprising revelation. I met countless individuals who chose to abstain from meat, not due to their culture, not due to their family traditions, but out of personal choice. And this community was spreading faster than I had imagined.

In every corner of the world I visited—be it California, London, the Netherlands, Germany, Indonesia, Mexico, Tel Aviv—I noticed the emergence of many restaurants proudly branding themselves as 'plant-based'. These restaurants refused to serve any animal products and instead offered dishes made primarily from grains, legumes, vegetables, fruits and nuts. When I observed this phenomenon, I wondered why I used to hide my vegetarian upbringing from my friends, when here, people were boldly advertising themselves as being plant-based, wearing it as a badge of honour.

In Florida, at the natural healing institute I visited, I met multiple people who had been consuming a lot of meat in their diets since childhood. Many arrived there with severe illnesses, some with advanced-stage diseases. Doctors had given up hope on them. However, the institute advocated a purely plant-based diet (alongside other healing therapies). Surprisingly, within a few months of following this approach, many were even able to heal their advanced diseases, including cancers.

I also came across stories of several top-level athletes: Novak Djokovic, the world's number one tennis champion; Lewis Hamilton, the seven-time world F1 racing champion;

Venus Williams, the tennis pro; Patrik Baboumian, a former bodybuilder, among many others, who had turned to plant-based diets to enhance their performance in their respective sports.

Witnessing all these instances led me to question: Was there more to this subject than what I had known? I learnt that people choose plant-based diets for one of three main reasons: for their health, for empathy towards animals or to protect the environment. But are these claims even true? Can going plant-based really make a difference to your health? Or is the lack of animal proteins and nutrients actually harmful to your body? Is this merely a new fad or is it the direction in which the world is headed?

Through life's experiences, I sought these answers, and want to share my learnings with you in the pages that follow. Given the depth and sensitivity of this subject, this topic of **plant-based** has been divided into two chapters. This one unravels the intricacies of meat, while the next chapter talks about dairy.

Before we begin, one important disclaimer: The goal of this chapter is not to convince you, enforce a belief or make you feel guilty about your food choices. Although Harshvardhan and I have embraced a plant-based lifestyle for many years and we're deeply passionate about it, we've always felt that beliefs and lifestyles shouldn't be forced on others. We are opposed to pushing ideologies or framing information in a way that instils fear or guilt. Instead, our intention is to simply share the knowledge and insights with you which we've gained over the years, which have had a deep impact on our lives, and then the decision is yours to make.

If you love consuming meat, you might wonder, 'Why should I read this if I have no interest in following a plant-based diet?'

Our answer is simple: so you can make a well-informed decision. The problem is that we aren't shown both sides of the story—the reality of animal agriculture is hidden from us or is disguised by marketing labels and public relations (PR) strategies. When we are shown both sides of the story, we are then able to make informed decisions for ourselves.

In this chapter, we'll delve into understanding the impact of meat on three levels:

- your physical health
- your mental health
- your spiritual health

The initial section on physical health dives into scientific research and evidence. We've tried our best to simplify the scientific jargon, but we understand it may come across as a little technical for some. Bear with us through this portion, because as we transition to the latter sections, exploring the more intangible effects on our mental and spiritual health, the tone will shift to become less technical and more reflective.

With that said, let's begin.

How Does Meat Impact Your Physical Health?

Everyone who includes meat in their diet does so for a different reason. Many consume it because it's a traditional practice that their families have been following, so they too adopted it from a very young age. Their grandparents ate it, their great-grandparents ate it, and so on.

But tradition isn't the only reason. Many continue eating it, or even start eating it, because it's a rich source of protein.

However, what we miss is that along with protein, it also comes with high amounts of saturated fat and cholesterol, which are both detrimental to our health. (In contrast, plant proteins, such as lentils and legumes provide us with protein, but have no cholesterol and negligible amounts of saturated fat.)

Terms like 'saturated fat' and 'cholesterol' might seem like jargon. Hence, let's understand what they do inside the body through the diagram that follows.

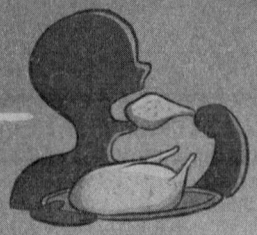

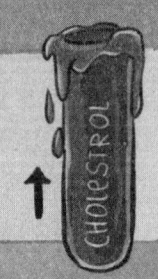

Meats, especially red and processed meats, are high in saturated fats. Over time, their consumption can elevate cholesterol levels in our blood.

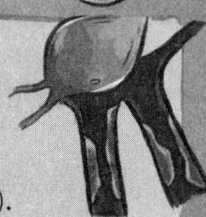

When there is too much cholesterol circulating in the blood, it forms fatty deposits on the inner walls of your arteries (arteries are the blood vessels that carry blood from the heart to the rest of the body).

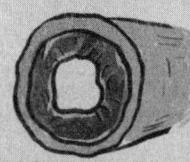

As these fatty deposits continue to build up in the arteries over the years (much like a clogged pipe), it makes them narrower and narrower.

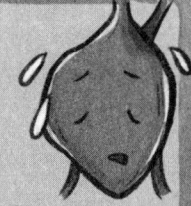

These narrower arteries restrict blood from flowing freely within them. So, the heart has to work harder to pump the blood through these tighter spaces, which often results in high blood pressure and heart disease.

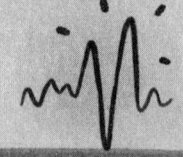

Sometimes, these fatty deposits in the arteries can also break suddenly and form a clot that causes a heart attack or stroke.

It is no surprise that in 2020 the *British Medical Journal* published a study concluding that men who consumed about one serving per day of either processed or unprocessed red meat had a **greater risk (upto 28 per cent) of heart disease**, compared to people who ate plant-based protein sources like legumes, soy and nuts.

This is just one among many studies showing that those who follow plant-based diets have a much lower risk of heart disease.

In a meta-analysis (from a scientific standpoint, a meta-analysis provides more robust evidence than a single study), researchers gathered the outcomes from thirty studies. They found that people who switched to a plant-based diet had a 10 per cent reduction in their LDL (bad cholesterol) levels, compared to their peers who continued eating a meat-based diet.

Interestingly, the World Health Organization (WHO) has also listed processed meat as a Group 1 carcinogen. They've found that there's sufficient evidence showing that it causes cancer, especially colorectal cancer.

Now that we've discussed how meat impacts our physical health, let's delve into how our bodies react when they're fuelled by a plant-based diet. Before we proceed, let us quickly clarify what 'plant-based' means. A plant-based diet involves consuming foods that come from plants, including vegetables, fruits, grains, legumes, nuts and seeds, while excluding animal products such as meat, fish, eggs and even dairy (dairy might be surprising to some, but we'll address it in the next chapter).

For the past many years of running Satvic Movement, we have been advocating a living, whole-food, plant-based diet. Through our observations, we've found that it is not only incredibly effective with helping people improve their health, lose weight and gain more energy in their day, but it's also a powerful tool to reverse and heal diseases. However, during the days of writing this book, we were surprised to find one more benefit of a plant-based diet, which we hadn't encountered before, and it involved a 100-year-old secret.

The Secret of the 100-Year-Olds

Live to 100 is a very interesting documentary by Dan Buettner. It features the Blue Zones—places around the world which are home to some of the world's oldest living people. What's striking is that these Blue Zones have high rates of centenarians (people who live to be over 100 years old). What we found most fascinating was that these aren't sick or feeble individuals; they are healthy and robust, with these regions having not only the highest life expectancy, but also notably low rates of chronic disease.

The five Blue Zones are located in: Okinawa (Japan), Icaria (Greece), Sardinia (Italy), the Nicoya Peninsula (Costa Rica) and among a group called the Seventh-day Adventists in Loma Linda, California (USA).

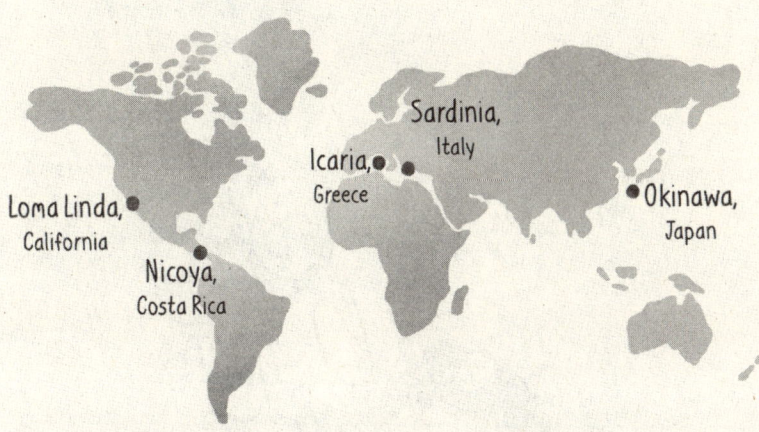

Interestingly, it was found that genetics only account for 20–30 per cent of one's longevity. Factors like diet and lifestyle play a huge role in determining lifespan.

Can you guess what was found to be one of the common patterns across these Blue Zones?

Well, people in these Blue Zones primarily eat a 95 per cent plant-based diet. Their diet consists of vegetables, legumes, whole grains, nuts and very low amounts of animal proteins. (Adventists in the Loma Linda, were the one exception—they ate no meat at all.) For instance, in Okinawa, Japan, the purple sweet potato is a regular staple, and in many dishes, they use tofu as a replacement for meat.

In essence, what the Blue Zone communities show us is that we don't need to win the genetic lottery to live a long and healthy life. Rather, longevity is deeply rooted in what we decide to put on our plates every single day, with a plant-based diet emerging as a vital contributor.

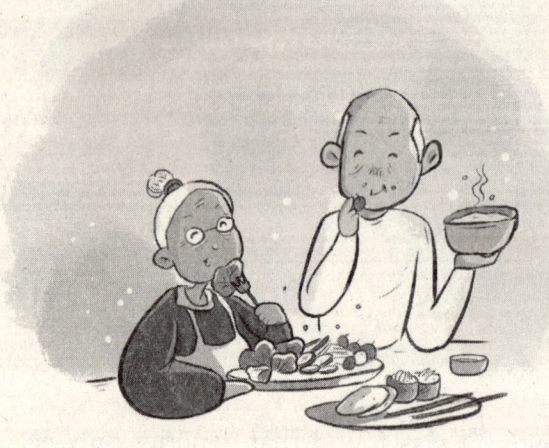

Another significant lesson that we've learnt from our journeys is that a plant-based diet holds the potential not only to extend longevity but also to effectively reverse chronic lifestyle diseases.

Plant-Based Diet as a Powerful Tool for Healing

In a study published in the *European Journal of Clinical Nutrition*, researchers conducted an eighteen-week experiment with 291 corporate employees. Half of them were given a plant-based diet to follow, whereas the other half made no changes to their diet. These were their findings:

- The plant-based group lost an average of 4.3 kg, compared to 0.1 kg in the other group.
- The plant-based group saw their bad cholesterol levels (LDL) drop significantly by 13 mg/dL, while the other group saw a drop of only 1.7 mg/dL.
- The plant-based group saw a 0.7 percentage point decrease in their HbA1c levels, while the other group saw a drop of only 0.1 percentage points.

In essence, this study shows that a plant-based diet is a pathway to a disease-free life, helping in weight management, cholesterol control and diabetes prevention. Perhaps this is why today, there are so many doctors emerging throughout the world who are using it not only to prevent, but also to reverse many diseases. Here is what some of the leading doctors across the world have said about it:

'A plant-based diet is like a one-stop shop against chronic diseases.'

—Dr Michael Greger,
A renowned physician and
New York Times bestselling author

'In the next ten years, one of the things you're bound to hear is that animal protein is one of the most toxic nutrients of all that can be considered. Quite simply, the more you substitute plant foods for animal foods, the healthier you are likely to be.'

— Dr T. Colin Campbell,
A biochemist, nutrition scientist
and author of the bestselling book, *The China Study*

'Some people think that the plant-based whole-foods diet is extreme. Half a million a year will have their chests opened up, a vein taken from their leg and sewn onto their coronary artery. Some people would call that extreme.'

— Dr Caldwell Esselstyn,
Renowned for his pioneering research in
preventing and reversing heart disease (also the doctor
whose programme the former president Bill Clinton
turned to, in order to reverse his heart disease)

As more and more people are experiencing the healing benefits of a plant-based diet, it is becoming increasingly popular around the world. However, when someone tries to transition to it, there is one real challenge that they almost always face: resistance from family and friends. If someone has health issues, others might still be understanding. But, for those who are perfectly healthy, a common question is,

'But won't you become weak? And where will you get your protein from?' In order to answer this question, come, let's explore if we can get enough protein without eating animal products.

If I don't eat meat, where will I get my protein from? Where will I get strength from?

This is a valid concern, as proteins play a crucial role in our body—they help build, maintain and repair our tissues.

Now, how much protein you need in a day depends on several factors: your age, activity level, muscle mass and more. However, as per a joint report by the World Health Organization (WHO), Food and Agriculture Organisation (FAO) and the United Nations University, for adults leading a moderately active or sedentary lifestyle, the protein needed is 0.83 grams per kilogram of body weight.

So, if you're an adult, to figure out your daily protein needs, just multiply your weight in kilograms by 0.83. This means that for someone weighing around 60 kg, their protein requirement will be around 50 grams in a day.

A variety of whole plant-based foods are easily capable of satisfying these needs. To provide some context:

One cup of cooked lentils has 18 grams of protein.
One cup of cooked chickpeas gives you 15 grams.
One cup of cooked kidney beans gives you 15 grams.
A cup of green veggies? About 8 grams.
A handful of nuts adds another 6 grams.
One cup of whole grains contributes around 5 grams.

Typical Indian meals are rich in lentils, grains and veggies, and can easily provide us the protein we need. Those who do intense workouts or need more protein can easily increase their intake of lentils, legumes, nuts, seeds, etc. to meet their requirement.

Lastly, while it's important to be aware of your protein intake, there's no need to obsess over the exact gram count daily. We believe that food is much more than just numbers, or fragmented nutrients. However, we have provided the breakdowns for those keen on understanding.

How Does Eating Meat Impact Your Mental Health?

To understand this, let's begin by exploring some interesting facts:

- Chimpanzees, when they fight, often mend their relationship with each other with a kiss.

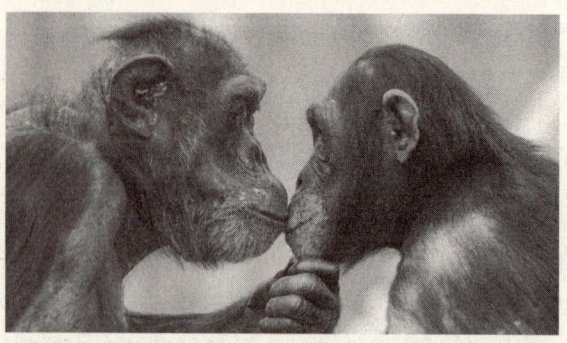

- Pigs, while sleeping, love to cuddle up close to one another, nose to nose. To greet other pigs whom they know, they rub noses with them, much in the way we humans would shake hands.

  In the 1990s, a fascinating study was conducted by animal scientist Stanley Curtis. He trained pigs to play a video game using a joystick. Impressively, these pigs not only mastered the game but also progressed from one difficulty level to the next.

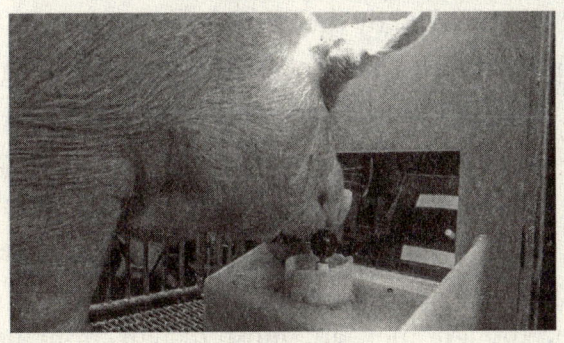

- Sheep, on the other hand, display an astonishing memory. They can recognize and remember human faces for years. They are also known to form strong maternal bonds with their lambs. Lambs, especially when they are young, are quite playful and can be seen frolicking, jumping and racing around fields—much like children in a playground.

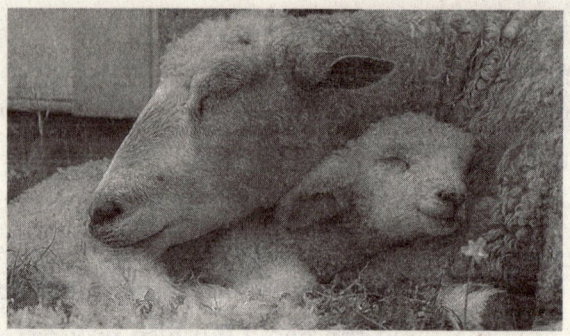

- Hens have a world of dreams as vivid as those of dogs and cats, marked by their rapid-eye movement (REM) sleep. Not only that, one of the sweetest things you'll ever hear is a mother hen chirp to her unborn chicks, and the chicks chirp back from within the egg! They also make around thirty different calls to communicate with each other, expressing everything from 'thanks for the food!' to 'there's a threat in the coop!'

- Fish, though they are most distant from us, have fascinating social lives. They talk to each other with sounds, body movements and chemical signals that we can't even see. And believe it or not, some fish choose one partner and stick with them for life. Together, they protect their home and help each other out when danger comes near.

You might be wondering why we're delving into the world of animals in a book centred on health and joy. It's because there's a prevailing notion that animals might not have the same depth of feelings as we do. Some might even say they're 'dumb' or 'emotionless' creatures who do not feel things. But is that truly the case? Could it be that they, too, are sentient beings? With a capacity to feel and perceive?

I understand this is a polarized topic and views can widely vary, but my heart says that they are not the unintelligent beings that society may have led us to believe. Sure, they may not be as intelligent as us, but it's clear that they experience many of the same emotions, bonds and feelings that we do.

How Does Death Feel?

Just as animals feel pleasure and joy, they also experience pain and terror.

When we conducted research on this topic, we came to understand the lives of these animals. In the next few paragraphs, we would like to share some details. While it may be uncomfortable to confront the entirety of their reality, we will share just enough for you to be informed. Everything we mention has been extensively written about and is covered in various videos online.

In a factory farm, animals are trapped in small cages or enclosures, where they are barely able to move. They have to pass faeces at the same place where they sleep and spend their days. Here, they're also pumped with artificial growth hormones, pushing them to grow unnaturally large. Why? You may ask. The larger they are, the greater the yield of meat, and consequently, the higher their market value.

Once they grow large enough, they are loaded on trucks and transported to slaughterhouses. When the truck arrives at a slaughterhouse, the animals don't even get off the truck. Why? Because they know what's coming next. They know that they're headed towards their inevitable death. So, the workers often use electric sticks to force them out of the truck.

Some animals, such as pigs and cows, watch their peers die in front of them, increasing their anxiety as their own time comes near. Soon, when it's their turn, they are shifted on to a moving belt and hung upside down (while they're still conscious). From there, they see the bolt gun or knife approaching, ready to chop them into pieces.

The mere thought of this scene can be deeply disturbing for many of us. But, in such a situation, what feelings do you think the animal goes through?

- FEAR
- TERROR
- INTENSE ANGER
- PAIN
- DEPRESSION
- EXHAUSTION

Isn't it?

Once their flesh leaves the slaughterhouse, chopped up into pieces, it's sent to the supermarkets and sold to us as food.

Is There Anything More to Food than Nutrients?

Is food all about calories, protein and nutrients? Or is there something more to it?

Well, food is not something inert. Each food possesses a certain energy, a certain vibration.

Now, when we eat the flesh of tortured animals, not only are we ingesting the animal, but we are unknowingly also ingesting their stress, their fear, their exhaustion and the anger that they went through before they were killed. As we continue to consume this negative energy, over time, it manifests within us in the form of stress, agitation, violence and illness.

This is not to say that eating meat will make you unhappy or agitated, as there are many factors contributing to our mental health. However, it's worth considering that your food has energy beyond its physical properties and nutrients. If the food comes from a place of pain and suffering, it may impact you in ways that are not immediately apparent.

There is an old adage in Indian culture: '*Jaisa ann, waisa mann.*' This translates to, 'As is your food, so is your mind', suggesting that the nature of our food imprints upon our thoughts and emotions.

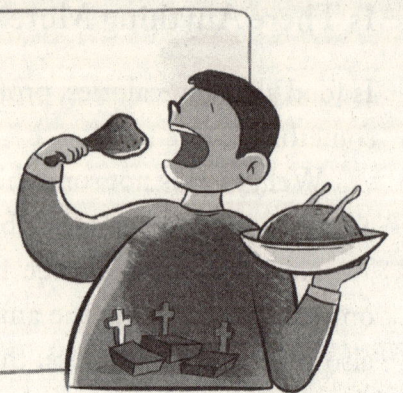

Food for thought:
Dead bodies are taken to graveyards to be buried or burned. So when we consume the dead bodies of animals and birds as food, are we not turning our stomachs into a graveyard?

While you read all this, you may be feeling a whirlwind of emotions. That's perhaps because we've all grown up with certain habits, traditions and beliefs surrounding our meals, and when these are challenged, it can disrupt the very foundation of our identity. In some of us, this can stir up a lot of sentiments, sometimes even provoking defensiveness or aggression, with every new detail prompting further questions.

It's perfectly natural to feel such emotions when faced with such revelations. We're all on our individual journeys, and it's okay to take your time, process this information, and decide what feels right for you. Remember, you don't have to change anything you don't feel ready for.

Now, there are two questions that invariably arise whenever we bring up this subject in front of an audience.

1. **How can you justify eating plants? Don't plants also feel pain? Aren't we ingesting their pain as well?**

From our current scientific understanding, plants cannot experience pain. In order to feel pain, a being needs to possess a brain and a central nervous system connected to different receptors—connected with the eyes, ears, skin, taste, smell. When an organism has a brain, a central nervous system and all these receptors, it can think, feel, touch, hear and taste. Plants neither have a central nervous system, nor do they have pain receptors.

2. **But weren't our ancestors hunters and gatherers? They hunted and ate animals all the time. What makes it bad for us today?**

It's true that our ancestors hunted and ate animals, but it's important to understand the context of their actions. For them, the consumption of animal meat was rarely about taste or pleasure—it was about survival. Their choices were very limited, and hunting was often one of the few ways they could secure any food.

Fast forward to today, and the scenario is completely different. We live in an age where we have abundant access to fruits, vegetables, nuts, seeds and grains. Unlike our ancestors, we're not stuck in survival mode any more. We have the privilege to make decisions based on knowledge and compassion, and not mere survival.

So, the question, really, isn't about what our ancestors did to survive, but about what we can do today to thrive.

Having explored the effects of meat consumption on both our physical and mental health, let's now turn our attention to the third, and very important aspect.

How Does Eating Meat Impact Your Spiritual Health?

While I was training to become an educator, I had the chance to learn under several teachers and masters. The topic of consuming meat often came up in their lectures. While some of my teachers approached it from a scientific and research-based lens, others approached it from an intangible spiritual lens, which I found even more interesting and thought-provoking. I want to share this with you.

The law of karma might sound familiar to you. This universal law, shared by religions such as Buddhism, Hinduism, Sikhism and Jainism, essentially states that all actions have consequences which will affect the doer of the action at some future time. It's like that line from the Bible, 'As you sow, so shall you reap,' or the law of cause and effect: 'What you do, comes back to you.'

In simple words, when our actions negatively impact another living entity—causing pain, suffering, hardship or even death—we're likely to experience similar repercussions in the future. This could mean more pain, suffering and hardship for us. On the other hand, positive actions towards others will bring us good fortune in return.

We are always under the influence of this law of karma, whether we believe in it or not.

So, what happens when we consume animals? In a spiritual sense, it's seen as creating substantial negative karma. According to the ancient text, Manu-Samhita (5.51–52), it's not just the person who does the killing, but also all those involved in the process—those who kill, transport, cook, serve or eat the meat. All of them are part of this karma.

Interestingly, these negative consequences often manifest in our health, as if each animal we consume takes its revenge on us. To quote Dr William C. Roberts, 'When we kill animals to eat them, they end up killing us, because their flesh, which contains cholesterol and saturated fat, was never intended for human beings.'

Reflective Activity

There are some questions that we often find ourselves thinking about. For the next few minutes, we invite you to reflect on these questions. After reading each one, pause for a few seconds, think about your answer, and then proceed to the next one.

1. Why do we only consume the meat of some animals and spare others? Would you be okay if you were served dog or cat meat? What makes it okay to consume the meat of a pig, sheep or hen, but not a cat or dog?

2. If you had to personally raise, feed and then slaughter the animal you consume, how might that affect your food choices?

3. Imagine explaining to a child where meat comes from. How comfortable would you feel describing the process from the factory farm to the table?

4. How much do your family's traditions or your culture influence what you eat, especially when it comes to meat? Do you believe that these traditions are reason enough to keep eating the same way, or do they need re-evaluation?

The questions you just read don't have a right or wrong answer. But what's for certain is that the lives of billions of animals every year and the health of the largest ecosystem on our planet hang on the answers we give to these questions.

Let us turn to the words of a couple of history's notable figures, who've pondered over similar dilemmas.

'To my mind, the life of a lamb is no less precious than that of a human being . . . The more helpless the creature, the more it is entitled to protection from humans from the cruelty of humans.'

—Mahatma Gandhi

'If a man aspires towards a righteous life, his first act of abstinence is from injury to animals.'

—Albert Einstein

'Non-violence leads to the highest ethics, which is the goal of all evolution. Until we stop harming all other living beings, we are still savages.'

—Thomas Edison

'I gave up eating meat at a very young age. The time will come when men such as I will look upon the murder of animals as they now look upon the murder of men.'

—Leonardo Da Vinci

'Animals are my friends, and I don't eat my friends. I choose not to make a graveyard of my body with the rotting corpses of dead animals.'

—Pythagoras

'All beings tremble before violence. All fear death. All love life. See yourself in others. Then whom can you hurt? What harm can you do?'

—Gautama Buddha

What about Eggs?

I know many people who exclude meat from their diet but include eggs. And what's wrong with that? There's no slaughter, no killing, no death. I also held that belief. Although much of my family didn't eat eggs, in my later teenage years, I would relish the taste of egg-containing pastries, cupcakes, donuts, breads and muffins when visiting bakeries.

Growing up in India, I remember a catchy TV commercial that had just been released: 'Sunday ho ya Monday, Roz Khao Ande' (if you know, you know). It appealed to both children and adults and showcased various ways to enjoy eggs—as omelettes, hard-boiled or even raw.

This was definitely an 'Egg'cellent' campaign by the National Egg Committee, because it took our country by storm. Many Indians who previously identified as vegetarians now dubbed themselves 'eggitarians'. (Never underestimate the power of quality jingles.)

While such commercials excel at marketing, they often omit the full picture. An organization named Animal Equality decided to investigate the conditions inside India's poultry farms, and conducted an investigation in 2019.

They discovered that it's standard practice to confine four to eight hens in cages so small they can barely move. This can be hard to conceive, but what it basically means is that in the typical cage, each bird has 67 square inches of space. To put this into perspective, it's only about two times the size of the rectangle drawn around this text. This is how much space one egg-laying hen has, for her whole life.

To understand this better, imagine you're in a crowded elevator. The elevator is so crowded that you cannot even turn around. If you were trapped in this elevator for a whole day, how would you feel? Some might become violent, others might lose their sanity. There's no escape, no break and no elevator repairman coming to help. That is the reality for hens in cages. But for them, the doors will only open once, at the end of their lives, to a place far worse.

Also, have you ever wondered what happens to all the male chicks in the poultry industry? If man hasn't designed them for meat, and nature clearly hasn't designed them to lay eggs, what function do they serve?

They serve no function. Hence, all male chicks are systematically destroyed.

Destroyed?

Most of these male chicks, while fully conscious, are placed on a conveyor belt that leads them to a giant revolving grinder, shredding them into pieces. Others are tossed into large plastic containers and left to suffocate slowly.

Is such treatment cruel? It depends on one's definition of cruelty.

Are eggs healthy? That depends on one's definition of healthy.

By now, we've discussed the impact of meat and eggs on various levels of your health. Perhaps, some of you are reconsidering your intake and feel that you would like to decrease it. Or maybe there are some of you who wish to shift to a completely plant-based diet. To support you in your journey, we've compiled some practical advice through some frequently asked questions.

How to Really Make This Practical?

I want to stop eating meat. Should I quit all at once or gradually reduce my intake?

Different approaches work for different people.

1. **The Immediate Cut-Off Approach:** This involves cutting out all forms of meat from your diet immediately and entirely. Even though this is a powerful approach, it also requires considerable willpower. Hence, we would suggest setting a goal to give up meat only for the next twenty-one days to begin with, as that is said to be the length of time it takes to form a new habit.

2. **The Gradual Approach:** This involves slowly reducing your consumption of meat over time. This could involve cutting down on the number of days per week you eat meat—for instance, going from six days a week to four, then to two, and eventually giving it up. Or,

if you're accustomed to having meat in almost every meal, start by eliminating it from just one meal a day, such as breakfast.

The choice as to which approach is better completely depends on your personality, lifestyle and family situation. Regardless of the approach you choose, remember that when eliminating meat from your diet, you should also add plant-based sources of protein, such as lentils, legumes, nuts and seeds. This is essential for ensuring you receive proper nourishment.

I'm considering a meat-free diet, but when I tell my family or partner about it, they just don't understand or support this choice. How can I handle this situation without causing tension in our relationship?

Here are some suggestions:

1. **Communicate openly with them.**
    Start by understanding why they might be resistant to you not including meat in your diet. Maybe their concern is rooted in tradition, concern for your health or simply a resistance to change. Understanding their concerns with empathy is the first step.

Once you've fully understood their concern, communicate your 'why' to them. Openly share with them why you're choosing a meat-free diet.

2. **Find common ground when it comes to food cooked at home.**

    For example, if there's a meat-based curry made at home, prepare another version of that curry, substituting the meat with vegetables, pulses or beans.

3. **When eating out, find plant-based restaurants in advance.**

    If you leave it to chance, they will probably choose the restaurant, and perhaps you may not find enough options for yourself there. So, whenever possible, simply search for a 'plant-based restaurant' online, and request your family or loved ones to go there instead.

4. **Most importantly, don't force them to change.**

    The key is to lead by example rather than by force. Understand that food habits, especially for your parents or grandparents, are deeply ingrained for so many years, and difficult for them to change. Instead of attempting to convert others to your way of eating, focus on living the change in yourself first. Then, let the benefits you experience speak for themselves. Over time, your family may become curious about the transformation they see in you. This can open the door to a dialogue based on their genuine interest, rather than them feeling pressured.

Every time I try to make a change to my diet, I find myself falling back into old habits after a few days or weeks. What can I do?

First off, give yourself a pat on the back for the efforts you've made so far; making changes to your deep-rooted food habits is not easy, especially if you've been eating a certain way for many years. If you find yourself struggling to stay consistent, here are two suggestions:

- **Educate yourself with documentaries.** Watching documentaries can be a powerful way to stay motivated. Films like *What the Health*, *The Game Changers* and *Food Choices* are highly recommended. They are widely available online and can provide a continued source of inspiration.
- **Be kind to yourself if you fall back into old habits.** It's highly likely that you feel inspired after this chapter, decide to give up meat, and then, after a few days or weeks, slip back into your old habits. At that moment, you may find the strength to rise up and try again, only to face another setback. Perhaps it takes you one, two,

three or even four tries before you can finally make the transition. Be prepared for this. Don't abandon your commitment if you fail. Instead, rise up and try again. Don't be hard on yourself; understand that you are on a journey, and with each time you get up after falling, your resolve is becoming stronger.

Concluding Thoughts about This Practice

Today, the plant-based lifestyle has become one of the most prevalent and discussed social movements of this generation. As more celebrities endorse it and mainstream restaurants adapt their menus, it's clear that what was once a fringe idea has now grown into a mighty social revolution, influencing industries and inspiring change on an unprecedented scale.

Every time we choose to consume a meal that is plant-based, we're not just nourishing ourselves; we're making a powerful statement about our relationship with the world. It's a loving message to our bodies, a caring whisper to the animal kingdom, and a heartfelt pledge to Mother Earth. This is a choice that extends compassion to all beings, recognizing that their right to life and freedom is as important as our own. Now, the choice rests in your hands. It begins with deciding what to place on your plate, but its impact ripples far and wide.

In the next chapter, we will cover another important topic within the 'plant-based' diet: dairy. This is something many of us consume multiple times a day, yet we know very little about it. Does dairy have a place in a plant-based diet, or is it better left out? Is it truly the nutritious nectar we've always seen it as, or are there overlooked truths behind it that no one is willing to see? These questions will be addressed in the pages that follow. The chapter you're about to read has taken us the longest time to write in this entire book. In it, we've shared stories and anecdotes— some that will make you laugh, some that might make you weep. So flip the page and prepare to uncover some 'moo-ving' truths about milk.

6

Moo-ving Facts about Milk

It was a bright Sunday morning when we were about to begin work on this chapter. I had just opened my laptop, clicked on the folder labelled 'our book', and created a new document titled 'Chapter 6'. Then, I just sat there, staring at a blank page for about ten minutes. The topic was 'milk'. There was so much to share from the insights we had gained over the past few years. Yet, there seemed to be a missing link. Most of what we had learnt about this topic was based on the experiences of others. I still felt that we hadn't seen the reality with our own eyes, and hence felt that we weren't fully qualified to write this chapter.

I shut my laptop, closed my eyes, and a few moments later, a thought came to me: 'Before writing this chapter on milk, Harshvardhan and I need to go to the very source of the topic. We need to experience first-hand where milk originates from. Milk, after all, starts its journey from the cow.' And so, I knew we needed to visit dairy farms before writing anything.

I quickly pulled out my phone, opened a search engine and typed 'dairy farms in Kolkata' (we had come to Kolkata to our family home for a couple of weeks while we were working on this chapter). I found a few dairy farms on the map, but when I called them, to my dismay, the conversations were short-lived. 'Why do you want to come?' they asked. When I explained we were writing a book and wanted to simply understand how milk production in our country works, they quickly said, '*Arre*, I'm getting another call . . .' before hanging up. After a full day of calling at least twelve farms I found online, requesting a visit, they either didn't pick up, or hung up, or said they would call back but never did.

As I was about to give up on the idea of visiting dairy farms, at around 9 p.m., I remembered an acquaintance who had visited multiple dairy farms himself. I called him and shared what we wanted to do and how nobody seemed receptive to the idea of letting us in. In response, he gave two pieces of advice:

1. Don't call. Just show up on their doorstep. You will be let in (in most cases).
2. Don't tell them you're writing a book. Just say that you are college students conducting research on this topic.

I thanked him for his time and hung up.

The thought of telling a lie that we're college students made me feel uncomfortable. Adventure wasn't in my nature, nor Harshvardhan's. Yet, this seemed to be our only ticket inside. Determined, we planned to leave at 6 a.m. the next morning to visit a belt of dairy farms that we had spotted on the map, about an hour and a half from our house. In the dimly lit room, as we prepared to sleep, I scribbled a few questions in my diary that we wanted to ask the workers and milkmen there. Then, turning off the lights, I drifted off to sleep.

The next morning, we woke up at around 5 a.m., got ready, and packed a bottle of ash gourd juice, lots of fruits and some nuts for the journey. We sat in the car, entered the GPS coordinates for the dairy belt, and set off. We weren't even sure if we'd be let in. In fact, we didn't even know for sure that these dairy farms even existed. What if they were just ghost locations on the map?

With only four minutes left before we arrived, and the sun just beginning to rise, we were far away from the hustle and bustle of the city, on the outskirts of a small town. The lanes were getting narrower and narrower as we moved closer to our destination. The buildings around us were dilapidated, the streets were littered with trash, and it seemed like a rather shady area. We also noticed that the streets were unusually empty, with only a few people in sight, going about their morning chores. As we drove past them, they stared suspiciously at us, as if we were aliens from a distant land. With a tinge of fear creeping into my heart, I asked Harshvardhan, 'Are you sure what we're doing is safe?'

'Don't worry. *Mein hu naa* (I'm here),' he responded, with a confident smile on his face, as he put his hand over mine.

'You have arrived at your destination,' interrupted the lady on the GPS. We got out of the car and started walking towards the first dairy farm on that belt. Enclosed within a big blue gate, it was about the size of a small house, not too big, with a large banner hanging outside that said 'Babu Ghaat Dairy Farm'. As we approached the gate, we could smell cow dung in the air and hear the sounds of workers chatting, cows mooing and milk splashing from one container to another.

Upon reaching the gate, Harshvardhan gave a strong knock on the giant blue metal door, only to realize that it was already unlocked. We called out, '*Koi hai*? (Is anyone there?).' No one responded. We stepped inside. Surrounded by at least twenty cows and the same number of buffaloes, all tethered by their ropes, we called out again, '*Bhaiyaa, koi hai* . . .?'

Before we knew it, a man appeared in front of us. He was heavily built, perhaps a foot taller than either of us. His arms were thick with muscle, and we could see his veins etched into his skin, probably from years of rigorous labour milking cows. His eyes, sharp and piercing, made it clear that he was the owner of the place.

With a thick voice, he asked, 'Who let you in?' I let Harshvardhan do the talking.

He replied, 'We're doing research for our college project to understand how milk production works in India so that . . .'

'Which college? You're not allowed here. Did no one tell you?' he interrupted, while rolling up his sleeves.

As we were attempting to answer the question, we saw four other men of a similar stature as him appear, entering one by one from behind him, walking towards us. The intense, warning glares in their eyes made it clear to us that danger was imminent. That's when Harshvardhan and I looked at each other, knowing we shouldn't have done this, and signalled to each other to walk out through the same blue door we entered. Our walk quickly turned into a brisk jog, and then a full-on sprint towards the car. Too scared to turn back and look around, I still did and realized that all five men were running behind us, each with a broom in their hand.

That's when suddenly my eyes opened, and I jolted wide awake, my heart still racing. I looked at the window— it was still dark outside. I turned my head—Harshvardhan was peacefully asleep beside me. With a huge sigh of relief, I whispered to myself, 'Thank God.' I quickly grabbed my phone and saw the time was 5.05 a.m. Our real journey to the dairy farms was about to begin in just about an hour.

Shaking Harshvardhan awake, I told him about my wild dream. 'Subsi . . .' he murmured, his usual nickname for me. 'See, this is why I tell you not to work right before sleeping. You keep thinking about it even while you sleep . . .' Not paying much heed to what he said, I quickly got ready, packed our food basket (for real this time), and we left for the journey.

Upon reaching the dairy farms, I was surprised to find how different reality was from my dream. The dairy farm owners were actually locals from the area and were really warm people, willing to share everything with us about the process. In fact, many of them were excited that two young people had come to their place and they transparently showed us every detail—the good and the bad, behind the industry that creates a drink which our country probably loves even more than water: Milk.

Our journey didn't end at Kolkata. In the coming few months, we went on to explore a vast number of dairy farms across various states of India, including Maharashtra, Tamil Nadu, Delhi-NCR and Karnataka. After all this, we finally felt ready to write this chapter.

In the pages that follow, we would like to share with you the most important things we learnt on this journey, which we feel are the most relevant for you. Alongside, we will also cover the following topics:

- Why do our parents and grandparents advocate so strongly that we drink milk?
- What are the four surprising changes that have happened in our milk—from our grandparents' time to our time?
- What does milk really do to our body? Is it good or bad?
- Are some types of milk better than others? What's the best type for your health?

With our foundation set, let's begin.

Why have our parents and grandparents always insisted on us drinking more milk?

Growing up, milk and its products were an indispensable part of my life.

Without a bowl of curd, my plate looked empty.

Without a big spoonful of ghee, I wouldn't eat my roti.

To see a pizza without a double cheese layer made me snappy.

And until I drank that glassful of milk before school, my mum wouldn't be happy.

Whether it was parents, elders in the house or grandparents, all advocated having at least two glasses of milk per day, plus the curd, plus the paneer, plus the ghee, and the white butter.

I'm sure this is not just my story. Perhaps you can relate to it too. Milk has been a major part of our culture since time immemorial. But I wanted to understand why it is so. Why has milk been revered so much by our ancestors, our grandparents and in our cultures throughout history? Where does the love for milk stem from?

I realized that a lot of knowledge about milk in our society today is passed down from historic texts and ancient scriptures, which are replete with references to milk. For instance:

- In the Mahabharata (Anu 65–46), cow's milk is referred to as 'Amrit'—the elixir of life.
- The Rigveda (1-71-9) says, '*Gashu Amrutam raksha mana*,' meaning 'cow milk is Amrit, it shields us from diseases.'
- Ayurveda also speaks highly of milk's virtues. As per the Charak Sutrasthana (27/217–218), milk is sweet, tasty, gives us calmness and increases vitality within us.
- In the Quran (Surah 16, verse 66), it is said that Allah has given us a drink from the cattle—pure milk, which is a palatable drink for those who take it.
- Even the Bible mentions milk about forty-eight times in the Old Testament alone, each time in high regard, as something to aspire for.

So much praise for milk in our scriptures is perhaps one reason why the love for milk flows through generations and why it's more than a mere beverage in our culture; it's a tradition, a ritual.

However, as shared in the previous chapter, today, a growing number of people are turning away from dairy, terming themselves as 'plant-based', 'lactose-free' or 'vegan'. There are restaurants, cafes and entire food product lines that proudly claim they use no animal products in their menus (not even milk, butter or cheese). Even top-level athletes around the world are joining this shift.

This brings up some important questions: If milk has been a revered drink since Vedic times, why are so many people moving away from it today? If it's as nourishing as our scriptures say, why are entire brands and communities being built that are proudly claiming not to use/drink it? Is there something about the milk we consume today that we're not aware of? Or is it merely a disregard for our cultural teachings?

As the two of us sought to unravel these questions, we discovered something striking. The milk we consume today is markedly different from the milk that our ancient texts spoke about. What we're getting today may look like milk, may smell like milk, and may even taste like milk, but it is simply not the same substance that our ancestors revered.

What, then, has changed from those ancient times to the present regarding this esteemed drink? The next section aims to shed light on just that.

Four Surprising Changes that Have Happened to Milk: From Our Ancestors' Time to Ours (and perhaps the fourth one is the most surprising)

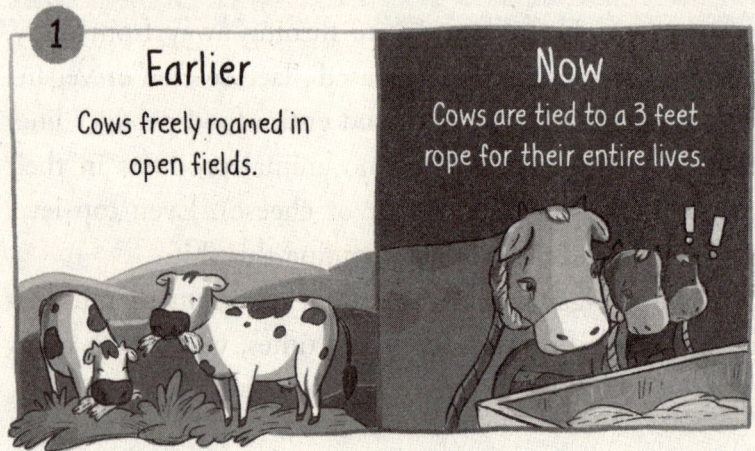

1

Earlier
Cows freely roamed in open fields.

Now
Cows are tied to a 3 feet rope for their entire lives.

In the olden days in India, people lived in rural settings; in villages where almost every home had a cow. Their homes may have been simpler, but they always had enough space outside their home where the cow could graze all day, freely. As the cow grazed from various places, automatically, she would also end up eating grass of a range of different varieties. Different grass species have unique medicinal values, so having access to a diverse range of grasses contributed to a balanced diet for the cow. Hence, this ability to freely graze not only made their milk more nutritious but also kept them active, and thus healthy and happy.

Let's compare this to today.

We saw that most dairy farms are located in cramped areas, with no access to grasslands or open fields. The cows are housed in a simple shed, which has brick walls on all four sides. (Note: Throughout this chapter, when we refer to 'cows', it includes cows and buffaloes, considering that in India, nearly 50 per cent of the milk production comes from buffaloes.)

In each shed, multiple cows were packed closely together. To prevent them from wandering or going outside, each of them was tied from their neck to a 3-ft rope. (To visualize this, look at the tip of your finger, and then look at your shoulder. The length in between is roughly the same length that the cow is tied to—morning, afternoon, evening and night, its whole life.) This means that the cows have no room to run, to walk, to move or even just to turn around.

During our visits, we asked the dairy workers, 'Do the cows really stay in one place all day? Don't they need to move around? Don't they need any exercise?'

'Yes, they need exercise, but what should I do, madam? There's no space outside,' said one.

'What's the need to open them? They're eating, drinking, sleeping, giving milk. Then why leave them open, needlessly?' asked another.

'Yes, they always stay tied up. The only time we'll open them now is when we give them out for sale,' said another.

We were surprised to hear such responses. But even more than that, we think they were surprised to hear our questions. The mere idea of letting the cows roam free sounded absurd to some of them.

As you can imagine, if the cows are never allowed to walk, where would they defecate and urinate? In the very same space they're standing and sitting all day. This not only makes their living space filthy and smelly but also turns it into a breeding ground for infections.

~

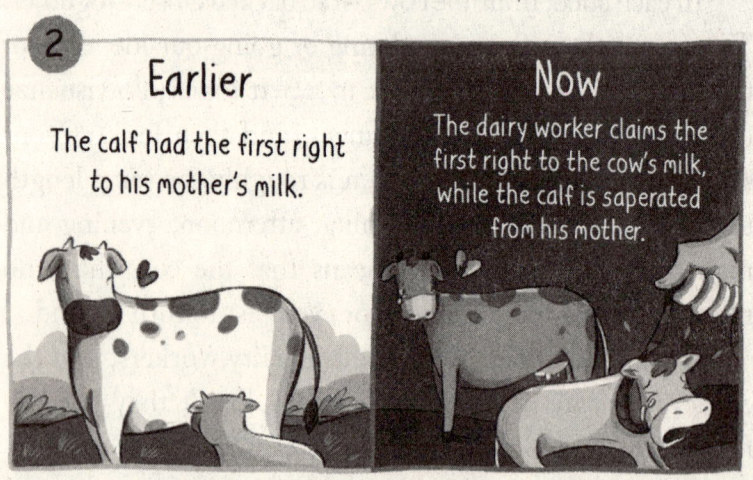

2

Earlier

The calf had the first right to his mother's milk.

Now

The dairy worker claims the first right to the cow's milk, while the calf is saperated from his mother.

In the olden days, the sacred bond between a calf and the mother cow was respected. Calves stayed with their mothers and were allowed to have sufficient milk. The farmer would only milk the cow after the calf had had enough. Typically, this milk was rarely sold. It was only distributed amongst the farmer's own family.

However, the situation we witnessed across multiple dairy farms around the country was vastly different. Based on our observations and interviews with multiple dairy farmers, we found the following:

A cow, just like a human, endures a nine-month pregnancy, bearing her baby with patience. This is probably the only time in her life when she actually feels happy, eagerly waiting to meet her baby.

However, as soon as the calf is born, in majority of the cases, he is immediately taken and tied up at a distance from his mother. In fact, as per the findings of Animal Equality India, the calves are separated from their mothers within just a few hours after birth.

Despite this, the mother still produces milk in her udders to feed her baby. When the time comes for milking, the calf is untied and allowed to come close to his mother. But, as soon as the calf reaches the udders to drink the milk, he is again taken away and tied apart. The farmer then proceeds to extract all the milk from the cow, to be used for commercial sale.

Throughout this, the helpless cow cries, while making desperate gestures to her calf, as if to say, 'Don't worry, I will bring you milk again in the evening.' However, when the evening comes, the cycle repeats and the cow is milked, once again. As the cow realizes she's being tricked, she tries to kick with her leg, as though to signal, 'Please let me go. I want to feed my baby.' But the human doesn't understand her plea. The cow's legs are tied up with a rope and she continues being milked, yet again.

Why do the dairy workers separate the mother from the child, you may ask? Well, the answer is simple: if the calf were allowed to remain near his mother, he would consume a significant amount of the milk—milk that could otherwise be sold. Consequently, the dairy farm's profits would be lowered. Therefore, to sustain the business, calves are separated early on, ensuring that the cow's milk is available for commercial sale.

This, dear reader, we saw happening in all the dairy farms we visited, across our nation, behind closed doors, unnoticed by the world outside.

Whenever we think about this harsh reality, it makes us ponder: if anyone ever did this to a woman—held her captive, took away her child and extracted her milk—the mere thought of it would be unbearable to society. We would be up in arms, demanding justice. Yet, when it happens to a voiceless cow, day after day, we remain silent. Why?

'We feel entitled to artificially inseminate a cow, and when she gives birth, we steal her baby. We take her milk that's intended for her calf, and we put it in our coffee and our cereal.'

—Joaquin Phoenix
American actor, in his Oscar speech

I remember a dairy farm we had visited in the rural countryside of Bengal. While entering the farm, we saw a small black calf peacefully sleeping outside, on top of a bed of dry grass. Surprisingly, he was loose—no rope attached around his neck. After a few minutes of conversation with the worker at that dairy farm, we pointed towards the calf near the door and asked, 'Why is he sleeping while everyone else is awake?'

'He's not sleeping,' the worker replied.

'Then what?'

'He's dead.'

We were shocked. 'Dead? But how?' we asked.

'Yesterday, a new batch of buffaloes came here in a truck. He was the child of one of the buffaloes. He must've been squashed under one of the big buffaloes in the truck,' responded the worker.

Harshvardhan, confused, asked, 'I didn't fully understand . . . Tell me again.'

The worker elaborated, 'Four or five new buffaloes were brought here in a small truck yesterday. The space in the truck is very tight. The animals often have to stand on top of each other. Sometimes, the smaller ones at the bottom, like that calf, get crushed by the weight of those on top and die.'

I went closer to the dead calf, offering a silent prayer while trying to hold back my tears. Seeing him lying dead, with his mother just a few blocks away, was perhaps the hardest thing to witness at the dairy farms that day. Later, we understood from the dairy farmers that this was not a one-off. It was common for calves to die in the long truck rides during transfers.

As we witnessed this heartbreaking separation of the mother and child, a thought occurred to both of us, 'Any mother gives milk for their child. If the child is no longer alive, would she continue producing as much milk?'

The answer to this was revealed to us as we continued our journey to the next few dairies.

~

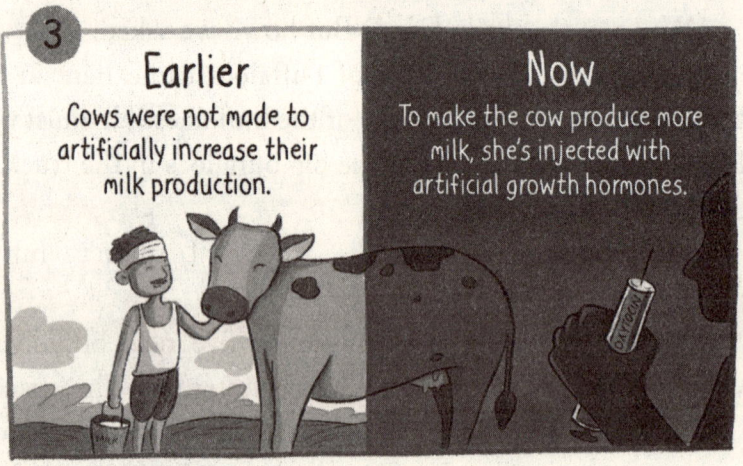

In times past, milk wasn't seen as a commodity or a source of income. The owner of the cow was satisfied with however much milk he or she got. There was no push to 'increase production' because their livelihood didn't depend on it.

Let's compare this to today.

When a calf is absent, cows and buffaloes naturally reduce or cease milk production. To counter this, they are injected with an illegal drug called oxytocin. The intent is to ensure these animals keep giving milk even when their natural tendency would be to cease milk production after the calf is no longer present.

We witnessed this process first-hand during a visit to a dairy farm in Maharashtra. It was about 2 p.m. when we arrived, and we saw a worker milking a cow with his hands. There was a row of cows closely placed next to each other. That's when we noticed something unusual. The cow next to the one he was milking had a stream of blood trickling down from the region beside her tail. Confused, I pointed towards the bleeding cow and asked the worker, '*Bhaiya*, how come this cow is bleeding?'

Chuckling, he replied, 'Because I just gave her the injection, na, *didi*,' as he continued milking the cow.

I asked, 'How many times a day do you give this injection?'

'Once in the morning, once in the evening,' he replied. 'Whenever I have to milk her, I have to give her this injection at least a few minutes before I start.'

'What does the injection do?'

'It makes her release milk,' he responded as he finished milking and moved to the next cow in the row.

'What's inside this injection?' I asked.

'Umm. How can we know that, didi? This comes from the industry. We just insert it.'

The farmer was now set to inject the next cow, as he took the needle and pushed it from behind. The cow trembled for a few seconds, as a thin stream of blood released from the newly made puncture on her skin.

Seeing all of this made us wonder: Do these growth hormones stay within the cow, or do they also get transferred to the milk that ends up on our tables? Upon further research, we found some leading experts shed light on this.

'In order to get the milk, dairy owners inject them with an illegal drug called oxytocin twice a day. Oxytocin comes into the milk and results in hormonal imbalances in humans, who get diseases like tuberculosis, cancer, etc.'
—Maneka Sanjay Gandhi,
Indian politician and former
member of the Lok Sabha

'Most factory-farmed cows are injected with a growth hormone to increase their milk production that also increases their udder size, sometimes to painful dimensions—a physical condition that promotes inflammation called mastitis.

Antibiotics are then required to reduce the resulting infections, increasing the amounts of antibiotics, pesticides, blood, and bacteria in the milk that we buy and consume. What a unique cocktail for human consumption!'
—Dr T. Colin Campbell, in his book, *Whole*.
Dr Campbell is a biochemist, nutrition scientist and
author of the bestselling book, *The China Study*.

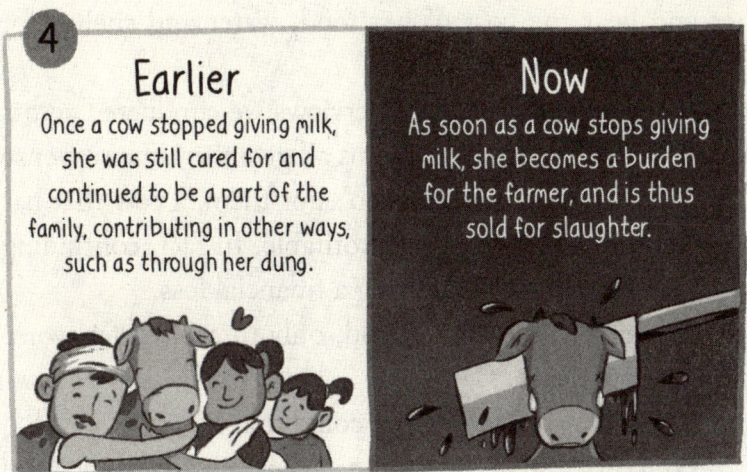

4

Earlier

Once a cow stopped giving milk, she was still cared for and continued to be a part of the family, contributing in other ways, such as through her dung.

Now

As soon as a cow stops giving milk, she becomes a burden for the farmer, and is thus sold for slaughter.

Today, in the dairy industry, in order to remain profitable, a cow is needed to continuously produce milk. To achieve this, she is made pregnant when she is only twenty-five months old. After she gives birth, the dairy worker lets two months pass, and then, she is again made pregnant. Essentially, a cow is kept pregnant for most of her life in the dairy industry.

A cow has a natural lifespan of about fifteen to twenty years if properly cared for. However, due to the cycle of repeated births, unhygienic living conditions, traumatic separation from their calves, and constant injections, the vast majority of dairy cows are considered 'spent' and no longer useful to the industry by the time they reach around eight years of age.

Now, imagine yourself in the shoes of a dairy owner. What would you do with a cow that has stopped producing milk and is no longer economically viable? Would you keep her and bear the cost of her food, water and shelter for twelve more years?

Based on the multiple interviews we conducted across India, we found that dairy farms all give the same response to this question, which was 'no'. For them, a cow that has ceased producing milk isn't profitable. In fact, continuing to care for her means incurring a financial loss.

As a result, the cow is sold, only to a place far worse than her own farm.

A place far worse? Where could that be?

Well, to a slaughterhouse. Here, she is killed and converted into beef.

You might know that India is the largest producer of milk in the world. But did you know that India is also one of the largest exporters of **beef** in the world? Do you think this is a coincidence? Surely, it isn't. The dairy and beef industries work hand in hand. The same cow, when she stops giving milk, becomes the raw material for the meat industry.

'The dairy, meat and leather industry are interdependent. The dairy industry churns out a large number of unproductive animals for slaughter every day, which in turn helps the meat and leather trade thrive. In other words, the meat and leather industry is heavily dependent on the dairy industry for its supply.'

—According to a two-year nationwide study conducted in 107 dairy farms across India by Animal Equality

As a child growing up, I was always taught not to hurt animals, to love them and never take their lives. But it never occurred to me that even as I enjoyed my glass of milkshake, my sandwich filled with cheese or my bowl of curd, I was unknowingly contributing to the meat industry.

~

As you've read the chapter up to this point, we have a personal request for you: please pause and watch this short, eye-opening video which provides a visual representation of our experiences of visiting dairy farms. You can access the video by scanning the QR code or by visiting satvicmovement.org/book/dairy

Our Reflections

Witnessing the realities of the dairy industry can be difficult and unsettling. We believe that the root of this issue stems from the fact that our fundamental relationship with the cow has completely changed today. Earlier, the cow was considered a cherished part of the family. She was given a special name. She was loved, cared for, even served, like a mother. She was even referred to as 'Gau Mata'. It's no wonder that the milk she provided was revered as pure and a life-sustaining nectar.

But what we saw is that today, a cow is no longer seen as a mother. Rather, she's viewed as a milk-making machine—to be fed, impregnated, milked and eventually sold for slaughter when she's no longer useful. All of this for what? To increase production and maximize profits.

The debate about whether milk is designed for human consumption or not will likely never end. However, we ask you, dear reader—if a cow lives a life of confinement, pain, sickness and distress, can the milk coming out of her really bring us health and vitality? Can we be healthy drinking milk from a suffering, sick cow? Deep down, we all know the answer. Yet, let us see what research has to say about this matter.

Is Milk Good for Our Bodies? A Scientific Perspective

Key Finding #1: Evidence of Stress Hormones in Milk: The Presence of Cortisol

A study published in the *Journal of Animal Science and Biotechnology* observed cows' milk production over the first twenty-two weeks (which is approximately five months) after they started producing milk. During this time, researchers collected samples of both milk and blood from the cows. They discovered that cows in pain showed significantly higher levels of cortisol (a stress hormone) in their milk.

Another study published in the journal *Animals* (Basel) revealed something similar. Researchers discovered that when cows experience increased stress due to higher temperatures or higher humidity in the dairy farm, it showed in the composition of their milk in the form of increased cortisol levels.

Now, in modern dairy farms, do you think stress arises solely from heat and humidity? Certainly not. Consider the emotional stress of the mother cows whose babies have been separated from them, the stress of living in cramped conditions, of constantly being milked, impregnated and injected with growth hormones. What these studies suggest is that the cow's stress is essentially transferred to the milk, as evidenced by the elevated cortisol levels. The same studies also confirm that cortisol is not broken down when dairy is sterilized and pasteurized. It remains in the milk and dairy products that we consume.

'Stress hormones like adrenaline are abundant in dairy due to the abhorrent conditions in which the cows are kept. Stress hormones in dairy naturally cause stress in the consumer.'

—Dr Nandita Shah,
Author of *Reversing Diabetes in 21 Days*
and awardee of the *Nari Shakti Puraskar*

Key Finding #2:
Three Quarters of the World's Population Struggles to Digest Milk

Besides the stress hormones, another problem with milk is that most people struggle to digest it. In a comprehensive meta-analysis published in the *Lancet*, researchers analysed 450 studies involving 62,910 people from eighty-nine countries. They discovered that a staggering **68 per cent of the global population suffers from lactose malabsorption.** In simpler terms, this means that 68 per cent of people globally cannot digest and/or absorb lactose effectively.

What does this mean for our bodies? Milk contains a key component known as 'lactose'. To break down lactose, our digestive tracts need to produce something called 'lactase'. Lactase is basically an enzyme that is vital for breaking down lactose present in milk, allowing the body to absorb and use it. However, the study reveals that a majority of people worldwide lack sufficient lactase, leading to lactose malabsorption, or in other words, improper digestion of milk and dairy. So then what happens to this undigested lactose? It remains in the gut, where it undergoes fermentation by gut bacteria (this is just like how yogurt or cheese is made). This fermentation in the gut produces gases that can lead to several symptoms, like bloating, acidity or abdominal pain.

Key Finding #3:
The Link between Milk Consumption and Acne

When dairy isn't properly digested within our bodies, it can manifest in various ways. One of those ways is through the channel of our skin, resulting in acne.

One meta-analysis of fourteen studies that included over 78,000 participants between the ages of seven and thirty years old found that dairy consumption increases the occurrence of acne breakouts. Researchers found that consuming any amount of dairy each day increases the odds of having acne by 25 per cent. And drinking two or more than two glasses of milk per day increases the odds to 43 per cent.

> 'You quit drinking milk and 50% of hospitals all across the world will be shut down. Consumption of milk has been responsible for the spread of numerous diseases in the world.'
>
> —Dr Kadar Vali,
> The millet man of India and also a
> recipient of the Padma Shri award

Now that you have learnt about the changes in milk and how it impacts the body, you might be reconsidering your intake and questioning whether you want to consume it. But perhaps there's still one question that remains unanswered:

'What if I find a genuinely trusted source of milk? One that comes from a clean, ethical, good-quality source?'

Well, our suggestion would be not to blindly trust any label. If you really want to consume animal milk, you have to ensure that:

1. The cow is loved and cared for.
2. She has ample space to freely roam and graze in open fields.
3. Her calf is kept with her and gets the first share of the milk.
4. There are no growth hormones injected in her to artificially increase her milk production.
5. That you yourself have the digestive strength to digest milk (as suggested by the studies mentioned earlier, today, most of us are not able to digest the lactose present in milk).

Now, let's be honest. For most of us, finding milk that meets these conditions is impossible! Most of us don't have access to such ideal dairy farms in our modern world. Hence, switching to plant-based alternatives is the wisest choice.

Today, there are alternatives to just about everything, which give you the same taste, the same texture and the same look. Come, let's learn more about what these alternatives are.

Substitutes for the Five Most Common Dairy Products

INSTEAD OF ✖	TRY THIS ✔	NOTE ✏
Animal Milk	Coconut or Almond Mylk	These are simple to prepare at home. Blend the nut with water, sieve and it's ready. Can be used as a milk substitute in smoothies, curries, chaas, desserts and everything else.
Butter	Nut-based spreads (made using peanut, almond or coconut)	Roast the nuts, blend them and your nut butter is ready. Can be spread on fruits to make delicious snacks or even in desserts.
Cheese	Cashew Cheese	This is easy to make at home with a few ingredients, in under five minutes. Can be spread on pizzas, used as a salad dressing or added to practically everything you want a cheesy flavour in.
Curd	Peanut Curd	Requires overnight fermentation but is a fantastic plant-based substitute for curd, to be used in chaats, kadhi, raita, etc.
Paneer	Tofu	This too can be made at home using soybeans. It's good for those looking for additional protein in their meals.

Our Satvic team has created a detailed document sharing recipes for each of these substitutions. You will find the link to these at the end of this chapter.

We encourage you to try at least one of these alternatives in the coming week. Starting with coconut or almond mylk is the easiest, and as you get comfortable, over the next few weeks or months, you can gradually incorporate more substitutes into your diet.

Before we close this chapter, it's important to address two questions that often arise when considering a plant-based lifestyle.

1. **If I stop consuming dairy, where will I get my calcium from? Won't my bones weaken?**

Let us first understand what calcium really is. It is basically a mineral that is found in the Earth's crust. Grass absorbs calcium from the earth. Cows eat this grass, which is how they get their calcium. When we drink that milk, that calcium is passed on to us.

But think about it—can't we obtain calcium directly from plants, without involving the cow?

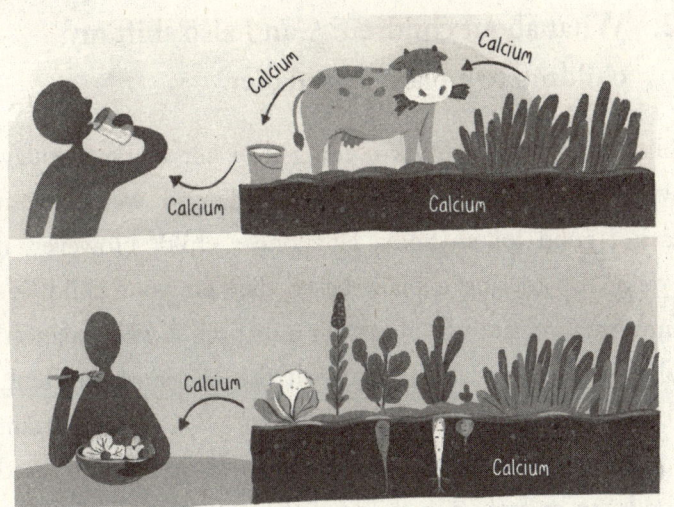

Most foods coming from the earth have some amount of calcium. However, there are certain foods that are especially rich in it, such as sesame seeds, poppy seeds, finger millet (ragi), drumstick, spinach, fenugreek leaves, oranges, chickpeas, broccoli, etc. If you're worried about your calcium intake, you can incorporate more of these calcium-rich sources into your diet.

'Calcium is a necessary nutrient, but we can easily get enough from plant foods. The most healthful sources are green leafy vegetables and legumes, or "greens and beans". And instead of harming our health like cow's milk, these plant foods boost our immune systems and help us avoid chronic illnesses. Just think how much healthier our nation would be if everyone traded their milkshakes for green smoothies!'

—Dr Neal Barnard,
physician and clinical researcher

2. **What about children? Can I also shift my children to a plant-based diet?**

Given the kind of milk coming into our markets today, which has already been discussed at length, we believe it is not good for anybody, let alone a child. However, if you're considering a plant-based diet for your child, it's important to carefully plan their nutrition. A well-balanced plant-based diet can provide all the necessary nutrients for healthy growth and development. But it's important to replace dairy with a variety of wholesome plant-based foods, to ensure your child's dietary needs are fully met. For guidance on this, we suggest seeking advice from a plant-based nutritionist or doctor.

Concluding Thoughts about This Practice

With this, our dear reader, we draw a curtain not only on our chapter on dairy but also on the second habit of this book: 'Eating Living, Wholesome and Plant-Based'. We've come a long way—from learning about living and dead foods, to journeying through wholesome and refined foods, to finally discovering the power of a plant-based diet.

This is the largest number of chapters we'll dedicate to any habit. This is because food is one of the most important elements in our journey to peak health. We think of food as just something to consume in order to fill our bellies. We eat it without much thought or presence. But the truth is that our food quite literally creates who we are. It's the architect of our being. It decides how much energy we wake up with each morning and the clarity of thought we experience through the day, and to a large extent, the overall quality of our life.

This being said, we understand that food is much more than just nutrition. Food is also about love, connection, celebration and joy. Often, it's not just an individual eating, but a family sharing a meal together. And thus, to change all our food habits at once, which we have been following for many decades, may feel difficult, and perhaps overwhelming as well. Remember, you don't need to flip everything in your life upside down all at once. Internalize what you've read and start with what feels most doable for you.

In the beginning, the weight of the change can feel immense. But as you progress and establish systems around it, it keeps becoming easier. Then, after a while, something remarkable happens: eating living, wholesome and plant-based doesn't require effort or too much thought; it simply becomes second nature.

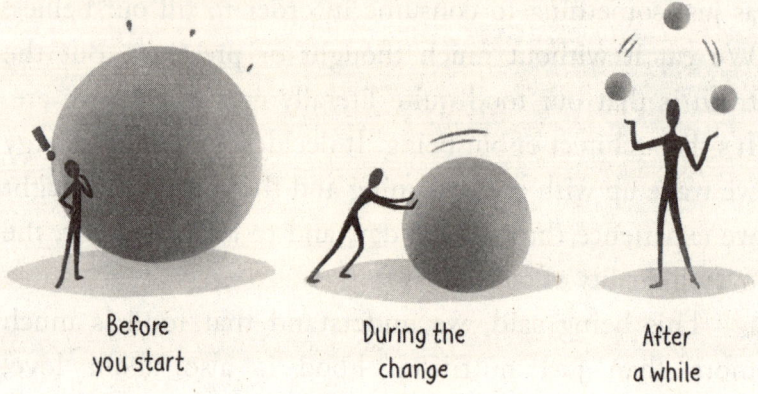

Before   During the   After
you start   change   a while

In the next chapter, we will learn about an activity that we spend nearly thirty years of our life doing! It's something that we're not taught much about while growing up. It's something that we probably never even stop to think about. But, the depth of this activity, to a large extent, determines the health and longevity of your life. Stay tuned as we uncover another hidden miracle.

To access the dairy replacement recipes, scan the QR code or visit satvicmovement.org/book/dairyreplacements

Habit 3

Sleep Like a Baby

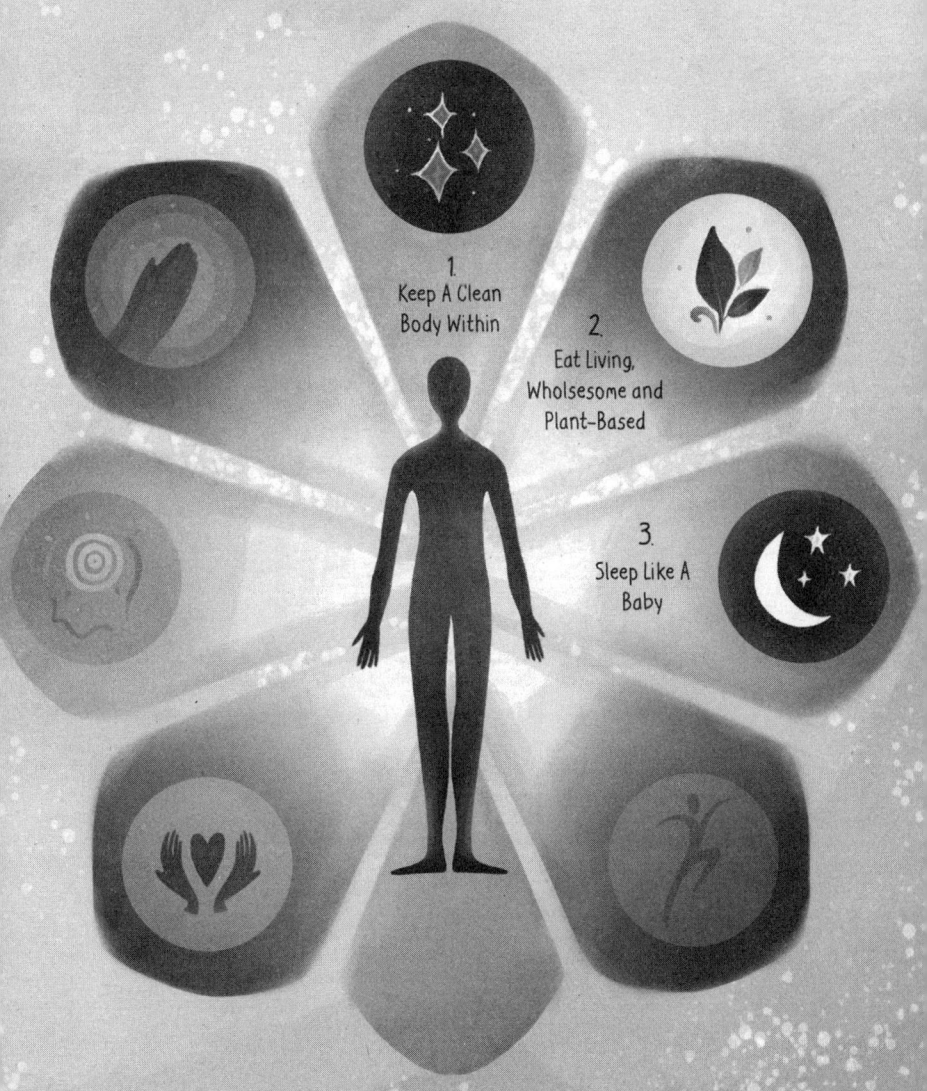

1.
Keep A Clean
Body Within

2.
Eat Living,
Wholsesome and
Plant-Based

3.
Sleep Like A
Baby

7

How to Sleep Smarter at Night to Achieve More in the Day

From the dinosaurs to the apes, from a fish to a bumblebee,
Every species that has ever been studied engages in me.

To repair, restore and recharge is my life's main purpose.
Without me, the world would be nothing short of a circus.

I come to you every night, a little after the sun goes to bed,
I bring with me the moon and the stars, which in the sky I
    widely spread.

I am the one who makes your eyelids heavy, and your
    mouth open in a yawn,
After all, I don't have much time with you, as I have to
    depart before dawn.

185

My hope is to have you with me in the hours that are prime,
So I can energize your mind, and refill your body's batteries
    for the next day's climb.

You spend with me more time than you spend eating,
Yet in your school and college, I was a subject quite fleeting.

Learn about me and you'll find great miracles in store,
Neglect my lessons, and chaos & destruction may knock at
    your door.

You can't miss me for too long, even if you try,
Can you take a guess, who am I?

Answer: Sleep

There's a new treatment in the market!

Researchers have discovered a groundbreaking new treatment that elongates your lifespan, helps heal all diseases, be it a cold or cancer, and lowers your risk of heart attacks and strokes, not to mention diabetes. It reduces food cravings and keeps you in shape. Taking this treatment keeps you looking young and attractive till the latter years of your life. It even sharpens your memory and enhances your creativity. It makes you feel happier, less depressed and less anxious. Would you like to give this treatment a try?

While this might sound like an exaggerated advertisement, nothing about it is inaccurate. If this were an ad for a new medicine, drug or treatment, most people wouldn't believe it. Those who would believe, would pay a large fortune even for the smallest dose.

Surprisingly, this ad is not describing a costly new drug or therapy. Instead, it reveals the proven benefits of something that has no prescription cost to it and is absolutely free: deep sleep.

Yet, despite its amazing benefits, many of us ignore the invitation to get a full dose of this natural treatment every night. Either we are never educated about it, or, in today's world, we don't respect sleep much at all. In fact, we are often programmed with the idea that to be successful, we need to work harder and sleep less. Little do we realize what a remarkable medicine deep sleep truly is.

Here's a question for you: If you were blessed with a long life, living up to the age of ninety, how much of your time would you have spent sleeping?

Pause. Take a deep breath and think about your answer.

Well, it would be close to thirty YEARS!

In other words, **we spend almost one-third of our lives sleeping!**

We find this a bit ironic. We dedicate one-third of our lives to this one activity, but rarely do we stop and think about its quality. Rarely do we stop and think about how we could improve it.

Well, this chapter is here to change that. In the next few pages, not only will you become aware of what exactly happens inside your body while you're asleep, but you will also learn how to reap all its benefits without compromising on your work time, family time or 'me' time.

Allow us to introduce you to habit number three—'Sleep Like a Baby'. Why 'like a baby'? Well, because they have the best and the deepest sleep. Have you ever observed a baby or a child sleeping so soundly that even if moved from the couch to the bed in the night, he/she would find out only in the morning? That's how deep their sleep is! Now, of course, as adults we cannot replicate their depth of sleep, but, even if we are able to achieve sleep close to that, we would accelerate our path to peak health and joy.

Here's what you can expect to learn from this chapter:

- Calculate your current sleep score. Find out whether you're getting deep sleep or light sleep.
- Why do we need deep sleep? What goes on inside us while we're in it?
- What's that one thing that robs us of this precious deep sleep every night?
- Steps to achieve deeper and more restorative sleep.

With that said, let's begin.

Calculate Your Sleep Score

While a clinical sleep assessment is needed to thoroughly understand your sleep quality, we at Satvic Movement have devised a short test that you can take in the next few minutes. The test covers seven different parameters. As you read each parameter, please circle the number that best describes your response (0=Never, 2=Sometimes, 4=Always). Mark your responses based on your experience in the last two weeks.

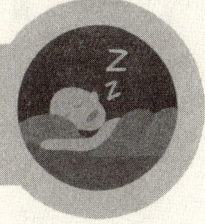

1 I fall asleep quickly after getting into bed. It takes me just a few minutes to fall asleep after my head touches the pillow.

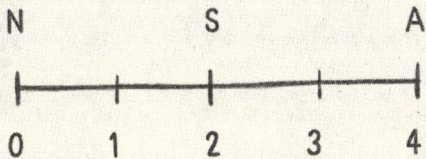

```
N           S           A
|---+---+---+---+---|
0   1   2   3   4
```

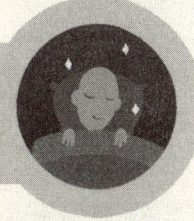

2 I get uninterrupted sleep at night. Once I close my eyes at night, I wake up directly in the morning.

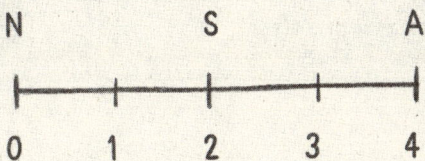

```
N           S           A
|---+---+---+---+---|
0   1   2   3   4
```

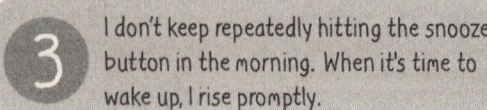 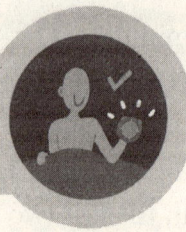

3 I don't keep repeatedly hitting the snooze button in the morning. When it's time to wake up, I rise promptly.

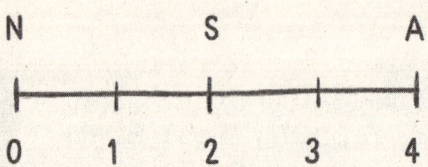

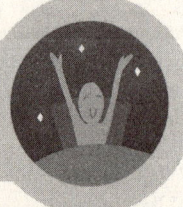

4 I wake up in the morning feeling refreshed and ready to tackle the day with a sense of enthusiasm.

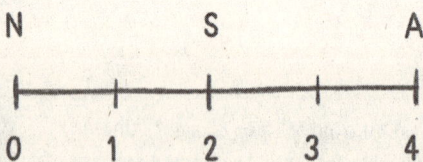

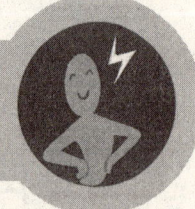

5 I have plenty of energy in the day without needing tea or coffee.

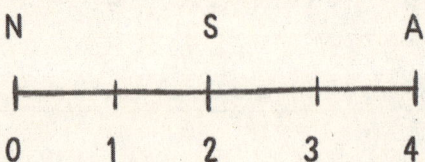

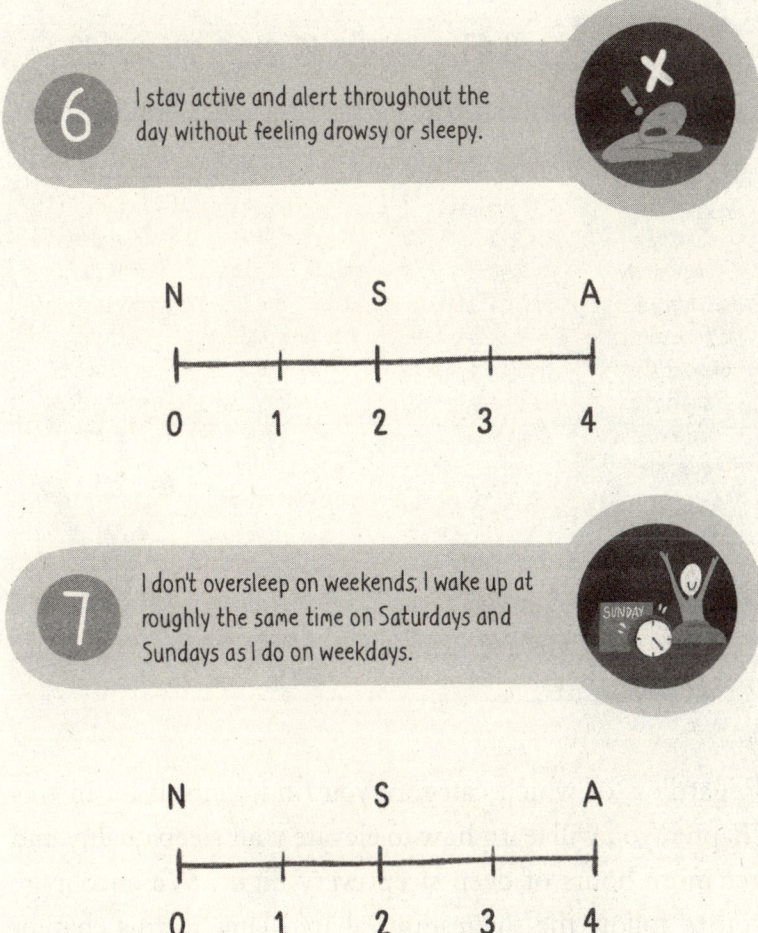

6   I stay active and alert throughout the day without feeling drowsy or sleepy.

N   S   A

├───┼───┼───┼───┤

0   1   2   3   4

7   I don't oversleep on weekends; I wake up at roughly the same time on Saturdays and Sundays as I do on weekdays.

N   S   A

├───┼───┼───┼───┤

0   1   2   3   4

Now that you've gone through the test, please add up your total score and measure yourself with the following key:

0–7	8–15	16–21	22–28
Zombie Zone	Alert Zone	Light Sleep Zone	Deep Sleep Zone
This means that your sleep quality is dangerously low. It's crucial to take control of your sleep situation as soon as possible.	This means that you are struggling to get solid rest at night, leading to tiredness through the day. It's crucial to take control of your sleep situation.	This means that you might experience disrupted sleep phases from time to time. Your sleep is satisfactory, but with a few changes, you can make it excellent.	If you're in this zone, congratulations! Your sleep quality is strong, with long stretches of amazing deep sleep.

Regardless of which category you find yourself in, in this chapter, you will learn how to elevate your sleep quality and get more hours of deep sleep every night. We encourage you to follow the suggestions shared later in this chapter for just twenty-one days, then retake the test. You will likely see a huge jump in your score.

Now, let us first delve into learning the two most critical processes that happen when we sleep.

The First Process:
Deep Cleaning and Healing

As we learnt earlier in this book, there is a self-healing and self-cleaning power within us that we call praanshakti. This is the inner force responsible for expelling toxins, eradicating illnesses and maintaining cleanliness within.

Now, when do you think our praanshakti carries out the majority of its healing and cleansing work?

Well, it's during sleep.

Why?

Because during sleep, many other functions are temporarily paused. Our body is in a state of complete rest. There's no energy (praanshakti) being spent on tasks such as talking, walking, thinking and so on. This means that after digesting the food, our praanshakti can fully focus on getting rid of accumulated waste from within. In essence, sleep provides a window for our praanshakti to engage in thorough inner-cleansing work.

You can think of sleep as a comprehensive check-up by your praanshakti for all your organs. It's as though your praanshakti pays a visit to your intestines, liver, kidneys, pancreas, blood vessels and all other organs to inquire, 'Is everything in order here? Any repairs required?' As a result, it is during sleep that wounds heal, old skin cells are replaced with new ones, our immune system actively defends against external threats, and the body undergoes thorough healing. Conversely, when you lack sleep or don't sleep deeply at night (indicated by a low sleep score), your praanshakti can't perform these crucial functions as effectively.

An article published in the journal *Sleep* performed a fascinating study on the impact of sleep on the immune system and its effectiveness in fighting off the common cold. In this study, 164 participants were given nasal drops that contained the active cold virus. They were monitored for five days to see what kind of symptoms arose. What the researchers found was shocking!

In the group of people who got less than five hours of sleep each night, the odds of falling ill with a cold were 450 per cent higher compared to those who slept more than seven hours. In other words, **those who got less sleep were nearly five times more likely to fall ill than those who got adequate sleep!** This directly shows how much our immunity and healing is dependent on good sleep. It's no surprise that when Harshvardhan and I look back, we notice that after a hectic travel, when we don't get enough sleep and are not well rested, that's the time we find ourselves falling sick most frequently.

Here's another interesting finding: sleep isn't just a time for the body to cleanse; even the brain clears toxins during sleep. You see, while we're awake, our brain performs various functions such as thinking, learning and processing. This generates waste products, which build up in the spaces between the brain cells. The flushing out of these waste products is essential for the brain to function optimally.

Now, as per researchers at the Centre for Translational Neuromedicine at the University of Rochester Medical

Centre, the brain has its own unique waste disposal system. It's called the glymphatic system. The researchers discovered that our glymphatic system actually becomes ten times more active during sleep, than when we're awake! As per the lead author of this study, during sleep, the spaces between the brain cells increase. This helps the brain flush out the toxic waste, as the cerebrospinal fluid washes over it.

So if we're sleeping less than our requirement, or if we're sleep deprived, or if we're in the zombie or alert zone, the brain is likely not able to remove these harmful waste products properly. This, in turn, can lead to various neurological disorders, starting from small problems such as fogginess in the brain and lack of focus in our work, to bigger disorders over time, such as Alzheimer's and dementia.

The bottom line is simple: good, deep sleep is just as crucial for our brain's health as it is for our body's.

The Second Process that Takes Place during Sleep: Recharging

Let's use a simple analogy to understand this concept better: Think of your body as a smartphone. We use our phones throughout the day, and at night-time, as the battery gets drained, we plug in our phones to charge. By the morning, the phone's battery is full again, and the phone is ready to be used for one more day.

Similarly, throughout the day, we utilize our bodies for various tasks—talking, walking, thinking, writing, watching, exercising—all of which consume our energy, our praanshakti. By evening, we feel tired because our daily quota of praanshakti gets depleted. This is where sleep comes in.

When we sleep, our praanshakti gets the chance to recharge itself back to 100 per cent, much like plugging in your phone to replenish its battery.

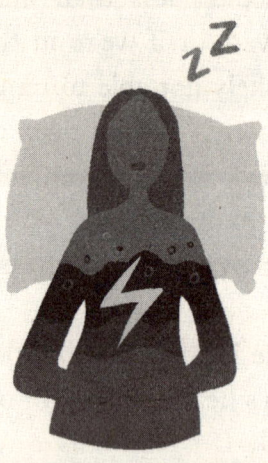

However, if we are not sleeping enough, or if we are lacking deep sleep, this battery that was meant to charge up to 100 per cent is only able to charge itself to 30 per cent, 40 per cent or 50 per cent. Consequently, we miss out on a fully charged battery. How does that manifest? When morning comes, the body feels sluggish. The mind isn't as sharp. There's a lack of mental clarity. As a result, we're not able to give our best to our work or to our tasks.

If you're stuck in the light-sleep zone, alert zone or zombie zone, **you're essentially navigating life with a half-**

charged battery—and the experience of course is not as pleasant.

How much you achieve with your eyes open depends on how deeply you rest when your eyes are closed. Everything you do in the day, you can do better with deep sleep at night.

We're sure that the points shared here are not new to you. But if deep sleep has so many amazing benefits, why, then, today, are so many of us not able to experience it? Why, according to a recent Nielsen survey conducted on over 5600 people across twenty-five cities, do 93 per cent of Indians suffer from sleep deprivation? Why is India the second most sleep-deprived country in the world? Have we, as a generation, simply forgotten its value? Or is a culprit robbing us of our deep sleep? Let's find out.

What's Robbing You of Your Deep Sleep?

We come to you in different sizes and shapes,
But unlike sleep, we never existed in the time of the apes.

Sometimes so small we can fit in your hand,
Other times we need a wall to ourselves 'cos we're so grand.

We beep, we buzz, we ring, we glow,
We keep you hooked to your friends' updates or that late-
    night show.

When you're with us, we shine so bright that we're all you
    can see,
Can you take a guess, who could we be?

Answer: Your gadgets

These include smartphones, laptops, TVs and tablets,
which we keep staring into long after the skies outside get
dark. Regrettably, in today's modern world, these gadgets
have become the number one obstacle standing between us
and the restorative power of deep sleep.

As we journey through this chapter, we want to reassure
you: We're not going to ask you to give up your gadgets.
Far from it. Instead, we'll share with you some practical
suggestions on how to use them in a way that doesn't rob
you of your precious sleep. But before we get into these
solutions, let's take a moment to truly understand how our
late-night scrolling affects our sleep.

Meet Melatonin—Deep Sleep's Best Friend

What is melatonin? Well, it sounds a bit technical, but
it's simply the sleep-inducing chemical our body naturally
produces. Melatonin has other names, too. These include
'the hormone of darkness' and 'the sleep hormone'.

As evening descends and darkness envelops the world,
our pineal gland, nestled deep in the back of our brain,
releases melatonin into our bloodstream. Melatonin acts
like a powerful siren, shouting out a clear message to the

brain and body: 'It's dark, it's dark!' This signal prompts our brain and body to gradually wind down and prepare for sleep. In simpler terms, **melatonin is like your body's internal sleep signal.**

However, while this process is supposed to unfold, many of us are absorbed in the digital world—scrolling through social media, binge-watching TV shows, engrossed in work on a laptop or playing Candy Crush. Unknown to many, it is a well-documented fact that these screens emit a blue light. When the blue light from gadgets hits our eyeballs, it's as if our brain receives an alternate message, 'Hold off on the melatonin! It's still daylight out there, not time to sleep yet!'

As a result, melatonin secretion is stopped. Our body's internal clock becomes confused as to what time it really is, and even at 11 p.m. or 12 midnight, we don't feel sleepy, as we're captivated by our digital companions.

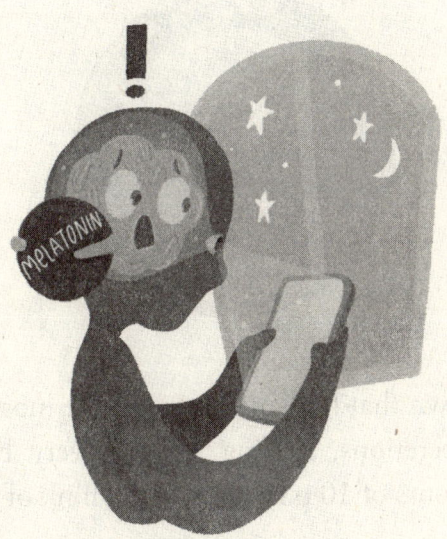

In short:

When we use gadgets at night → Blue light hits our eyeballs → Brain gets tricked into thinking it's daytime → Melatonin (sleep hormone) production gets interrupted → We don't feel sleepy until late in the night.

Now that you understand how using gadgets before bedtime causes delayed sleep, you might be thinking, 'But what's the issue with sleeping late? Whether I go to bed at 11 p.m., 1 a.m., or 2 a.m., as long as I'm getting my eight hours of sleep, does the timing really matter?'

Well, the answer is yes. You see, not all hours of sleep are equally replenishing for us. Remember the line from the poem at the beginning of this chapter, 'My hope is to have you with me in the hours that are prime.' The prime sleep hours are known to be from 10 p.m. to 2 a.m.

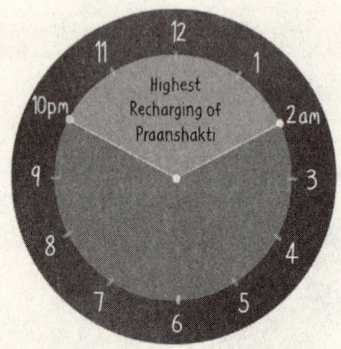

It's been shown that human beings get the most beneficial hormonal secretions, healing and recovery by sleeping during the hours of 10 p.m. to 2 a.m. Think of this period as the phase when your vital life force, or praanshakti, undergoes the highest recharging—a time when your body is in its peak battery-charging mode. So, for instance, you may be sleeping from 12 to 8 a.m. and getting eight full hours of sleep, but you are missing out on the prime sleep hours.

> 'Timing your sleep is like timing an investment in the stock market— it doesn't matter how much you invest, it matters when you invest.'
>
> —Kulreet Chaudhary,
> Renowned neurologist and MD

In summary, using gadgets before bedtime confuses our body's internal clock, thereby keeping us awake during prime sleeping hours, leading to lesser healing, slower recovery and compromised cleansing at night.

Other than interfering with melatonin production, using gadgets at night poses another threat to our sleep. Let's understand what it is.

Overloading the Brain with Information before Sleep

When we scroll through Instagram, Facebook or any social media, our minds get bombarded with content. Here's something interesting that Jim Kwik, the author of *Limitless* shares: **we now consume as much data in a day** as an average person in the fifteenth century would have absorbed in an entire lifetime!

What's worse is that much of this data exposure happens right before we sleep. In other words, we overload our minds with an unrestricted bombardment of information when it should really be winding down for rest. What happens as a result? Afterwards, our body may sleep, but our mind remains active.

'If we fill our minds with work-related thoughts, messages and emails, before we sleep, then, when we sleep afterward, the body might be asleep, but our minds continue to work, not allowing us to experience true rest.'

—Sister Shivani,
Renowned spiritual teacher

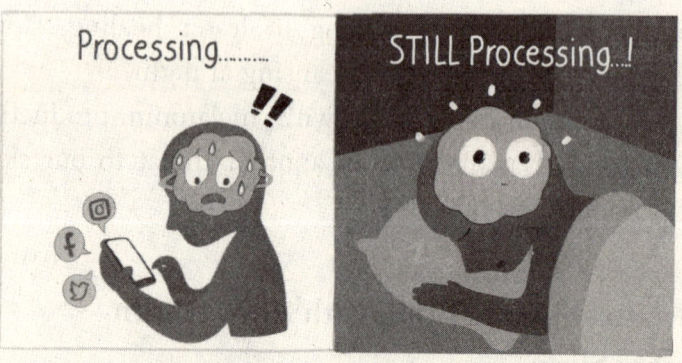

Have you ever experienced that the last thought you had before sleeping continues to generate random thoughts throughout the night? For example, watching a late-night horror movie often leads to a nightmarish dream, or if you happen to stalk someone on social media just before bed, their presence may find its way into your dreams. I must confess that I've encountered this phenomenon frequently, as you may recall from my rather bizarre dream in the previous chapter. But why does this happen? Because the last visual or audio input we expose our minds to before sleep leaves an impression that we carry forward with us to our sleep.

Regrettably, many of us go to sleep after watching world news or dramatic TV shows that showcase chaos, and families and homes breaking apart. What we don't realize is that we take this emotional residue (the lust, greed, jealousy, hatred, pain and fear) with us into our sleep. This not only keeps our minds on high alert, preventing us from sinking into deep sleep, but also makes that negativity seep into our subconscious mind.

In essence, **how deeply you sleep at night depends largely on how you spend the last one hour before sleep.**

Now that we've discussed how gadgets get in the way of achieving deep sleep, let's look at what we can do instead in that last one hour before sleep.

Creating a Wind-Down Routine

What really is a wind-down routine? We can understand it using a simple analogy: **just as we remove our belt, coat and jewellery before sleeping, we also need to remove the inner chatter and the buzzing thoughts from our mind**

before bedtime. In other words, we need to quieten the mind before we sleep. This process of quieting the mind is what we are referring to as 'a wind-down routine'.

In order to do this, the first thing we need to do is to disconnect from technology at least one hour before going to sleep. We need to set a designated cut-off time— whether it's 8 p.m. or 9 p.m.—after which we put away our gadgets, and don't look at any more screens.

How do we practically implement this? Do we just get off our laptop, phone and television and then just sit there looking at the wall? Well, that's a sure-fire way to get internet jitters and find yourself on your device a few minutes later. If we really want to be off technology before bed, it has to be replaced with something we enjoy equally or even more than being on our device. Simultaneously, this should be an activity that brings us peace, pacifying the mind rather than stimulating it.

Here are three examples of low-stimulation activities that you can replace scrolling/watching/working with (you may experiment and find what works best for you):

Reading a Book:

You could pick up a physical book on a subject you wish to learn more about. Reading allows you to enjoy a great story, inspiration or education without overwhelming your brain. Alternatively, you could even journal. This involves putting pen to paper and expressing your thoughts, feelings and experiences from the day. It's a mindful activity that allows you to unload the day's mental baggage before heading into a restful night's sleep.

Engaging in a Recreational Hobby:

This could involve anything that you have a natural interest in, whether it's knitting, crocheting, painting or playing an instrument. You could choose a hobby that you've been wanting to start but haven't found the time to.

Hot Foot Baths:

To take a hot foot bath, fill a bucket with comfortably warm water and soak your feet for twenty minutes. As you allow yourself those uninterrupted twenty minutes, you experience the absence of stimulation, signalling to your brain that it's time to wind down. Additionally, this practice improves blood circulation and immediately helps you feel more relaxed.

To summarize, in order to sleep like a baby, set a designated cut-off time for yourself—whether it's 8 p.m. or 9 p.m.—after which you put away all digital devices. Replace them with one of the calming low-stimulation activities during that final hour before sleep. This may seem too small of a switch to make any difference, but within a few days of implementing it, you will notice your sleep become deeper and your mornings much more energized.

Making It Practical

To help make this habit practical, you can use the golden rule of habit formation (which you learnt about in Chapter 4). The rule is simple: **If you want to build a habit, make it more visible in your environment. If you want to break a habit, make it invisible.** Here are a few examples of how you too could actually do this.

Make Your Gadgets Invisible:

- **Place Your Phone Out of Reach:** If your phone is within arm's reach in that last one hour before sleep, the temptation to check it will easily overpower your willpower and motivation to not use it. If you find yourself spending too much time on your smartphone before going to sleep, you could try placing it in another room, or at a distance where it's not within arm's reach.

- **Turn Off Notifications:** Adjust the settings on your cell phone and on your laptop, desktop or tablet so that you don't receive any automatic notifications. Automatic notifications are said to be a wonderful feature for any app, but they keep you feeling compelled to constantly check your phone, creating a cycle of distraction that's hard to break.

- **Remove the TV from Your Bedroom:** If you have a habit of watching TV before bed, the sure-fire solution is to remove the TV from your bedroom entirely. If it's not within reach, the temptation to switch it on will automatically go.

Make Your Low-Stimulation Activity More Visible:

- Suppose you've opted for reading as your low-stimulation activity. Instead of keeping your book on a distant shelf, keep it right on your bedside table. By doing so, when you settle into bed at night, you'll be naturally drawn to pick it up and read. Similarly, if playing a musical instrument is your chosen activity, make sure it's easily visible and accessible in your room, instead of being hidden inside your cupboard. Having it there in sight will act as a subtle reminder, so that you incorporate it in your pre-sleep routine.

Behind all these suggestions, the essential concept to grasp is this: Many of us in today's world believe that we can just jump into bed, turn off the light and quickly fall into deep sleep, similar to a light switch which we can instantly turn on or off. Unfortunately, deep sleep isn't quite like that. It's more like an airplane landing. Your brain requires time to descend through a good wind-down routine, in order to transition into good, deep sleep. It doesn't happen suddenly.

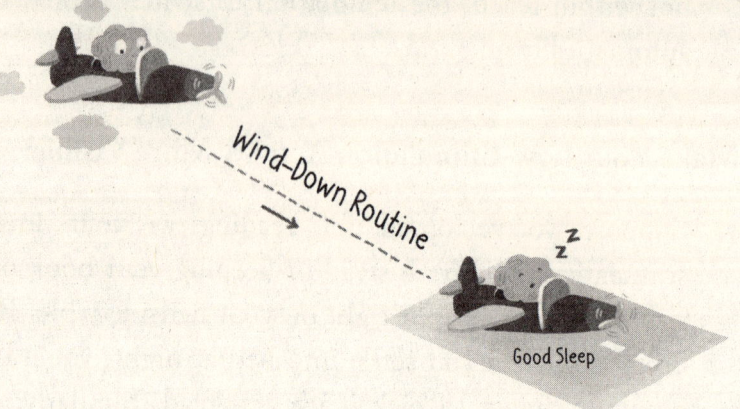

Good Sleep

How many hours of sleep do I really need at night?

Each person's sleep needs vary depending on their lifestyle, energy expenditure and age. You have to find what works best for you. On average, the body usually thrives on seven to eight hours of sleep.

However, also remember that it's not just the number of hours that counts, but also the depth of your sleep. If you sleep for less hours compared to others but meet all seven parameters discussed at the start of this chapter, you are likely getting sufficient sleep.

Nevertheless, avoid extremes of oversleeping or under-sleeping; neither is advised. This is also shared in the Bhagavad Gita: 'There is no possibility of one becoming a yogi, O Arjuna, if one eats too much, or eats too little, sleeps too much or does not sleep enough.'

Activity—Design Your Personal Wind-Down Routine

Let's turn learnings into action by designing a personalized wind-down routine. You could either create one for just tonight, or for the whole coming week. Take a moment to think of the following points and write your reflections in the space provided. (Tip: don't create a perfect plan, but rather a practical one.)

- **Choose Your Ideal Sleep Time:**

  _____

- **Set Your Technology Cut-Off Time:**

  _____

- **Make Technology Invisible:**
  Can you do something to keep technology out of sight in your environment?

  _____

- **Select a Low-Stimulation Activity:**

  _____

- **Make Your Chosen Activity More Visible:**
  Can you do something to increase the visibility of this activity in your environment?

  _____

As we're approaching the end of this chapter, we want to address an important point. Often, when we talk about the importance of deep rest and early sleep in our seminars, our participants ask, 'Ok, I get it. Creating a wind-down routine and sleeping early is good for me, but we live in the real world. I have to stay out late sometimes, go partying with friends, watch movies in the theatre which end at midnight, and attend late-night family gatherings. How can I practically make this change? It's impossible.'

We would like to answer this question by sharing an interesting experiment.

The Monkeys and the Ice-Cold Shower

Once, a group of scientists placed five monkeys in a room, and in the middle, they placed a ladder. On top of the ladder, they placed a bunch of delicious, ripe bananas.

Obviously, as soon as the monkeys saw the bananas, one of them went up the ladder to fetch the bananas. But as soon as he went up, the scientists soaked the rest of the monkeys on the ground with ice-cold water.

After some time, another monkey went up the ladder to take the banana and once again, the scientists soaked the rest of the monkeys on the ground with ice-cold water. After a few times of this repeating, the monkeys understood the pattern. And then, as soon as any monkey from the group even tried to climb the ladder, the other monkeys would beat him and not let him go up because they didn't want a cold shower. After some time, none of the monkeys dared to go up the ladder, regardless of their temptation to eat the bananas.

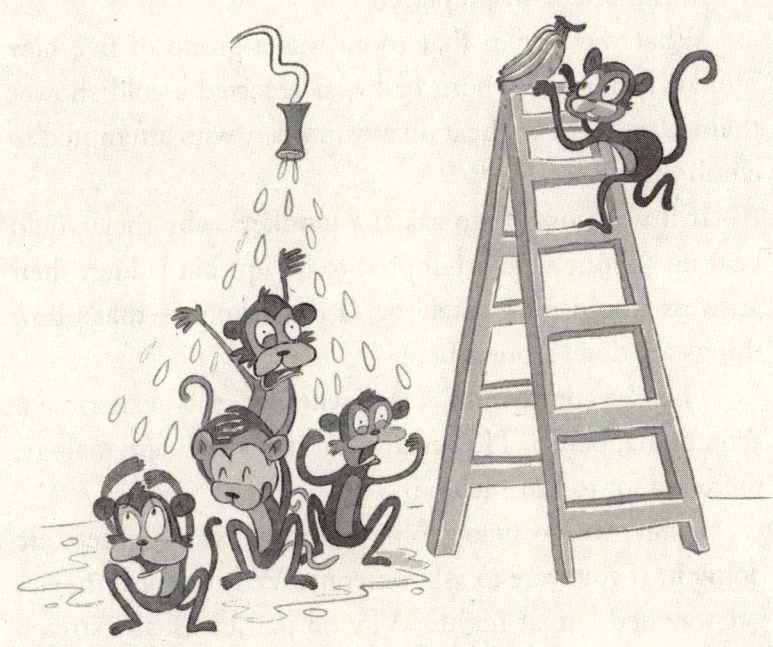

Then, the scientists decided to substitute one of the monkeys in the group. What do you think this new monkey would have done? Unsurprisingly, the first thing this new monkey did was to go up the ladder. Immediately, the four older monkeys beat him up. The new monkey learnt not to climb the ladder even though he never understood why.

Then, the scientists replaced a second monkey from the group. And predictably, the same thing repeated. This time, the first monkey even participated in beating the second monkey.

A third monkey was replaced and the same beating repeated. Soon, the fourth was replaced, and finally, even the fifth monkey was replaced.

What was left in that room was a group of five new monkeys, none of whom had ever received a cold shower themselves, yet they beat up any monkey who attempted to climb the ladder.

If it was possible to ask the monkeys why they would beat up anyone who attempted to go up that ladder, their answers would most likely be, 'I don't know—that's how things are done around here.'

There's controversy over whether this experiment actually happened. However, even if it's only an analogy, there is a lot to learn from it.

Today, we do many things simply because others are doing it. If you were to ask someone, 'Why do most movies get watched late at night? Why do parties usually stretch until the early morning? Why do many of our social events today begin at a time when we ideally should be in deep sleep?' A common response would be, 'I don't know—that's how things are done. Everyone does it this way, so I too do it this way.'

However, have we ever questioned who set these norms? Why are they done this way? If something interferes with one of our most prized possessions in life, our sleep, should we really continue to adhere to norms that destroy it, day after day, night after night?

Others who follow these norms, whether it's late-night partying or attending late-night gatherings, do so without much thought. And in the process, we've become a society that, just like the monkeys in the room, follows norms without understanding their origin or purpose.

However, we always have a choice. We could either say, 'No, I can't. I'm just stuck in this cycle. I have to do what everyone's doing. I need to fit in.' Or we could say, 'No, I want to be the first one to change norms that don't feel right. I don't want to blindly follow norms which take away my sleep and my health.' No choice is right or wrong, but each leads to very different destinations.

Personally, for both Harshvardhan and I, we've made the second choice. We try to meet our family, friends and community in the day, rather than at night, simply shifting the timing to start a bit earlier in the evening or even during the day.

Of course there are always exceptions, such as weddings or late-night gatherings which are beyond our control. But an **exception** doesn't become the **norm**. An exception loses its meaning if it happens every week.

If peak health and performance are what we seek, we have to reserve our nights for something far more precious: **deep sleep.**

Concluding Thoughts about This Practice

We know from common belief that a good diet and exercise are of vital importance to health. But we now know that deep sleep is just as important in this health trinity.

We hope this chapter has inspired you to embrace darkness, let go of gadgets in the final hour before you sleep, create a wind-down routine, and welcome your praanshakti to repair and recharge, both of which your body and brain need.

When you do take charge of your sleep, you experience massive benefits in your life. But, you also open a window to something extraordinary. Something that you have neither so far read about, nor may have even thought about. The most magical benefit of deep sleep—what is it? You'll find out in the next chapter.

8

Three Unknown Secrets of Waking Up Early

It was the last day of the year 2022. We were in a town called Auroville, in the south of India. We had been living there for two months in a quaint home, surrounded by a lush forest. In the evening, a thought had struck me—I didn't want us to spend the first day of the new year following our usual routine. Instead, I had a yearning for something different, something memorable. It was then that I recalled a suggestion from one of our friends who had mentioned a beautiful experience happening at Matrimandir (a spiritual building, in the shape of a large golden sphere, in the centre of Auroville). Eager to be a part of this experience, we asked our friend to arrange passes.

As the morning of 1 January dawned, we woke up at 4.30 a.m., got ready and made our way towards Matrimandir on our scooty. Harshvardhan was the one driving, navigating the quiet streets, while I sat behind him. I held his waist tightly, not only to steady myself on the bumpy road but also because the streets were pitch dark and silent, with not a soul in sight.

Finally, we reached our destination. The golden globe was even more majestic than it appeared in the photos, its shiny surface gleaming in the moon's gentle glow. After parking our scooty, we walked into the premises with anticipation. However, our excitement turned to dismay when we discovered that the building was closed, and the doors wouldn't open for a few more hours. But we didn't want to go back after coming all this way.

Just then, a volunteer approached and gently tapped my shoulder. Leaning in, he whispered, 'That's where you have to go,' pointing towards a large Banyan tree a short distance away. Before I could inquire further, he had walked away. Left with little choice, we made our way to the tree, finding a few small benches scattered under its canopy. While there were some people already seated there, both of us found one bench each, and sat cross-legged.

It was still dark outside. There was a sense of stillness all around, with no noise or distractions. It was so quiet that I could almost hear the silence. I gently closed my eyes. As soon as I did, my head filled with chatter—'What time is it?', 'When will we be allowed to go inside?', 'There are so many mosquitoes here, I should have applied my insect repellent oil.' Noticing this internal chatter, I tried to quiet my mind. In the beginning, the silence felt strange. But after a while, I don't know why but I found myself asking a question: 'What do I want to accomplish before I depart from this world?' It was a question that had occasionally surfaced during my everyday life, often at the end of a busy workday, but this time, it felt different, as if the stillness of the morning had opened a gateway to my innermost thoughts.

As I let the question sink in, something remarkable began to happen. Visions, both immediate and distant, began to flash vividly in my mind's eye. I saw a world which was very different to the present. A world where health, joy, compassion and wisdom were the norm. This world was called the Satvic world. I saw an image with thousands of health centres across the world, dedicated to supporting people in adopting a more conscious way of life, each having a Satvic cafe of its own. I saw a dedicated team of hundreds of health educators tirelessly spreading this knowledge to every corner of the globe. In the midst of it all, I also had a vision of a book, a tangible embodiment of these ideals, destined to go on the shelves of bookstores and introduce countless more people to the Satvic Revolution. (By the way, you're currently holding that very book.)

What surprised me was not merely the emergence of these visions, but the accompanying sense of crystal clear clarity that revealed how to actually bring them to life in the real world. It was as though all the fragmented thoughts, ideas, confusions, questions and uncertainties that had plagued my mind over the past several months had converged into a single cohesive thread, transforming chaos into clarity and dreams into blueprints. In those moments, the greatest ideas flowed into my mind with an effortless ease.

When I finally opened my eyes, I observed that the sky had transitioned from a dark shade of blue to a much lighter, brighter hue. An hour must have passed since I had closed my eyes.

I got up from the bench, the weight of these new ideas too much to keep to myself any longer. We continued with the rest of the experience as planned, and during our journey back, I couldn't help but pour out every thought, plan and idea to Harshvardhan. To my surprise, he shared that he also had experienced a similar inflow of ideas.

Upon our return home, I eagerly opened the notes app on my laptop and spent the next two hours meticulously documenting all the ideas that had unfolded to us in the dawn. This vision, which had emerged beneath the Banyan tree, continues to shape much of what we do at Satvic Movement to this day.

To be honest, this entire experience didn't come as a surprise to me. On various occasions in life, I had been blessed with these episodes of unclouded clarity and profound insight—whether I was confused about a decision at work or utterly bewildered about what to do in a personal relationship. In those moments, it was as if clarity would wash over my mind like a bucket of water washing a stained glass window.

Upon further contemplation, I came to realize that there's a common thread running through all these moments in my life when I've experienced such remarkable clarity, when I've been able to access these creative, extraordinary and brilliant thoughts. The common thread was that all such moments occurred in the hours before sunrise, during those early-morning hours when the rest of the world was still sleeping.

I was also certain that this common thread was not a mere coincidence. Because shortly after embarking on my healing journey, I had learnt about a special period of time that starts around one and a half hours before sunrise, every day. In our Vedic scriptures, this period of time is referred to as the Brahma Muhurta. 'Brahma' signifies the Creator, and 'Muhurta' translates to Time. In simpler terms, these early-morning hours form the Brahma Muhurta, which is the Creator's Time. It is said that during this period, we can actively shape and create the life we want. It's a period when the universe's energy is most accessible to those who are awake and alert.

When I first came across this concept of Brahma Muhurta, I found it strange. You see, even though my parents had named me 'Subah' (meaning 'morning' in Hindi), growing up, I was never an early riser. Every weekend or holiday, I would seize the chance to sleep in, not waking up before 10 a.m. The idea of rising before the sunrise seemed odd, impractical and, frankly, impossible for someone like me.

But shortly after embarking on my healing journey, I initiated the practice of rising early in the morning. Today, I can confidently say that this practice has, quite literally, helped me reinvent my life, and infuse each day with added purpose, energy and depth. In fact, the greatest benefit I gained from habit three—'Sleep Like a Baby'—wasn't merely experiencing deeper sleep at night, but it was that it helped me develop the powerful practice of waking up early.

When you also incorporate the practices we discussed in the previous chapter—having a calming wind-down routine, and prioritizing sleep during the prime sleep hours of 10 p.m. to 2 a.m.—a natural consequence will be that you will start rising early, possibly as early as 5 a.m. And that's what this chapter is all about.

In this chapter, you will learn about:

• The three miracles that can happen in your life when you wake up at 5 a.m.
• The two practical ways to translate this practice from motivational talk to real-life application

Before we begin, we want to say that it doesn't matter what your current wake-up time is. Maybe you don't consider yourself a 'morning person', and are accustomed to waking up at 8 a.m., 9 a.m. or even 10 a.m. Or perhaps you've tried waking up early many times before and failed each time. Either way, this chapter is designed to handhold you along a new path, a path to something extraordinary. We will not only discuss the lesser-known benefits of being an early riser, but also share insights on how to make the transition easier and more comfortable. Ultimately, whether you decide to embark on this path and to what extent—that's a choice you can make once you've gained all the tools and knowledge.

Three Miracles that Happen When You Wake Up at 5 a.m.

1. You Gain Access to Your Creative Genius Thoughts

When we read the word 'genius', many of us think of names like Albert Einstein or Isaac Newton, leading most us to consider our own intelligence as merely ordinary. Yet, Albert Einstein famously said, 'Everybody is a genius,' and he certainly wasn't joking. The truth is that each of us has a spark of genius within us. But because we're fast asleep when these brilliant, creative and extraordinary thoughts come, we fail to access them.

Here is an example to understand this better. Imagine you opened a south Indian breakfast shop. Your idlis and dosas are famous all over town. But your most valued, high-paying and loyal customers come to you with a special request—they need breakfast at 5 a.m. What would you do in such a situation? Would you respond with, 'No, I can't wake up that early; I love my sleep too much'? Certainly not! You'd open your shop at 5 a.m., ready to greet and serve your most valued customers.

In much the same way, your most brilliant, powerful and creative thoughts knock at your mind's door during these early-morning hours. If you're a business leader, these thoughts may be groundbreaking business strategies. If you're a student, they may be solutions to challenging problems. If you're feeling lost about something, these thoughts may be answers to your confusions. These thoughts are basically your most innovative, extraordinary, powerful ideas. However, if you're asleep during this time, you unknowingly shut the door to these powerful thoughts and ideas, letting them go to waste.

Science has told us that creativity is a function of connections between many different networks throughout the brain. In an insightful study conducted by scientists at Aachen University, researchers conducted brain scans on fifty-nine people. Among them, sixteen were early risers, twenty-three were night owls who slept late, and twenty fell somewhere in between.

The researchers found that people who wake up early have more of something called 'white matter' in their brains. White matter is fatty tissue in the brain that helps different nerve cells connect and communicate. Reduced white matter in the brain has been linked to reduced cognitive function. In simple words, the study shows how waking up early helps improve brain function. This, in turn, helps us to be more creative, focus more, and have an unparalleled mental clarity.

Perhaps this is why many of the world's greatest writers, poets and thinkers never waste the morning golden hours in sleep. Apple chief executive officer (CEO), Tim Cook starts his day at 3.45 a.m. Disney CEO Robert Iger also gets up at 4.30 a.m. Michelle Obama rises at 4.30 a.m. These successful people understand that early in the morning, the mind is a powerhouse of creativity, and so, they use that time to think and get things done.

2. You Gain Three Extra Hours Every Day for Your Personal Growth

Do you often find yourself creating a long to-do list or setting personal goals? 'I want to start exercising', 'I want to start reading books', 'I want to finally begin meditating', 'I want to learn to play the guitar', 'I want to listen to that podcast'. You have big dreams and a burning desire to pursue them. But somehow, time slips away. Your job takes up most of your day, or perhaps you're responsible for taking care of your family. We get it—life is busy and hectic.

However, we have something to tell you—you actually have time for everything. You have time for exercise, for reading, for meditating, for learning a new skill, for pursuing all that you wish to for your personal growth. There is more than enough time. The issue is not lack of time but an inability to access it, because it's hidden. Where is it hidden? In the first few hours of the day, at dawn, while you may still be asleep.

You see, your current routine probably involves waking up, getting dressed, making breakfast and rushing off to work or doing your daily chores. You return home in the evening, feeling drained and tired. You have dinner, watch some TV, go to sleep, and the cycle continues the next day. Eventually, life starts feeling boring, dull and monotonous. Without knowing it, you find yourself settling for a mundane, mediocre existence, with little energy to pursue your passions, to exercise, or to go the extra mile to take care of your loved ones.

Why does this happen? One reason is that you're navigating life with an empty cup. Each of us has a cup of intrinsic vigour. This is like your cup of internal energy. If your cup is empty, how much can you offer to your work, your partner or your children? Not much. But when you rise early and spend time re-energizing yourself through practices that you resonate with—be it reading to grow your mind, exercising to energize your body or meditation to nourish your spirit—you basically fill your cup at the start of the day. When you start your day with a full cup, you automatically have so much more to give to your work and your loved ones.

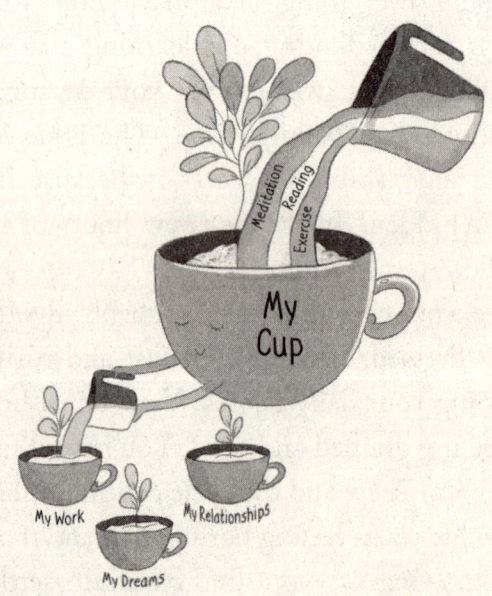

By waking up early, you gain approximately three extra hours (from around 5 a.m. to 8 a.m.) to do whatever you believe fills your cup—develop a new skill like singing, painting or writing, or getting fit. An extra three hours each day adds up to a lot of time!

An extra three hours per day
= twenty-one extra hours per week
= 1095 extra hours a year
= forty-five extra days per year to get more done in your life!

Remember, you don't have to sacrifice sleep to gain these three extra hours. You'll sleep the same, but gain three extra productive hours each day. How? You convert those late-night unproductive hours to morning super-productive hours.

This is why we genuinely believe that **waking up early is the mother of all good habits**. It paves the way for all other good habits, including the ones you've learnt in this book and those you're about to learn.

Remember, **you don't feel exhausted because you're doing too much. You feel exhausted because you're doing too little of the things that energize you,** that fill your cup. Early waking brings back those three hidden hours to fill your cup, to work on yourself.

3. You Unlock Your Flow State

The idea of being in a 'flow state' was popularized by positive psychologists, Mihaly Csikszentmihalyi and Jeanne Nakamura. But even before they came up with this term, similar concepts existed in various philosophies and schools of thought worldwide.

A person is in a state of flow when they become completely engrossed in an activity. When a person is 'in flow', they may not notice time passing, think about why they are doing the task or judge their efforts. Instead, they remain completely focused on what they're doing. Even if a task is hard, it feels easy when one is in a state of flow. They feel a sense of control and joy, as the activity itself brings immense satisfaction.

Imagine a skilled pianist playing the piano. As their fingers dance across the keys, they lose themselves in the music. Time loses its grip, and they play without conscious thought, as the notes flow naturally. So absorbed are they in the melody that even applause from the audience doesn't register. In such a state, the pianist is in a 'flow'.

Another example is of a person deeply engrossed in watching a movie. As the film plays, the rest of the world seems to fade away. They become so absorbed in the storyline that they might not even notice someone calling their name. If someone were to walk in front of the TV, they'd instinctively shift their gaze to keep the screen in view, barely registering the person's presence.

Have you ever experienced a flow state yourself when you were fully immersed in an activity? It could be while playing sports, practising a hobby or working on a project. Pause and take a moment to reflect.

One fascinating discovery made by psychologist Csikszentmihalyi in his research is that people are at their most productive when they are in a state of flow.

Reading a book? If you can read five pages in a regular state, you can perhaps read ten pages in a flow state. Not only that, you're even able to absorb the knowledge better. Preparing for exams? Remembering information becomes easier. Acquiring a new skill such as playing the guitar? The flow state allows you to master the skill in days, not weeks or months. Even for spiritual practices, we have realized that being in the flow state allows you to go much deeper into your practice. In essence, the flow state multiples the impact of any action.

Now, the natural question that may come to mind is, 'How do we enter this state of flow?' Well, you don't have to do something extra to enter this state. The early-morning hours hold the key to this state of flow. In the early morning, you can effortlessly slip into the flow state. Wondering why?

It's because the hours before sunrise are Zero Distraction Hours. There are no interruptions. No notifications popping up on your phone. No yelling children. No phone calls coming. No traffic noise. No honking. No chatter of people around you. Just silence, as the rest of the world is still asleep.

It's not that you can't enter a flow state at other times of the day, but in the early morning, it is the easiest to do so.

I've personally experienced this as well. One of the most challenging tasks in my role at Satvic Movement is script writing for our videos. As someone who isn't naturally spontaneous, I prefer to carefully plan and craft each word in the videos that go out on Satvic Movement's channels. However, I always found script writing daunting and often found myself procrastinating.

However, one morning I decided to start my writing work at 5 a.m. To my surprise, that morning, my experience of script writing completely changed. I became so deeply engrossed in the writing that nothing else mattered. What used to take me two days was completed in just four hours because of the early-morning flow state.

Today, Harshvardhan and I choose to do the bulk of our thinking and writing work, including working on the book that you're reading, in the early-morning hours, because that's when we can effortlessly transition into the state of flow.

To summarize, early waking offers three incredible miracles:

- Access to your creative genius thoughts
- Three extra hours daily for self-growth
- A state of flow that supercharges your productivity

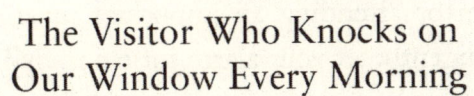

The Visitor Who Knocks on Our Window Every Morning

In Indian culture, the Sun is known as Surya Dev (meaning 'Sun God'). The Sun God is revered as the deity of health and vitality. According to our age-old traditions, one should leave one's bed before the Sun God arrives. The philosophy behind this is simple yet profound.

Imagine this scenario: You're expecting guests at your home. What do you do? You tidy up, clean and prepare to welcome them with open arms. The Sun God, too, is like an honoured guest who visits us each morning. He gently knocks on our windows through his soft sun rays.

However, if we're sound asleep when our celestial guest arrives, we unknowingly show Him disrespect. As a result, we miss the most precious gift brought by our guest—abundant health and boundless vitality.

~ Adapted from the teachings of
Acharya Mohan Gupta Ji

Turning Theory into Action

Now that you've learnt about the miracles of early waking, here are two steps to help make it practical:

The First Step: Establish a Strong Morning Routine

Think back to those days when you had an important event lined up in the morning—catching a train or a flight, sitting for an exam or attending an important meeting. Before bed, you diligently set your alarm for 6 a.m. Miraculously, however, you woke up at 5.58 a.m., unassisted, right before the alarm. Has this ever happened to you?

The reason behind this is that when you plan an event or task before going to bed, it gets registered into your subconscious mind, which prompts you to automatically wake up at the planned time the next day.

If you struggle to wake up early, it's likely because you don't have a compelling reason to do so. Even if you're highly motivated, lacking a strong 'why' can lead to hitting the snooze button when the alarm rings.

Therefore, it's so important to find your 'why' for waking up early. Is it a skill you want to master? A book you've been longing to read? A fitness routine you want to follow? A new project you're excited to start? A spiritual practice you want to begin? **The intensity of your drive to work on this 'why' will decide whether or not you are able to wake up early.**

For many people in the Satvic community who we've spoken to, their morning routine itself becomes their 'why'. You too can create a morning routine so motivating that it becomes your reason to wake up at 5 a.m. every morning. A holistic morning routine contains three M's:

The first M:
Meditation
This refers to any spiritual practice that connects you with your spirit or with the Higher Power. Different people resonate with meditation differently. It could involve mantra chanting, worship, introspection, visualization or focusing on the breath.

The second M:
Movement
Engage your body in physical activity, be it yoga, brisk walking, jogging, dancing, swimming or any sport. Move your body to invigorate yourself physically.

The third M:
Mastery
Dedicate time to mastering a skill or acquiring knowledge relevant to your personal or professional life, whether through reading books, taking courses, watching videos or listening to podcasts on that particular subject.

We discovered the concept of the three M's in Robin Sharma's book *5 AM Club*, and it has added immense value to our own lives. Most mornings, we devote thirty to sixty minutes to each of these activities, depending on the time that is available. Meditation nourishes our spiritual self, movement invigorates our physical body, and mastery enriches our mental and intellectual faculties.

Over time, our morning routine has become our 'why' for waking up early. In the process, what we've realized is this: **take excellent care of the first few hours of your day and the rest of your day will take care of itself.**

Another way to understand this is using the analogy of an archer. An archer's goal is to hit the target. Ironically, the first movement he has to do is to pull back the arrow. When he pulls back, it may seem like he's going away from his target, but that backward motion actually allows him to set the right target and generate more power. Similarly, when we take the time in the morning for the three M's, we are like a bowman pulling his arrow back. It allows us to generate a lot more momentum and power for the rest of our day.

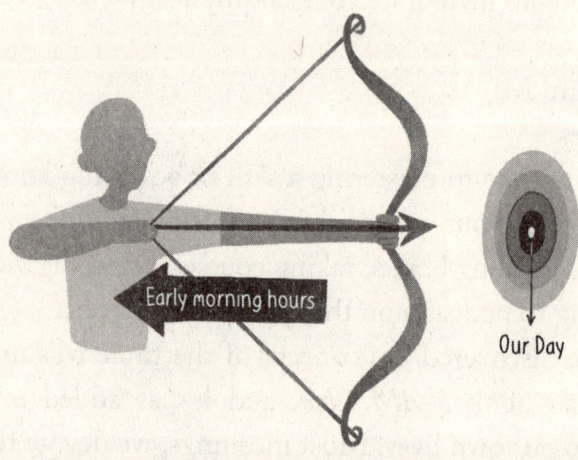

Early morning hours

Our Day

By embracing the three M's in the morning, even if it's for just thirty minutes each, not only do you generate a lot more power for the rest of your day, but you also fill your cup to the brim, allowing you to give much more to your work, to your family, to your children and to your purpose.

The three M's are simply a framework to make it easier for you to remember. If beginning with all three seems too overwhelming, begin with just one or two. But ensure that you choose activities that genuinely inspire you. That motivate you. That you feel strongly about. You'll be surprised at how much easier it becomes to wake up early when you have a strong 'why'.

Design Your Three-M Morning Routine for the Next Week

Before we move on to the second step to help you wake up early, let's reinforce this first step with a short activity.

In the table below, fill in the following details (to begin with, think about only the next seven days):

1. **Identify Each M:** Write down what you plan to do for meditation, movement and mastery, starting from tomorrow. Be specific about the activities you'll engage in.
2. **Set Clear Times:** Assign timings for each activity. Note down the precise hour when you will engage in meditation, movement and mastery.

3. **Designated Space:** Assign specific areas for each activity
    within your living space. Identify where you'll meditate,
    where you'll perform your movement exercises, and
    where you'll immerse yourself in mastery activities.
    Commit to not practising meditation, movement or
    mastery on your bed. The energy of your bed is best
    suited for sleep. If you engage in any of these activities
    on your bed, you'll likely find yourself sleeping a few
    minutes after.

Now, take a moment to pause and fill in the table below.

	Specifically what I will do	Timing	Space
MEDITATION			
MOVEMENT			
MASTERY			

Your Mind Is Like a Mattress

Throughout the day, your mind can be compared to a mattress covered with a protective sheet. Even if you spill something on it, the sheet acts as a barrier, preventing the substance from soaking through. However, in the early-morning hours, when you've just woken up, your mind is like a bare, uncovered mattress. Any liquid you pour on to it will be readily absorbed and internalized. In other words, your mind is more permeable in the early-morning hours. If you start your day by scrolling through celebrity gossip, World news or politics, you're essentially staining your mental canvas for the day ahead.

Now, the question is—when your mind is more permeable, what would you choose to pour into it? Value-based education, enriching books, spiritual insights or mindless distractions, frivolous gossip and negative news? The decision is yours to make.

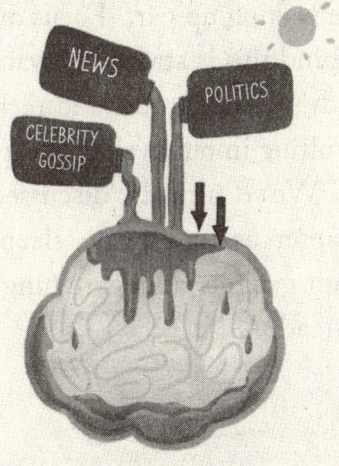

The Second Way to Make the Habit of 5 a.m. Waking Practical

Set Your Alarm Right

If you aim to wake up at 5 a.m., what time do you think you should set your alarm for?

4.30 a.m.?

4.45 a.m.?

Or 5 a.m.?

What's your guess?

The answer is—none of these! More important than setting an early morning alarm is your reminder for sleeping on time. By 9 p.m. each night, remind yourself to be in bed. If you want to wake up early, don't focus so much on the waking up part. Focus on sleeping early. The principle behind this is straightforward: when we sleep on time, our body's need for rest and recharge is also fulfilled on time, resulting in our eyelids naturally opening at 5 a.m.

We've already discussed in depth in the previous chapter as to how to sleep on time—by disconnecting from gadgets and switching to low-stimulation activities instead.

Quick Activity:

Open the alarm app on your phone right now.

- Set an alarm for 9 p.m. (or whatever you consider your sleep time) and make it repeat every day.
- You can name the alarm 'get into bed for 5 a.m. magic' if you like.
- Now, when this alarm goes off in the evening, regardless of what you're doing, simply respond by getting into bed. This is the time to engage in any winding-down activity that helps you relax.

These two steps—establishing a strong morning routine and an early bedtime—have proven highly effective, not only for us but also for countless members of the Satvic community, in regaining control over their mornings. If you decide to embrace these two steps, please remember that in the beginning, when you first start, you will experience setbacks. You might successfully wake up early for a day or two, only to slip back into old routines a few days later. But that's okay; remember, developing new habits is a gradual process. Try again, and soon, after a couple of attempts, early waking will become the new rhythm for your body.

Here's an additional suggestion if you find yourself hitting the snooze button in the morning: place your alarm clock or phone away from your bed. By doing so, you'll need to physically rise and walk to turn it off, ensuring you're on your feet and, in the process, you'll become wide awake.

Concluding Thoughts about the Practice

So far in this book, we've covered three of the seven habits. First, we learned how to keep a clean body within (by eating an early dinner). Then, we learned about the highest quality fuel for our bodies (living, wholesome and plant-based foods). And finally we learned how to take full charge of our routine (by sleeping like a baby, and consequently making the most of the early morning time). Now, there's a chance that you might be wondering how you can possibly juggle so much change. Questions could be coming: Is it necessary to adopt all seven habits? Is it even possible to do so in our modern, fast-paced world?

We want you to know that embracing all seven habits from this book immediately is nearly impossible. Our advice to you would be to start with what feels most doable for you. If getting up at 5 a.m. feels like too big of a leap, try setting your alarm just an hour earlier than you do right now. These small steps themselves will start showing you results in your life. When you see those results, you'll want to take one more step, then one more, and then another.

Also remember that adopting any one of the seven habits in this book will create a positive ripple effect, making it easier to incorporate the others. For instance, when you start having dinner by 7 p.m. and eat wholesome, plant-based foods that your body can easily digest, you'll discover that waking up early becomes effortless. Each habit feeds the other. Eventually, these habits will become easier and easier.

Until then, our dearest reader, keep revisiting this book often. Don't read it once and then never look at it again. The learnings will fade away from your mind. Rather, think of this book as a constant companion, offering guidance when you need it most—when motivation dips or when you're seeking further growth in your life.

Our concluding message from this particular chapter is this: **Every new morning is a blank page in the story of your life. Don't waste it by hitting snooze.** Every day, when you wake up, remind yourself, 'Today I am fortunate to be alive. I have a precious human life. I am not going to waste it.'

With that, we conclude this chapter and also habit three: 'Sleep Like a Baby'.

The next habit is about something that makes your skin blush, and leaves your heart racing faster. As you turn the page, you'll delve into its biggest myths, meet two new characters—Mr Perfect and Mr Reps—and uncover the five great elements residing within you.

Habit 4

Celebrate Movement

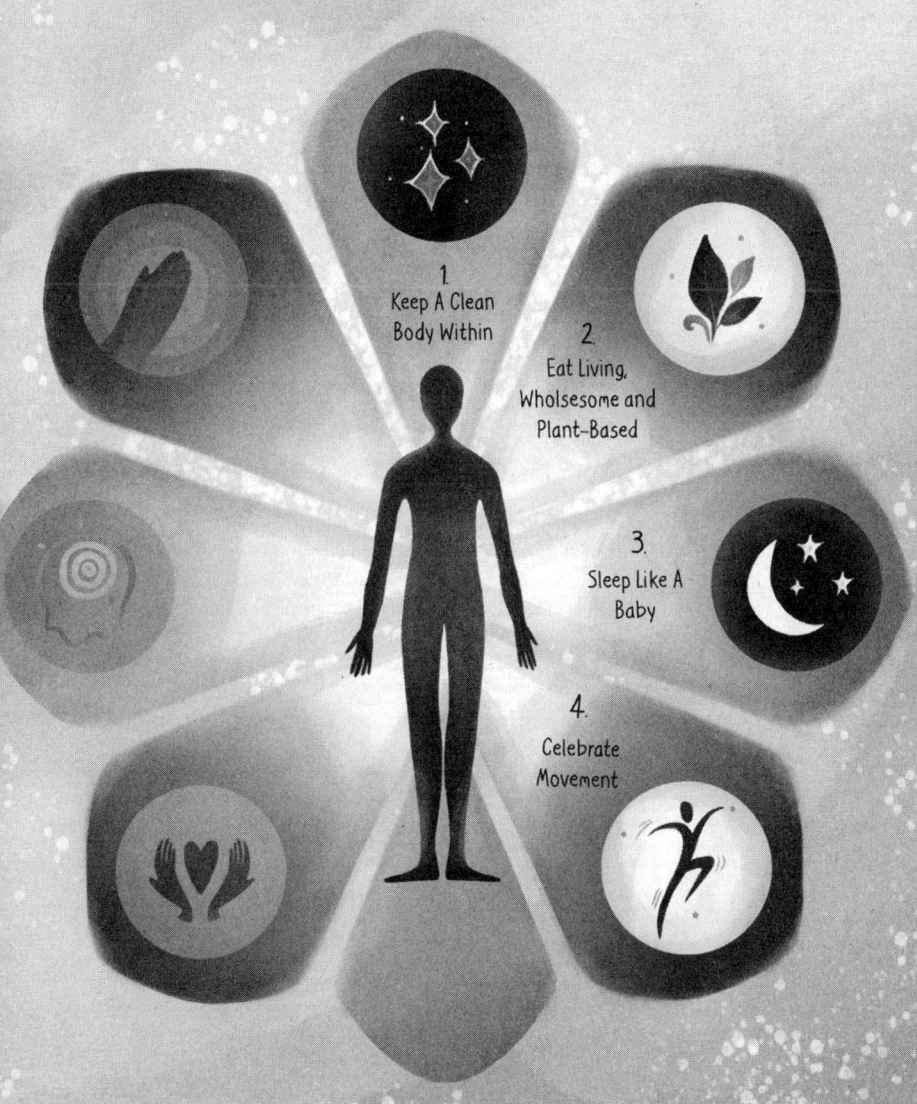

1.
Keep A Clean
Body Within

2.
Eat Living,
Wholsesome and
Plant-Based

3.
Sleep Like A
Baby

4.
Celebrate
Movement

9

Move, Breathe, Celebrate

We would like to begin this chapter with a question. Imagine you're in a room. It's an empty room. On a chair in front of you are some items: a packet of cigarettes, a bottle of alcohol, a big hamburger and a crispy fried samosa.

If we asked you to pick one item that is the unhealthiest of all, which one would you choose?

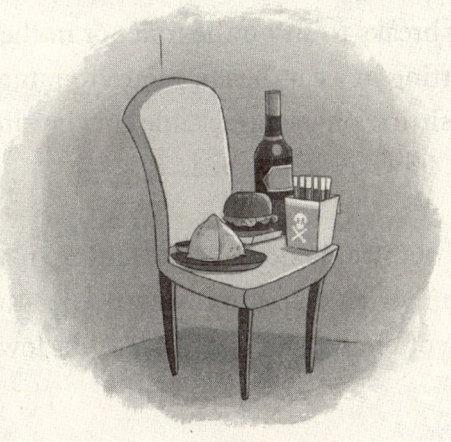

Many of us would point to the usual suspects—the cigarette or the alcohol, maybe even the hamburger or the fried samosa.

Well, these are all pretty bad for you. But you most likely know the harmful effects of cigarettes, alcohol, hamburgers and fried samosas, right? And hence, you might try to avoid them or limit their intake. But, there's one thing in this room you may not have even thought about, which might be the biggest obstacle stopping you from achieving peak health.

What is that one thing?

Well, the real culprit is . . . the chair!

We, in modern times, spend our whole day sitting down. We go from:

Sitting on the bed
→ to **sitting** on the toilet,
→ to then **sitting** at the breakfast table,
→ followed by **sitting** in a car, bus or metro to get to work,
→ where we spend the entire day **sitting** at a desk,
→ with brief breaks to **sit** on the toilet or in the cafeteria,
→ to then **sitting** in a car, bus or metro to return home,
→ to finally **sitting** on a comfortable couch watching TV,
→ before we crawl back into bed.

When we go out, we spend our time **sitting** in a restaurant or **sitting** at a movie theatre. Even at social gatherings, the first thing we often look for is a place to **sit** down!

In essence, today many of us are living a life where we are just moving from one chair to another. It's like playing musical chairs, not in a birthday party, but in life.

Pause for a moment. Think: how many hours do you think you spend sitting each day? Write your answer here:

Most people who fill the box report about ten to twelve hours of sitting each day. But here's the thing: The human body simply wasn't designed for so much sitting. If you go back to any period in the past, people were constantly on the move. They were engaged in daily household chores like farming, ploughing fields, grinding grains, drawing water from wells, walking long distances for trade, participating in communal dances and ceremonies, and playing outdoor games. In other words, our ancestors, to a large extent, lived in accordance with nature's laws. One of these intrinsic laws of nature is **movement**. But today, our ratio of movement to sitting has become the opposite of what it once was.

Even when you look at nature, everything is in movement all the time. Trees sway from side to side. Ocean waves are in constant motion. Planets are constantly spinning around the sun. Birds migrate across vast distances. Butterflies fly from flower to flower in search of nectar. Animals are constantly moving in search of food and shelter. Movement is a fundamental attribute of every living organism on this planet.

So when everything in nature is constantly moving, why are we humans always tied down to our chairs and couches? If we humans are a part of nature, shouldn't we also move, if not always, at least from time to time?

This is where our journey in this chapter begins. Dear reader, welcome to habit four: 'Celebrate Movement'. We'd like to warn you: this chapter may make you fall in love with movement (and by 'movement', we mean any form of daily physical activity or exercise of the body).

Here's what you can expect to learn from this chapter:

• What really happens in your body when you engage in movement?
• The three golden steps to make this habit a consistent part of your life
• How to get more out of each movement session

You probably know that movement, or physical activity, is good for you. With this habit, the problem isn't the lack of awareness; it's maintaining consistency. We've all started a new exercise routine with lots of energy. And from wanting to do it every day, we eventually end up doing it only when we find 'the time', which, let's be honest, we rarely find. So in this chapter, we will place a lot of emphasis on how to actually make movement a **consistent** practice.

But first, let's learn about those unexpected benefits of movement which you may have never heard about.

What Really Happens in Your Body When You Move?

From an external perspective, you might just seem to be jogging, jumping or dancing. But just a few minutes into your movement routine, a carefully choreographed process is initiated within your body, which is not apparent from the outside. It is invisible to the naked eye.

Your heart quickens its rhythm. The heart rate of an average adult at a restful state is about 60–100 beats per minute, but during intense exercise, it can surge to approximately 150–180 beats per minute. As your heart beats faster, it begins to pump more life-giving blood. This newly pumped blood then flows like a river through your veins, through your arteries, to every corner of your body.

You can even see this for yourself. Have you ever noticed the 'pinking up' of your skin after a few minutes of exercise? It's a sign that blood has circulated through your entire body, including beneath your skin's surface, and hence your skin turns a little pink.

This boost in blood circulation during exercise is actually a powerful process that leads to many other processes inside your body. Let's understand the four most important ones:

1. **More Oxygen for Your Cells:** This circulated blood carries oxygen. In other words, exercise essentially

delivers more oxygen to every cell of your body. Remember, oxygen is like food for your cells, keeping them active and healthy. So, through exercise, each cell of your body gets bathed in oxygen, getting its proper nourishment.

In fact, research studies clearly show a direct correlation between a person's health and the level of oxygen in their bloodstream.

Dr Otto Warburg, twice Nobel Laureate, awarded the Nobel Prize in Medicine for his research on cellular respiration, discovered that unlike all other cells in the human body, cancer cells do not breathe oxygen. He explains how the growth of cancer cells is initiated by a relative lack of oxygen, and how cancer cannot live in an oxygen-rich environment.

2. **Getting Rid of Toxins:** As your blood circulation increases with exercise, waste products and toxins inside the cells get dislodged. In other words, toxins, which were once stationary, are stirred from their resting places and set into motion.

Then, as you sweat, the body often expels these toxins. Sweat is not just your body's cooling system; it's also a waste disposal service. Through sweat, you're getting rid of toxins and waste products, creating a cleaner internal environment.

3. **Digestive Boost:** As your blood circulation increases with exercise, your digestive organs, including

the stomach, receive more blood, improving their efficiency. Your digestive fire becomes stronger. As a result, when you consistently exercise, your praanshakti can digest food faster and more effectively.

Today, many of the diseases that we suffer from, as a society, such as diabetes, obesity and thyroid imbalance, are metabolic disorders, which stem from sluggish digestion. Movement is a direct way to drastically improve digestion.

4. **Uplifts Your Mood:** All our lives, we're made to believe that exercise is needed for physical fitness. However, today, society has come to realize that exercise isn't just for physical fitness but also for our mental well-being. In fact, movement is one of the most transformative things that you can do for your brain. A single workout makes your brain immediately release dopamine, adrenaline and serotonin. These are also known as 'happy hormones', and they instantly improve your mood.

    To better understand this relationship, an interesting study was conducted by the University of Vermont in 2015. In this study, researchers analysed data from approximately 13,000 high school students. They discovered that exercising for four or more days per week was linked not only to significant reductions in sadness among these students but it also resulted in a 23 per cent reduction in suicide attempts among bullied students!

Astonishing, isn't it?

> 'If you are in a bad mood, go for a walk.
> If you are still in a bad mood, go for another walk.'
>   —Hippocrates, the Father of Modern Medicine

To summarize, movement improves the functioning of every part of your body. On the other hand, if you're not getting enough exercise in your week, chances are that you will have a weakened digestive fire and, consequently, slow and sluggish digestion. This gives rise to bloating, lethargy and tiredness in the day. It will also lead to reduced efficiency of the organs, which may manifest as increased symptoms of any chronic health problem. Remember: **A body in motion stays alive. A body without motion decomposes.**

> 'Those who think they have no time for **exercise**
> will sooner or later have to find time for **illness**.'
>   —Edward Stanley

The Biggest Myth about Exercise

Before we dive into practical suggestions, it's essential to clear up one common misconception. Many of us believe that exercise is meant for weight loss, that if we don't need to lose weight, exercise is not *that* important for us.

This is actually a big myth.

Sure, if you're carrying excess weight, exercise greatly helps in shedding those extra kilos. But, if you're underweight, exercise is just as important. It is essential to build strength in your muscles which eventually helps in weight gain. It also greatly enhances your body's ability to absorb the nutrition from your food.

That said, the type of exercise needed varies for different body types. If you're on the heavier side, movements that increase the heart rate and make you break into a sweat may be more beneficial. If you're lean or underweight, exercises that focus on muscle building, using external weights or just your body's weight, may be more suitable.

The bottom line is that movement is essential for everyone, irrespective of age, health or weight. It's a universal health booster.

Now, let's understand how to apply this in our daily routine so it can become a habit.

Practical Ways to Build Consistency: Three Golden Steps

We believe that the number 1 problem when it comes to movement is consistency. We all WANT to do it. We all know that it's good for us. There's no debate on that. We even try to do it. But somewhere down the line, we lose consistency. We're simply not able to maintain our discipline.

We tell ourselves, 'Okay, tomorrow morning I'll definitely exercise.' When the morning comes, we tell ourselves, 'Ah, I have too much to do; I'll definitely do it in the evening.' When the evening comes, we say, 'Now it's too late. I'll start tomorrow morning. In fact, I'll do an even more intense workout to compensate for the lost day.' Before we know it, three days, then a week, and eventually a month slip away without us engaging in any exercise routine.

We say we'll start it 'Someday'. The irony is that there are seven days in a week and 'Someday' is not one of them!

Despite knowing its benefits, why is maintaining consistency so hard?

Well, based on our findings, there are three main reasons why we're not able to make movement a consistent habit:

1. We don't genuinely enjoy the process. Some of us even hate the process. And so, we have to really push ourselves to do it.

2. We have an 'all or nothing' mindset. We think, 'If I cannot do a full hour of exercise, what's the point?'

3. No one's keeping tabs on us. We are inspired initially, but when the actual moment comes to do it, we simply get lazy and talk ourselves out of the workout, because it's so easy to justify to ourselves why it's okay to skip. This happens because no one else is checking in, who we are answerable to.

We have observed these to be the three major reasons why we're not able to make exercise an everyday part of our lives. However, it's easy to overcome each of these obstacles and turn movement into a habit, something we pursue regularly and automatically, without a second thought.

Here are the three golden suggestions that have helped us and thousands of Satvic community members:

The First One:

Choose a Movement that Feels Like a Celebration, Not an Obligation

Ask yourself: Why do I want to exercise? To shed calories? To burn off those extra kilos? To compensate for that extra dessert I ate?

If these are your primary motivators, sustaining the habit will be difficult. Why? Because these motivations stem from a place of obligation, not joy.

To truly be able to sustain it, consider changing your perspective to this:

Movement should be a celebration of what your body is capable of, never a punishment for what you ate.

Mark this down, underline it, highlight it.

We need to stop viewing movement as an obligation but rather as a celebration of what this beautiful human body, that we've been given, is capable of.

In each movement session, celebrate the ability to move.

Celebrate the fact that you have legs to run.

Celebrate that you can dance to any tune you want.

Celebrate that you have a body that can swing and twirl.

Celebrate that you have arms that you can lift high up in the sky.

Celebrate that you can crawl, climb, walk, jog, run.

Make each movement session a celebration of your aliveness. Never just a way to burn off calories.

So far in your life, have you been seeing movement as an obligation or a celebration? As something you do just for health? Or also because it brings you joy? Pause, think and write your answer in the space below.

For me, up until my teenage years, I saw movement as something I 'had to' do. Often, I even viewed it as compensation for indulging in my favourite foods from the previous night. At that time, my preferred way of movement was going to the gym and running on the treadmill. But

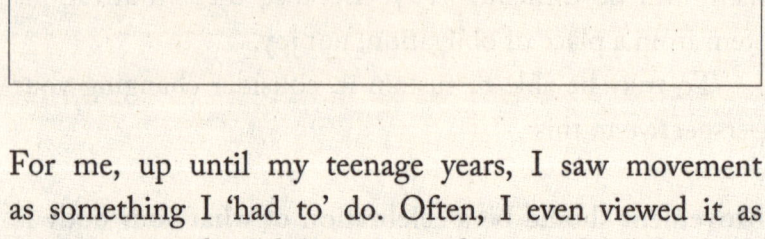

when I turned nineteen, I met my first yoga teacher. I practised with her one day, and for the first time in my life, I thoroughly enjoyed that one hour of movement. I started practising with her more often, and I found myself looking forward to the next session and then the next. I found what I could celebrate as a movement.

For some people, practising yoga asanas might be the kind of movement that sparks joy, while others may find this sense of celebration in jogging, running or playing a particular sport. When you engage in an activity and feel, 'Wow, I **get to** do this', rather than 'I **have to** do this', it's a clear sign that you've found a form of movement that feels like a celebration, not an obligation.

The Second Practical Step to Make Movement a Habit

Don't Break the Chain—Even if You Can't Do It Perfectly, Just Show Up

When it comes to building a habit, **it's more important to be consistent rather than perfect**. In fact, we'd even say, don't try to have a 'perfect workout'. Why? Let us illustrate this with the example of two characters: Mr Perfect and Mr Reps.

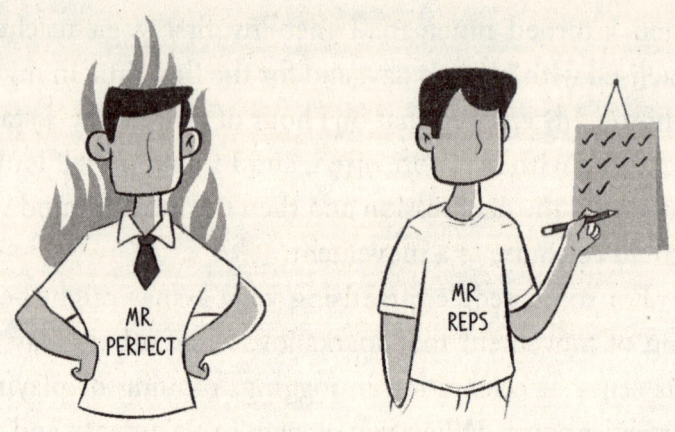

Meet Mr Perfect:

Initially, he's overflowing with enthusiasm and determination. He commits to a perfect hour-long full-body workout every day, aiming to drench his clothes in sweat.

Day 1: He's on fire, completing his hour-long workout and marking it off on his calendar.

Day 2: The momentum continues.

Day 3: The thought creeps in, 'Who would work out for a full hour?' Yet, he pushes through and completes his workout.

Day 4: His energy starts to dip. The thought, 'Ah, it's too strenuous. Let me take just one day off,' convinces him to skip his workout.

Day 5: He thinks, 'Who has the time for a full hour?' Feeling overwhelmed by the thought of his intense workout, he tells himself, 'I'll take another day of rest and catch up later.'

Day 6: Reflecting on the previous few days, he thinks, 'I've already missed two days; might as well start fresh next Monday.' Once again, he skips his workout.

Day 7: He spends the day planning to restart his regimen the following Monday.

Does Mr Perfect's routine feel all too familiar?

Now, Meet Mr Reps:

His full name is 'Mr Repetitions'. His approach is different. He goes by the motto of 'consistency over perfection'. His goal isn't to have the perfect workout but to show up every day, no matter how long or short his session is. No lofty ambitions of soaked shirts, just a commitment to being regular.

Day 1: Brimming with energy, he completes an easy thirty-minute workout and proudly ticks it off on his calendar.

Day 2: The momentum continues.

Day 3: With his energy still steady, he completes another straightforward thirty-minute workout.

Day 4: Just like Mr Perfect, his energy starts to dip on this day. But he recalls his guiding principle: don't break the chain. Choosing a shorter workout of just twenty minutes, he nonetheless shows up, completes it and adds another tick to his calendar.

Day 5: Mr Reps, taking inspiration from his unbroken chain for the last four days, sticks to a thirty-minute session and keeps the momentum going.

Day 6: Reflecting on his week, he thinks, 'I've been showing up daily; now it's time to level up my workout.' He challenges himself with a slightly tougher routine, lasting forty-five minutes. Another day, another tick on his calendar.

Day 7: Proud of his consistent efforts throughout the week, Mr Reps levels up his workout slightly more, marking yet another tick by the day's end.

Mr Reps' approach is quite different from Mr Perfect's approach. Mr Reps doesn't chase perfection. Yet, by showing up every single day, he continuously improves, getting better and better over time. In the long run, Mr Reps can make movement a habit. Mr Perfect cannot.

If we aspire for consistency, we need to be like Mr Reps, not Mr Perfect. All too often, we trap ourselves in an all-or-nothing mindset with our habits. We mistakenly believe that if we can't execute something perfectly, we shouldn't bother doing it at all. As a result, we end up giving up the habit altogether. We don't realize how valuable it is to just show up, even if it's for less duration, with less intensity, on a busy or hectic day. **Once we simply start showing up consistently, perfection automatically follows.**

The Magic Mantra: Don't Break the Chain

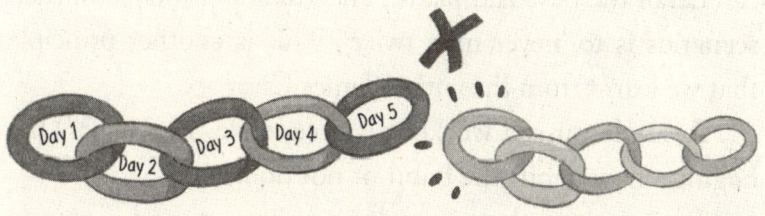

This is the mantra that Mr Reps used to stay consistent. The aim? Maintain your chain.

Life, with its unpredictable nature, will always present reasons to break the chain. Sometimes, you'll have an extremely busy schedule. Other times, you might wake up late or face an unexpected event. It becomes tempting, almost effortless, to break the chain, thinking, 'Does missing just one day really matter? I'll resume tomorrow.' However, those are the crucial moments when showing up matters the most.

You don't realize how valuable it is to just show up on not-so-smooth days. Commit to doing your chosen movement every day, even if it's only for twenty minutes. Don't break the chain.

Once you start showing up daily, you'll gradually perfect the habit. But remember, **the habit needs to be rooted first; only then it can be perfected.**

A Safety Net: Never Miss Twice

Despite our best efforts, there will be times when life interrupts. Emergencies, sickness, travel or family obligations can derail the best-laid plans. The guiding principle in such scenarios is to 'never miss twice'. This is another principle that we learnt from the author James Clear.

A single missed workout is acceptable. But two? That begins a new habit: the habit of not doing it.

Remember to keep the chain unbroken, and if you do miss a day, ensure you never miss two in a row.

> Note: The concepts of 'don't break the chain' and 'never miss twice' are aimed at maintaining consistency in your workout routine. However, it's important to note that there are times when your body genuinely requires rest, and exercising can actually be harmful. This is particularly true in cases such as injury, illness or extreme fatigue.

The Third Practical Step to Make Movement a Habit

Find an Accountability Partner

Having an accountability partner can be a game changer when aiming to maintain consistency in habit four, 'Celebrate Movement'.

Who is an accountability partner?

This is someone who ensures you stay true to your commitments. They could be a workout buddy, a family member joining you in your exercise routine or a professional coach or trainer. Their primary role is to hold you accountable, to be the observer of your actions.

There's a lot of power in knowing someone is watching and expecting you to show up. Such a presence reduces the chances of procrastination. If you falter, it's no longer just about disappointing yourself; now, someone else is involved. They might perceive you as unreliable or lazy. Suddenly, you're not only failing to meet the promises you made to yourself but also the ones you made to someone else. And this in turn helps you to be consistent.

Some might say that relying on an accountability partner creates dependency and that we should be self-sufficient. Well, if you have the willpower to stick to your movement routine independently, without any accountability, that's excellent. But the reality is that for most of us, having an external push is actually very helpful.

This approach works wonders for the two of us. Practising with a teacher or trainer makes a massive difference. We try to find trainers or teachers for whatever form of movement we wish to do. Then, we schedule our sessions in advance. As the scheduled session nears, even if our motivation dips and we think of cancelling, we're bound by our prior commitment. Inevitably, after the session, we're elated that we didn't cancel.

Reflect on this: If you tend to delay or avoid your movement routine, how can you establish an accountability system? Here are a few options:

- **Group Classes:** Try signing up for a group session of your preferred type of movement. Ideally, choose one that is conveniently located near your home. The collective commitment of the group can serve as a powerful motivator, making the entire group your accountability partner.

- **Online Trainers:** Nowadays, you can find trainers for almost any kind of movement you wish to master. Booking sessions in advance commits you to a specific schedule, making it harder to cancel based on temporary moods or excuses.

- **Personal Trainers:** If you have the resources available, why not have a dedicated trainer come to your residence? Guided sessions, even if it's just three times a week, can be transformative.

- **Family or Significant Others:** Consider making a family member or your spouse your accountability partner. But a word of caution: Ensure your chosen accountability partner is as dedicated as you. A partnership where you're the only driving force will not help.

In Summary:

To make your habit of movement shift from a 'sometimes' activity to an 'everyday' ritual, remember these three golden steps:

1. Choose a movement that feels like a celebration, not an obligation.
2. Don't break the chain. Even if you can't do it perfectly, just show up.
3. Find an accountability partner who can keep you on track.

Craft Your Personal Movement Routine

To keep reading this book without applying the learnings is futile. Thus, we encourage you to create and commit to a movement routine at least for the next seven days. In order to do this, contemplate on the following points, and jot down your answers in the space provided:

1. Identify Your Joyful Movement:

Which movement feels celebratory to you? One that you genuinely relish? That your heart is drawn towards? When you do it, time seems to fly. It doesn't come across as a chore but as pure enjoyment.

- It could be practising yoga asanas
- Or a sport, such as tennis, badminton or basketball
- Or brisk walking, jogging or running
- Or even activities like weight training or dancing

Write whichever form of movement resonates with you in the space below. You could even note more than one.

_____

_____

_____

2. Find an Accountability Partner:

Now that you know which movement feels like a celebration to you, it is time to think of who your accountability partner could be. This could be a coach or personal trainer who keeps you committed, or a friend or family member who is already consistent with their routine, or perhaps joining a group class. Write down your ideas for potential accountability partners.

_____

_____

_____

By now, you've successfully learnt the three golden steps to make movement a daily part of your life! Before concluding this chapter, we'd like to explore a topic that still remains unaddressed—**how to maximize the impact of each**

movement session. Are there any adjustments you can make in order to make your exercise routine much more powerful? Let's find out.

How to Get More Out of Each Movement Session

Have you noticed how being in nature—amid oceans, mountains or beaches—brings us a deep sense of peace and serenity? You may have noticed how just being in nature tends to make us feel calmer. This connection stems from a fundamental truth: **We humans are a part of nature and not apart from nature.** What does that mean? Well, more concretely, our bodies are made up of the same five elements that everything in nature is made up of.

Perhaps you're familiar with these five elements already, or perhaps this is a completely new concept. Either way, to truly improve the effectiveness of the movement routine you have just designed, it's important to have a basic understanding of the five elements that your body is made up of.

Almost every ancient culture talks about these elements. From yoga, to Ayurveda, to Indian philosophy, all share that everything in the universe is made up of five great elements:

Earth   Water   Fire   Air   Space

The five elements are also known as the '*pancha mahabhutas*' in Sanskrit ['pancha' means five, and 'mahabhutas' refers to the elements]. They form the basic building blocks of the universe, encompassing every person, animal, plant and object. Each object and body contains a varying degree and combination of the five elements, providing its unique features.

Where, you might think, do these five elements really exist? Let us see.

	Where it exists in nature	Where it exists within our own bodies
Earth Element *Prithvi*	All solid structures in nature are primarily made of the earth element: mountains, trees, soil, rocks, sand, plants, etc.	All solid structures within our body are primarily made of the earth element: bones, flesh, skin, tissues, nails, hair, etc. We absorb the earth element in our body when we eat food that comes from the earth.
Water Element *Jal*	In nature, the water element is found in oceans, rivers, lakes, glaciers, groundwater, moisture in the air, etc.	Within our body, the water element is basically all the fluids: saliva, urine, blood and sweat. We absorb the water element in our body when we drink water, or eat juicy foods rich in water.

	Where it exists in nature	Where it exists within our own bodies
Fire Element *Agni*	In nature, the greatest source of the fire element is the sun. Additionally, flames of fire, volcanic lava and geothermal heat are also composed primarily of the fire element.	In our body, the fire element is what keeps it warm and transforms the food we eat into smaller digestible molecules. Our digestive fire is a manifestation of the fire element.
Air Element *Vaayu*	In nature, the air element is present in the form of wind, breeze and various gases such as oxygen, nitrogen and carbon dioxide.	Within our body, this element governs respiration. It is the life-giving breath that we inhale and exhale, flowing continuously through our lungs.
Space Element *Akasha*	In nature, the space element is the vast expanse of the universe beyond Earth's atmosphere. It is also found in natural voids, such as in the cavities in caves, hollows in a tree and gaps in rocks.	Within our body, the space element is represented by the various empty areas. These include the nasal passages, the hollowness inside our intestines, the space within our blood vessels. Additionally, at a microscopic level, our

	Where it exists in nature	Where it exists within our own bodies
	Interestingly, the other four elements actually reside within the space element.	cells themselves have spaces between them. Among the five elements, this is the subtlest of all, and thus, the hardest to perceive.

Essentially, our bodies are more connected with Mother Nature than we may know. These five elements form the building blocks of everything in the universe, as they do of our own physical bodies.

When studying under the guidance of our teachers, another profound learning that they shared with us was this:

When the five elements are in balance within our body, it results in health.
When the five elements are in imbalance, it leads to disease.

So far in this book, we have discussed the earth element in depth. The entire focus of habit two, 'Eat Living, Wholesome and Plant-Based', was dedicated to understanding and incorporating the highest quality of the earth element into our lives, and as a result, also balancing it within our bodies.

We've also delved into the water element to a certain extent. When we start to eat more fresh living foods, such as fruits and vegetables, which are naturally high in water content, we automatically help balance the water element within our bodies.

We've also learnt one way to balance the space element. By eating an early dinner, as taught in habit one, we automatically undertake a mini-fast every night. Fasting is one of the most powerful ways to create a void, or space, inside our bodies.

Now, the two elements we haven't yet discussed how to incorporate are the **fire and air elements**. But guess what? Your movement routine actually presents a perfect opportunity to obtain these two elements. 'How?' you might ask. Well, by **taking your movement outdoors**.

Instead of exercising in a closed, stuffy space, if you simply shift your movement outdoors, you can reap abundant benefits. You could choose any open space where you have access to fresh air and sunlight. This could be a park near your home, a balcony, a terrace, a veranda or any other open space. When you do so, you gain the triple advantage of:

1. **The exercise itself.**
2. **Exposure to sunlight (fire element):** Sunlight not only provides free vitamin D but also strengthens your bones and acts as an instant mood lifter.
3. **A wealth of oxygen (air element):** This air element improves the functioning of your lungs, increases your energy levels and also enhances brain function.

So as often as you can, **try to shift your movement routine to an open, sunlit space**. This may not always be possible, due to inclement weather or high levels of pollution outside. However, whenever you can, take the opportunity to exercise outdoors.

The second way to substantially increase the intake of the fire and air elements during your movement routine is by **wearing natural fabrics instead of tight, synthetic ones**. You see, our skin is the largest organ in our body. It is covered with thousands of tiny pores throughout its surface. We often think that we only breathe through our nose. But the truth is that we are also constantly breathing through these innumerable pores on our skin.

Now synthetic fabrics such as polyester, nylon, spandex, and rayon might look trendy but they often suffocate and block the flow of air to our skin. Instead, natural fibres like cotton, linen, hemp, bamboo or jute are breathable fabrics. They allow air and sunlight to pass through them.

To summarize:

Here are the two steps to gain the maximum benefit from your movement sessions:

- Exercise outdoors, in the open air.
- Choose natural, breathable fabrics over synthetic ones.

Concluding Thoughts about the Practice

Habit four aims to remind you to celebrate movement once more. As children, we naturally did this. We genuinely found joy in movement—running, climbing trees, playing catch, engaging in sports. Movement actually filled us with happiness. However, as we age, we drift from our inner child and start seeing movement as a duty, as an obligation, as a chore rather than a privilege.

Today, most of us have the ability to jog, to run, to dance, to even climb mountains, and yet, we often remain glued to our chairs. We not only fail to realize the potential that our bodies hold but also miss the countless physical and mental benefits that movement brings to us.

So, we encourage you, dear reader, to re-establish your relationship with movement. Start with any practice you love. Do your best to not break the chain, and whenever possible, take it outdoors, so you can embrace the angels of fire and air. Every cell in your body deserves this. By doing so, you also celebrate your wonderfully functioning body, one of the most invaluable gifts that nature has given us.

With that, not only do you conclude this chapter, but you also complete the fourth of the seven life-changing habits in this book. In the upcoming habit, we'll delve into another fascinating aspect of our health: our relationships with others. Prepare yourself for an exhilarating story of a woman named Amy, life lessons from a running air conditioner and wisdom from Buddha's burning coal.

Habit 5

Nourish Relationships

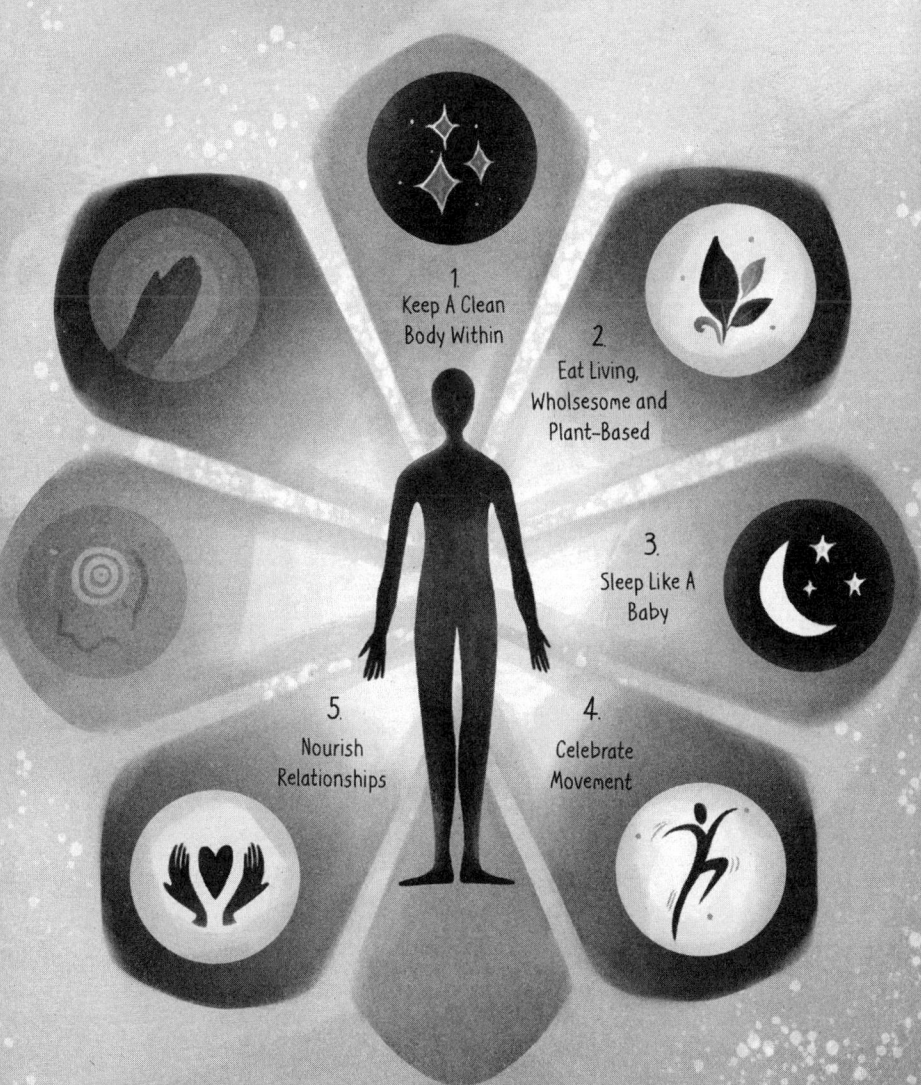

1.
Keep A Clean
Body Within

2.
Eat Living,
Wholsesome and
Plant-Based

3.
Sleep Like A
Baby

4.
Celebrate
Movement

5.
Nourish
Relationships

10

Switch Off That
Running AC inside You

I want to start this chapter with an eye-opening incident I had during my visit to a health institute in the United States. Early in my journey, having been guided by many experts and masters in India and having read extensively about health, I truly believed I understood the subject in depth. However, upon setting foot in the institute, it was as if a divine voice whispered, 'Subah, there's still so much more to uncover.' Consequently, my time there fundamentally shifted my understanding of health.

Located in Florida, this institute is a place where people from around the world come to learn how to heal their health problems naturally. When I went there, this institute had been in operation for the last sixty years. People suffering from various health challenges would come, and a team of doctors and healers helped these people heal themselves using food, lifestyle and various therapies. No, it wasn't a boring place. In fact, what I loved the most about this institute was that it made healing fun!

However, the food regime followed there was intense. For lunch and dinner, we were served sprouts. Lots of sprouts—broccoli sprouts, sunflower sprouts, alfalfa sprouts, fenugreek sprouts, and many others. It was a buffet of sprouts. Apart from that, there were also some salads and side dishes. Overall, the food was extremely nutritious. They even served green juice and wheatgrass juice, which was an essential part of their daily routine. They had great facilities, qualified natural health doctors, and a vibrant energy throughout the institute.

During my first nine-week stay there, there was one experience that left a lasting impression on me. A woman (who I'll refer to as Amy in this chapter, to respect her privacy) came in. She had been diagnosed with breast cancer. After she arrived, she quickly adapted to the programme, adopting every recommended practice from the institute. She switched to a wholesome, plant-based diet and diligently followed an array of healing techniques, including regular yoga classes, a tailored exercise routine, special green juices and mindful meditation sessions, among various other therapies.

A few weeks later, Amy underwent a series of medical tests and scans to evaluate how she was doing. The results were astonishing: there was no improvement in her condition. This was baffling to everyone. Here she was, in what was considered a sanctuary of health and healing, meticulously following all the prescribed advice, yet her health showed absolutely no signs of improvement. As days passed, Amy began losing hope.

When I heard her story, I became curious: Why hadn't Amy seen any changes despite her efforts? The question lingered in my mind, seeking an answer.

That answer began to unfold when I learnt about a unique session conducted by the institute every Thursday, called a 'healing circle'. In it, around twenty-five participants sat in a circle, led by a trained psychotherapist. I was fortunate to have witnessed two healing circles in my time there, and quite honestly, they were intense! In one of them, I had Amy in my group. During the healing circle, the psychotherapist would invite people, one by one, to share any emotional issues or pain they were holding on to. It wasn't easy; sharing deep-seated pain in front of an unfamiliar crowd is scary. Initially, most people were silent, hesitant to open up.

A few minutes later, the therapist invited Amy to voice how she was doing. She began by saying that she was doing okay, with nothing disturbing her emotionally. But as the therapist made her feel more and more comfortable, after a while, Amy started opening up.

Soon, she spoke of a traumatic event from her past. She shared an experience from her youth when she was physically abused by a member of her family. As she was speaking, tears began rolling down her face. She was talking about this episode after keeping it buried inside her for twenty years. Her voice was trembling as she recalled the specific details of the event: the identity of the person, the exact location where it occurred, and how it left her feeling. This was a pain she hadn't shared with anyone for over two decades before this healing circle, but with every word, it seemed that layers of suppressed pain were being peeled away. Later, the therapist explained how this unresolved pain, it seemed, was a significant weight that was coming in the way of her healing.

A few weeks after this healing circle, coupled with several sessions with the psychotherapist, a remarkable change occurred in Amy's health. It started showing signs of significant improvement. And a few months later, her cancer began to heal! Everyone at the institute was surprised and taken aback.

This experience was an eye-opener for me, because until then, I believed that health was all about eating the right food, cleansing from the inside, sleep, rest and exercise. But Amy's transformation led to a powerful realization: **Many of us can't reach our peak health because we're burdened with unresolved emotional baggage.** This is years-old baggage that still today, may be weighing us down without us even knowing about it.

Does this mean that the nutritious food, the juices, the exercise didn't benefit Amy? No, not at all. Those practices helped greatly in releasing physical toxins from her body. But that wasn't enough, because ultimately, she was also carrying emotional toxins that were not allowing her to heal.

Now this is true not only for Amy. Just like her, many of us also carry these emotional toxins within us. According to a WHO study conducted in twenty-four countries, 70 per cent of people reported experiencing one or the other kind of emotional trauma in their lives.

Unless these emotional toxins are also cleared out, we can't reach the full potential of our human existence—it's like something will always be weighing us down.

Just like for good physical health, we have to remove the physical toxins, and simultaneously nourish our bodies with the right food, in much the same way, for excellent emotional and mental health, we have to remove the emotional burdens that we carry, and simultaneously nourish our hearts with positive emotions. This habit is here to help you with both of these goals.

Welcome to Habit Five—Nourish Relationships

Through this habit, you will learn how to make the most of the greatest, most beautiful part of your human existence: your relationships with others. Over the course of two chapters, we will delve into this habit in depth. In this chapter, our focus will be on helping you identify if there are any unresolved relationships weighing you down emotionally, and then guiding you through effective methods to release them. In the next chapter, we will shift our focus to learning one of the most powerful human values to nourish and strengthen your existing relationships with others.

Here's a more detailed glimpse of what you'll learn in this chapter:

- What's the connection between your emotions and health?
- What are those relationships in your life that may be unknowingly depleting your praanshakti?
- A short exercise to identify if you do have any such relationships in your life.
- How to let go of such relationships to experience lightness, both in the body and mind.

This chapter is going to be quite different from the ones you've read so far. You'll be engaging in some inner work, and if there are distractions around you, you might not be able to enter the right mind space. Therefore, we request that you read this chapter in a quiet environment, free from any disturbances or distractions.

With our foundation set, come, let's begin.

Why Discuss Relationships in a Health Book?

Often, when we host face-to-face seminars for our community and delve into this topic, people question, 'Why are you talking about relationships in a health seminar?'

The assumption behind such a question is simple: health is just about the body. But as you might know by now, health is more than just physical. It also encompasses our emotions, mind and spirit.

Moreover, our emotions directly influence our bodily functions. **Our emotions actually have the power to change the biology of our body**. Let's understand this through an example.

Picture yourself seated at a dining table. You didn't eat much all day. Now you're quite hungry. Your stomach is grumbling, and you're prepared to enjoy your dinner. Just as you're about to start, your phone buzzes. You receive news that a loved one has been in an accident.

What happens to that intense hunger? Will it still persist? Most likely not—in fact, you'll lose your appetite. Even if others at home suggest that you take your meal, you'll probably respond by saying that you're no longer hungry.

What changed? An emotion you felt (sadness) created an impact on your body. It literally altered something in your body (because your praanshakti, your vital energy, shifted from preparing for digestion to dealing with the mental stress).

Here's another example. Imagine an auditorium with over 100 people seated in it. You're standing behind the stage, and you're afraid of public speaking. Your turn has just come to step on to the stage and address the audience. What's the first thing that will happen to you? Your heart rate will increase. What next? As you become nervous, even your palms will begin to sweat.

This isn't some random occurrence. It's a direct reflection of how the emotions that you feel in your heart, in this case, anxiety and fear, actually change the biology of your physical body. Sure, stage fright is temporary. It comes, we do what's needed and we move on. But even in its brief appearance, it alters your physical state.

The *Proceedings of the National Academy of Science* performed a fascinating study that demonstrated how impactful our emotional state can be on our immune system (which is a reflection of our physical state). In this study, researchers divided people into two groups. One group was asked to think about an extremely positive incident that had happened in their lives—an experience when they felt intense happiness or joy, specifically the best time or experience of their life. Participants in the other group were asked to think about an extremely negative incident— an event during which they experienced the most intense sadness, fear or anger. Then, participants in both groups were asked to focus on the emotion experienced, and then write about that event for five minutes. After that, each group was given a flu vaccination. In other words, a virus was inserted into their bodies through a vaccine. Then, researchers measured how many antibodies their bodies produced against the virus (antibodies are basically proteins produced in the blood that fight diseases by attacking and killing harmful bacteria or viruses).

What the researchers found was astounding! The group that were in a negative emotional state during the experiment had a significantly poorer immune response— their bodies produced fewer antibodies to protect them against the external disease-causing virus. This was not just a momentary effect; even six months post-vaccination, their immune functioning was impaired. The study shows how greatly our emotional state influences our immunity to illness, as well as our overall physical state.

If merely recalling a negative experience from the past can cause a dip in our health, imagine the impact of emotions that stay with us—like pent-up anger, chronic anxiety, suppressed grief or bottled-up guilt. These emotions can build up and persist not just for a couple of hours, but possibly for days, months or even years, without us even knowing it, causing alterations in our physical bodies.

Now, what do you think is one of the biggest contributors to this suppressed anger, fear, guilt and grief that we often carry?

Well, it is often an **unresolved relationship**.

What does this even mean? Come, let's learn.

What Is an Unresolved Relationship?

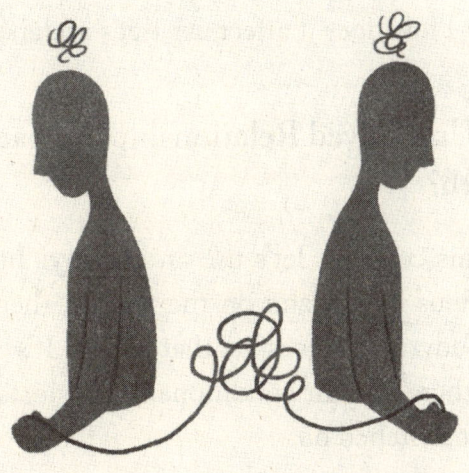

An unresolved relationship is one that ended on a bitter note, with negative feelings in either one or both of the people involved. Instead of understanding and reconciliation, this is a relationship that ends with lingering misunderstandings or conflicts.

The reasons for this unresolved state could come from either side: you might have hurt them or they might have knowingly or unknowingly hurt you, leading to bitterness in the relationship.

An unresolved relationship could be just a few months old, or it could be three years old, or it could even be twenty years old. Alternatively, it might be an ongoing relationship where you regularly interact or communicate with the other person, yet internally, you harbour negative feelings towards them. It could be with anyone—a friend, a family member, a distant relative, a teacher. It could even be with your own parent, your spouse or your child.

But why does it matter if some relationships remain unresolved? How does it affect us? Let's understand.

How Do Unresolved Relationships Impact Our Health?

To grasp this concept, let's use an analogy. Imagine you own a spacious house, and on the terrace, there's a small room. Nobody really goes to that room. It's rarely ever used. But, there's an air conditioner (AC) installed there, which is left switched on.

Now, even if you've forgotten about that room and its AC, will it continue to run and consume electricity? Of course it will. You'll still have to pay the electricity bill for that AC every month.

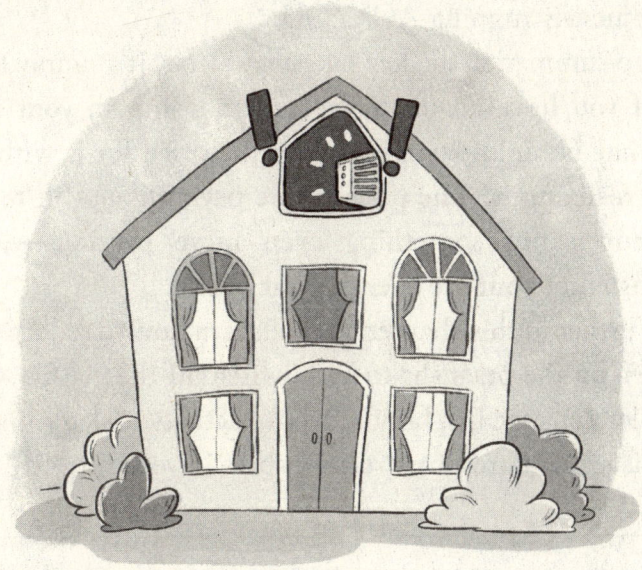

Just as a running AC continues to consume and drain the electricity of the house, similarly, when you have an unresolved relationship with someone, it continues to consume and drain your energy, your praanshakti.

If it's a past relationship, you may feel that you've entirely forgotten about it by now, that you don't even think about that person any more. But, if it was strained when it ended, then for the past two, three or however many years, your praanshakti is still being spent and wasted in that unresolved relationship. In other words, the AC of that relationship is continuously running in the background, day after day, without you even knowing it.

And guess who's responsible for settling the bill of that continuously running AC? YOU.

To summarize the key takeaway so far, it's simply this:

If you have an unresolved relationship in your life, you may be unknowingly paying the price for it without even realizing it. The price you're paying is not in terms of money but something even more precious—your praanshakti, your life energy, your health.

Further in this chapter, we will learn how to reduce this burden on the praanshakti and 'switch off these ACs'. But first, let's engage in a brief reflective activity to determine if you have any unresolved relationships in your life.

A Reflective Activity

As you read each of the questions below, take a few seconds to reflect, and then proceed to the next one.

- Do you recall any relationship in your life that was once amicable, but due to certain events, you stopped communicating with that person?
- Is there someone in your life who you believe wronged you? Whether it's a friend, a brother, a sister, an in-law

or anyone else. Thoughts like 'Why did they do that to me?' or 'What they did was unfair' come when you think about them.

- Is there someone who you feel you treated unfairly? Someone you believe you caused hurt to through your words or actions?

Even thinking about these individuals can be uncomfortable, because it impels you to come face to face with emotions that may have been suppressed somewhere deep within. However, try to recall the names. Once they start coming to mind, note them down. Use an empty piece of paper or a notes app on your phone to list them.

Please make this list with honesty. Don't worry, it will never be shown to anyone else. It's a private list that only you will see.

Begin with your family and extend to friends and distant relatives. Don't be surprised if you find seven to eight people, or even more. Once you've written your list of names, proceed with the reading.

A Note about the Reflective Activity

Through the reflective activity, there's a chance that you might not have recalled any names. You might have thought, 'But my relationships are all fine. I don't have strained relationships; I'm a friendly, affectionate person.' However, if no names surfaced in your mind, it's worth taking a deeper look. The majority of us have unresolved relationships in our lives.

When I first tried to do this reflective activity, like many, I couldn't initially think of any names. But as I spent some more time reflecting, I began to remember instances and relationships that I hadn't thought about for years. I realized that although I didn't face big issues like Amy, there were definitely relationships in my past that concluded on a sour note. So if you haven't identified any names yet, our suggestion would be to think a little deeper.

The Cost of Holding on to Unresolved Relationships

During the reflective activity, you may have thought about certain people who you believe did something wrong to you, who you find yourself carrying feelings of anger, bitterness or resentment towards.

But while we carry these suppressed emotions within us, there is something we often forget, and that is that while we may have carried that incident within us for **ten years,** the other person might not have held it even for **ten seconds.** They may have wronged us or even verbally abused us. But do we realize that by not letting go of it, we have been abusing ourselves for so long? They did something *that day* that caused us pain, but by holding on to it, we've allowed that pain to continue to affect us and drain our vital energy, for months or even years.

This realization can be summarized beautifully by the wisdom shared by Lord Buddha:

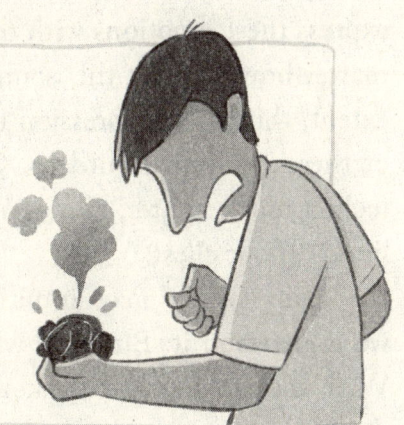

'Holding on to anger is like grasping a hot coal with the intent of throwing it at someone else; you are the one who gets burned.'

~ Lord Buddha

In many cases of unresolved relationships, we might hold on to anger or resentment, thinking it will teach the other person a lesson. However, we often forget that this resentment, much like holding a hot stone, ends up burning our own selves as we cling to it.

Now, the natural question may arise: How do we let go of these burning coals? How do we release these suppressed emotions? Let's proceed and learn.

Releasing Unresolved Relationships: A Path to Inner Peace

When we closely look at unresolved relationships, there is a common theme that emerges: In most cases, we are left with **unexpressed emotions and thoughts** within ourselves. However, when we take the courageous step to **share and express these emotions with the other person** involved (no matter how difficult this sounds), we find that, to a great extent, this act of expression naturally enables us to let go of these emotional burdens. Consequently, this leaves us feeling much lighter, almost as if a heavy weight has been lifted off our chest.

Many of us may intuitively know this. Logically, we understand it. But then why are we not able to do it? Well, the moment we think about expressing our feelings, the immediate thought that arises is, 'What will the other person think?' or 'Will he or she think I'm crazy?' or 'What if he/she reacts in a way that makes things even worse?' And then it seems easier to just keep those feelings stored in some corner within us and continue with life, not realizing that those suppressed emotions are always affecting us internally.

In the next section, you will learn an effective method for expressing these emotions in an easy and compassionate way, which helps you 'switch off that running AC'. But before we delve into this method of expression, I'd like to share a personal experience that had a profound impact on my life.

Over the past seven years, once every few months, I would wake up feeling slightly unsettled due to a recurring dream. This dream was about an old friend from my school days. We were good friends in school; however, circumstances led to them suddenly moving to another city. The transition was abrupt, and shortly after the move, they stopped communicating with me.

The sudden end of the relationship deeply hurt me, but I kept it inside and never discussed it with anyone. Over the next seven years, every two to three months, I would have a dream about this friend. The dreams varied, but a common theme was always there: I wanted to communicate with them, yet they were unwilling to talk. I never even thought about them during my waking hours. I felt so confused as to why I was dreaming about them, even though we hadn't spoken for seven years.

One morning, when I woke up from another such dream, Harshvardhan sensed that something was bothering me. When I shared my experience with him, he suggested I call the friend up. I told him that what he was suggesting was ridiculous and impossible. I didn't have the courage to do so. It had been over seven years since I had last spoken to that friend. I couldn't even think about calling. I tried convincing Harshvardhan that it was okay and that the situation would just resolve itself, without my intervention.

But he patiently explained to me that even though I believed all was well, a thought or memory of this person remained trapped in my subconscious. Soon after, he suggested that I not only call this friend up, but also ask them to meet me in person. I thought it was an absolutely terrible idea. I thought it was impossible, but then, I remembered the analogy of the running ACs. I didn't want an internal air conditioner continuously running in me. And more importantly, I didn't want to not practise the concepts that we taught others.

Thus, I finally gathered the courage and called this old friend one morning. We talked, and surprisingly, it went well. He was in good spirits, and I suggested we meet.

Eventually, Harshvardhan and I travelled to Mumbai to meet this individual. Throughout the journey, I felt as though I were navigating through a dense fog of anxiety. The closer we got, the faster my heart started beating, and the tighter my hands clasped each other, as if trying to squeeze out that nervous energy that buzzed through my veins.

Finally, I met my friend for dinner at a Mediterranean restaurant, and the meeting was quite pleasant. We laughed about our school days, and I shared my desire not to leave our relationship unresolved.

Following that meeting, we did not become best friends or resume regular communication. That was never the intention. However, the weight I carried for years was lifted. Post this meeting, the dreams stopped coming. This was quite unexpected for me. Essentially, I felt that the AC that had been running for several years within me was finally turned off after our communication.

I always knew about the power of addressing unresolved relationships but it took me years to truly practise it. For so long, I could not muster the courage to act upon it. It was many years after learning about this concept that I finally took the step, and today, I am so happy that I did. Through this process, I realized that when you release unresolved relationships, even with just one person, you start to experience a significant lightness and joy in your being.

Now, you don't need to experience dreams about a person to know that your relationship was left unresolved with them. That was just my personal experience. If a past or current relationship in your life matches any of the criteria mentioned in the reflective activity earlier in this chapter, it indicates that you may be carrying emotional baggage.

Now that you have a basic understanding of this topic, let's move forward with a practical activity designed to help you let go of these unresolved relationships.

A Guided Letter-Writing Activity for Emotional Release

There are two practical, yet powerful methods to do this:

1. Writing a letter to the other person.
2. Writing a text message to them.

As you read this, your mind might be protesting, saying, 'Absolutely not. I'm not doing that! Sending a message is absurd.' The very thought of reaching out might stir a whirlpool of emotions, from anxiety and uncertainty to a sense of vulnerability and fear of the unknown, making it seem like an insurmountable task. Remember, it's normal to feel this way, and it's a brave step to even consider releasing an unresolved relationship. Please stay with us as we guide you through the three-step process of composing your message—what to write, how to write it and what to expect in response—to make the process less stressful and as easy as possible.

Step 1:
Choose the Person to Write To

Begin this activity by thoughtfully reviewing your list of unresolved relationships. The key here is to select one individual with whom you feel prepared to 'turn off the internal AC'. Choose someone to whom the prospect of writing feels manageable and not overwhelmingly distressing.

A Word of Caution

It's important to distinguish between relationships that ended bitterly and those that are deeply traumatic.

If there is someone on your list with whom the relationship was seriously traumatic, or who evokes intense hatred, please do not write to them. **Such relationships require the personalized guidance of a qualified professional, which is beyond the scope of what this book can offer.**

Take a moment now to identify the person you wish to write a letter/message to, keeping the foregoing caution in mind. Once you have made your selection, you may continue reading.

Step 2:
Understand the Dos and Don'ts of the Letter-Writing Process

What TO WRITE in Your Message:

1. **Acknowledge that things didn't end well**
   Acknowledge that the relationship did not conclude on a positive note. Alternatively, if you're writing to someone with whom you have an ongoing unresolved relationship, you could acknowledge that there is tension in the relationship.

   You could express, for instance, 'I understand that our relationship ended after a disagreement', or 'We had a misunderstanding that has affected our relationship'.

2. **Express how it makes you feel today**
   Express your present emotions about the situation. Focus on how you feel today, not on how you felt back then. For example, you might say, 'No matter how difficult our relationship was, today I feel grateful for

the memories we shared', or 'I feel that hurt is still left in my heart'.

3. **If you believe you made a mistake in that situation, ask for forgiveness**
    You could say, 'I sincerely apologize that my actions caused you sadness. I'm deeply sorry.'
    However, if you feel that the other person was at fault, then release the hurt. You could say, 'I want to let go of the hurt that I have been carrying.'

4. **Clearly state your intention behind writing to them**
    You could say, 'I'm writing to you because I know that somewhere this bitterness is affecting me, and I want to clear it out so we can both have peace in our hearts.'
    Remember, the intention of writing may not always be to start talking to them again or becoming friends. The intention is simply to let go **of the knots in your own heart.**

Sample Letters

(For a situation where you want to ask forgiveness)

Dear Rahul,

It has been over three years since we have spoken to each other. We used to be so close but, unfortunately, our relationship ended after certain misunderstandings led to a fight.

> Acknowledging things didn't end well ✓

Even though it's been three years, I still feel sadness in my heart when I look back at what happened.

> Expressing how it makes you feel today ✓

I know I didn't stand by my commitments and made mistakes. I sincerely apologise that my actions caused you sadness, Rahul. I just want to say. I am deeply sorry for what I did.

> Asking for forgiveness ✓

I am writing to you because I still carry this bitterness within me and I want to clear it, so we both can have peace in our hearts.

> Clearly stating the intention behind writing ✓

I hope you can understand my emotions. I genuinely wish the best for you.

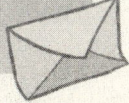

(For a situation where you want to release the hurt)

Dear Priyanka,

I hope you're doing well. I was reflecting if I have any strained relationships in my life and your name came to my heart.

I am aware that our relationship didn't end on the best terms. We shared a close bond, but due to whatever reasons, things fell apart between us, leaving a trail of bitterness.

Acknowledging things didn't end well ✓

We may not even speak to each other anymore, but the hurt from the past still lingers in my heart.

Expressing how it makes you feel today ✓

But today, I want to let go of whatever hurt, frustration or anger that I have been carrying towards our relationship. I have realized that holding onto these feelings serves neither of us.

Releasing the hurt ✓

The reason I'm writing to you is not to reopen old wounds, but simply to release what I have inside me. This is a step towards my own healing and peace.

Clearly stating the intention behind writing ✓

I wish you all the best in your journey and hope only the best for you!

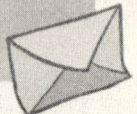

While these samples may be helpful, please remember, the essence of writing this letter lies in its sincerity and authenticity. It's a personal letter, not a formal document. The most important thing is to write from your heart. Don't worry too much about perfect grammar or textual errors; what matters more is the genuineness of your words.

What NOT TO WRITE in Your Message:

✗ Do not portray yourself as right, and them as wrong

When composing your message, aim to express your feelings without placing blame or labelling the other person's actions as bad or wrong. Avoid using phrases like 'Even though what you did was bad . . .' or 'You could have handled it better', as these imply blame. While it's true that the other person may have wronged you or genuinely made mistakes, it is important not to accuse or criticize them in the letter.

✗ Avoid justifications or demands for justifications

The intention of writing this message or letter is not to dig up old baggage or discuss the details of the damage. Not at all. So, do not write sentences like 'Explain why you're angry with me' or 'Please tell me what I did wrong'. Do not justify your actions or ask for justification for theirs.

While writing your message, be mindful of the dos and don'ts shared above. The purpose of writing this letter isn't to change the other person's perspective. It's only to let go of the burning coal in your hand, to turn off the AC that's been draining your vital energy. If you end up even indirectly blaming them or making them seem wrong, it might be best not to write the letter at all. That could make things more bitter, which we don't want.

So, don't write this letter unless you can write it with compassion in your heart. If you believe that writing the letter might cause more harm than good, or if you don't feel prepared to do it yet, that's perfectly okay. Hold off until you're comfortable and ready.

For some of you, you may even prefer to directly call the person instead of writing to them. That's a great idea too. In that case, instead of proceeding to step three, you can directly call them. Just keep in mind the same principles while having that conversation.

Step 3:
Finally, Write Your Letter

Now that you've familiarized yourself with the dos and don'ts of the letter-writing process, it's time to put pen to paper or fingers to keyboard. To guide you through this process, we've prepared a follow-along video that is designed to help you get into the right frame of mind, take you through the writing process, and even offer direction on what to do with the letter once it's complete.

Once you're prepared, simply scan the QR code or visit satvicmovement.org/book/letter to start the guided video.

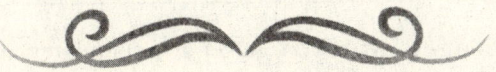

If you've completed the letter-writing activity, congratulations! This may not have been easy, but you've made it through, and that's truly commendable. For those who couldn't complete the activity but plan to do it later, we strongly encourage you to find some time and complete it today.

Frequently Asked Questions

I just can't gather the courage to send this letter. I don't think it's a good idea. Can I simply write it and not send it?

As shared earlier, unresolved relationships fall into two categories: some which ended unpleasantly and you're simply holding bitterness, and others which are deeply traumatic ones. It's difficult for us to guide you through this book as to which category your unresolved relationship falls into. You have to use your own judgement to decide.

However, we sincerely urge you that if your unresolved relationship is from the first category, where the situation was unpleasant but didn't leave you in deep trauma, then please go ahead, write and send the letter, because that's when the most healing takes place.

If, for any reason, sending it feels absolutely uncomfortable and there's no way you can do it, the next best option is to write your letter and then later, tear it up, burn it or bury it as a symbolic act of release.

On the other hand, if you feel that your unresolved relationship falls into the second category, characterized by traumatic experiences such as abuse (especially of a sexual nature), abandonment (such as a parent leaving without contact), or being victims of war, crime or other deep-rooted traumas, then we sincerely advise **not** to reach out to that person. In such cases, it's not as simple as writing a letter, and the guidance of a psychotherapist or mental health professional will be needed.

What if the person I've written to is no longer in this world? Or there is absolutely no way to contact or reach them?

In situations where the person you wish to communicate with has passed away or there is absolutely no means of contacting them, you can still benefit from the therapeutic process of writing the letter. After writing it, consider burning, burying or tearing up the letter as a way to release your emotions and find closure.

What if the other person doesn't reply? Or replies negatively?

If you chose to send the letter or message to the person, remember that any of these three things can happen:

- They might respond positively.
- They might not respond at all.
- They might respond negatively.

If they respond positively, you can simply say, 'Thank you for your understanding', or, 'I'm happy to hear that we've cleared our hearts'.

If they don't respond at all, it's okay. You don't need to take any specific action. Remember, your intention is not to get a specific response from them. Once you've communicated from your side, that AC has been automatically turned off. Whether they reply or not, it doesn't matter. By simply doing your bit—writing to them—you have fulfilled your responsibility. You have done your duty. You can't take responsibility for the outcome. That is in the hands of the Divine.

If they respond negatively, then you have to handle the situation carefully. While it may be tempting to counter their points and prove yourself right, doing so can increase the conflict, which will go against what we are trying to achieve here. Instead, the first step to regain control of the situation is to clarify that your intention was not to hurt them or stir up negativity, but rather to bring peace. If you feel like it, you could even apologize for the fact that your message triggered negative emotions within them.

Chances are that the person you're writing to will most likely understand your intent behind writing to them.

Concluding Thoughts about This Practice

With that, you've reached the end of one of the most challenging chapters in this book. Congratulations! Our hope is that it has encouraged you to let go of at least one coal from your hand, and turn of at least one running AC in your life, so ultimately, you can lead a life that's more free, joyful and compassionate.

In the upcoming chapter, we will move on to the second pillar of habit five, 'Nourish Relationships'. You will learn about the most precious gift you could ever give anyone—a gift that holds the power to heal wounds, uplift people's spirits and deepen connections like nothing else can. As we go through the pages, you'll encounter a crazy optician, interesting roleplays between a girl named Bulbul and her mother and even timeless wisdom from none other than Lord Krishna himself. So, what exactly is this gift? There's only one way to find out, flip the page and continue the journey.

11

The Most Precious Gift You Can Ever Give Anyone

Here's a question for you: When you were growing up, which of these did you receive training in?

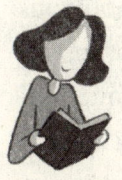 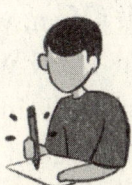 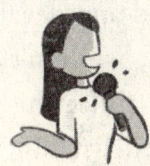 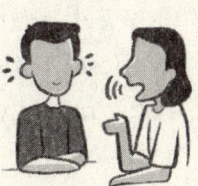

Reading   Writing   Speaking   Listening

Take a moment to pause and reflect on the above question before reading on.

Well, for most of us, our schools spent years teaching us how to read and write. They also helped us hone our speaking skills. But what about listening? Did you ever receive training in learning how to listen? How not to just hear the other person but actually listen?

The reality is that for most of us, the answer is no. The skill of listening is never *really* taught to us growing up.

So instead, what do we tend to do in our conversations? We don't genuinely listen to people. Remember those times when someone is sharing an important story about their day and you just can't wait to check the notifications popping up on your phone? You nod at what they're saying, but deep down, you're not absorbing a word they're sharing! Or consider those times when a loved one opens up about a sensitive topic and instead of truly listening, all you find yourself doing is thinking about what to say next.

When we don't truly listen to people, as a natural consequence, we end up interrupting them, giving unsolicited advice or passing judgement without understanding them. We end up making them feel unheard, unattended and devalued. Often, we're oblivious to these tendencies; we don't even know we're doing it. Yet, gradually over time, this seemingly inconsequential habit of half-hearted listening can weaken many of our relationships.

You may have even, knowingly or unknowingly, experienced the effect of this. Think about it.

Do you find yourself in frequent conflicts or disagreements in any of your interactions? It could be with anyone: your partner, parent, child, sister, brother or colleague.

Do your conversations ever end on a bitter note, where it ruins either your or their mood for the rest of the day?

Do you find yourself in situations with others where you get into pointless fights over the silliest and smallest of things?

Harshvardhan and I have been there and have experienced it all. However, there's one practice that has transformed our relationships with our families, friends and team members. It has prevented many fights, dissolved disagreements, and enriched almost every interaction in our lives. The practice we're referring to is **deep listening**.

Sounds a little unbelievable, right? How can something so simple do so much? We were surprised as well at how powerful it is. And therefore, in this chapter, we want to share this practice with you, so you too can use it to elevate every relationship in your life, and consequently, your emotional and mental health.

Here's how you can expect this chapter to unfold:

- First, you'll learn what happens when you don't fully listen to people during conversations.
- Then we'll do a quick reflective activity to understand how good of a listener you really are.
- Next, you'll learn a golden rule to actually practise deep listening in your relationships.
- Last, we'll cover some commonly asked questions about this practice.

What is about to come is not a superficial quick-fix technique, but a practice that works on the very roots of our relationships. It takes time and it needs conscious effort. But ultimately, if you master it, you can prevent so much stress and conflict in your life. You can save so much time and energy that might otherwise be lost to unnecessary relationship strains. And most importantly, you can deepen your connections with the people you love in leaps and bounds, and in turn, enjoy a more blissful and healthier life.

With our foundation set, let us move to our first topic.

How Shallow Listening Affects Our Relationships

To understand this, let's look at a conversation between two people: Bulbul and her mum.

Scene: Bulbul, a seventeen-year-old girl, has just come home from school looking visibly upset. Sensing something is amiss, her mother tries to understand the cause of her daughter's worry.

Mother: *(noticing Bulbul's expression as she enters)* You seem upset, Bulbul . . . What happened?

Bulbul: *(mumbling, avoiding eye contact)* Nothing, Mum . . . Just, uh, leave me alone, please.

Mother: *(steps closer)* What's wrong, my dear? You can share anything with me. I'm your mum. I'm here for you.

Bulbul: I . . . I don't think you'd understand.

Mother: Who loves you the most in this world? Your mum, right? Come on, tell me . . . what's bothering you, my dear?

Bulbul: Can I . . . can I just tell you the truth?

Mother: Of course, my dear, tell me.

Bulbul: *(confiding)* I . . . I just hate school, Mum. I'm just so tired of it.

Mother: What's wrong, beta? Is something troubling you?

Bulbul: *(frustrated, raising her voice slightly)* It's just . . . school doesn't make any sense to me. It's not helping me in any way.

Mother: You know, at your age, beta, many students feel the same. I didn't like school either. But now, my child, I understand how important education is for every stage of life.

Bulbul: I've already dedicated so many years to it! How has it helped me, really? This calculus and algebra I'm learning—how will it ever help me in the real world, Mum?

Mother: *(pointing towards a family photo)* Bulbul beta, look at your sister. You have a role model at home. She has studied hard, worked hard, and look at her now! She is doing so well.

Bulbul: *(assertive)* But I don't want to be like my sister, Mum! I just . . . I just don't like school!

Mother: *(raising her voice)* Do you hear what you're saying, beta? Do you know how many sacrifices your dad and I have made for you? Just so you could go to school? And now you're saying you don't want to go?

Bulbul looks away, disappointed, giving up.

Mother: *(gently)* My child, my sweetheart, you're an incredibly intelligent girl. I've seen it. You're so sharp. Don't let these thoughts hold you back. Focus on your studies. Try to find enjoyment in it. I'm confident you'll do well, my dear.

Bulbul simply nods, her feelings bottled up inside, realizing her mother will never understand.

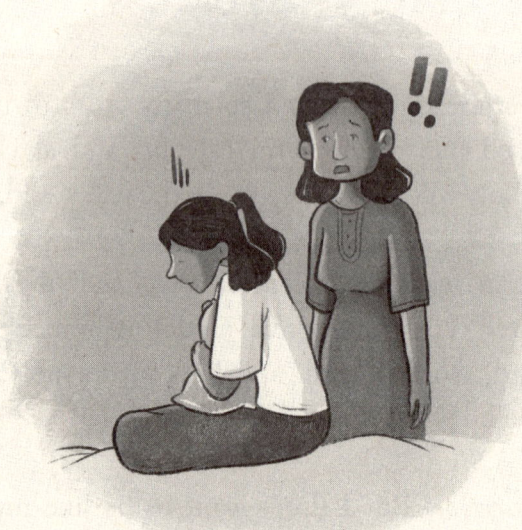

Decoding the Conversation: Who Was Right?

Having gone through the conversation between Bulbul and her mother, do you think that the mother's intentions were wrong? No, certainly not. She loved her daughter and wanted the best for her. Therefore, from her perspective, she was offering the best advice possible. She was doing what any caring parent would do—trying to guide her child through a difficult time.

Yet, by doing this, how did Bulbul feel? Despite the mother's well-intentioned words, Bulbul still felt isolated and unheard, so she closed off. By the end, she went further into her shell. To Bulbul, it seemed like her feelings were being overlooked. She felt that nobody understood her. And the more her mother tried to explain, the more Bulbul felt her own voice being drowned out.

So, where might the mother have gone wrong? Well, in her eagerness to help, there were three mistakes she ended up making in her conversation with Bulbul.

1. **She was quick to give advice.**
   The mother quickly offered advice like 'education is important' and 'focus on your studies'. This advice, undeniably, came from a place of love and concern. It was in her daughter's best interest. But, let's pause and consider: Did Bulbul truly want advice when she shared her school struggles with her mother? No. **Bulbul simply wanted to be heard.** She simply wanted her mother to understand what she was going through.

She wanted her mother to empathize with her stress, her pressure.

So even though the mother's intentions were pure, advice is not what Bulbul was seeking at that moment, which made her feel further closed off. Basically, Bulbul's mother was in a *fixing* mode, when her daughter needed a *hearing* mode.

2. **She started comparing.**
The mother began to compare Bulbul's situation to her sister's achievements, saying, 'Look at your sister. You have a role model at home.' Moreover, she also compared Bulbul's feelings to her own past, saying, 'You know, at your age, beta, many students feel the same. I didn't like school either.'

From the mother's perspective, these comparisons were coming from an eagerness to help Bulbul, by giving her perspective, by showing that others have gone through similar experiences.

However, let's delve a bit deeper: How might these comparisons have affected Bulbul? They took the focus away from Bulbul's feelings, which could have made her feel that her emotions aren't valid, that she shouldn't feel what she's feeling.

Comparisons, though intended to inspire or console, can sometimes have the opposite effect. Instead of feeling uplifted, the other person may feel their struggles are being sidelined. **Comparisons, though meant to console, often alienate.**

3. **She only saw the problem through her own lens.**

When the mother spoke about the sacrifices she and Bulbul's father had made to send her to school, she was looking at the problem exclusively from her own viewpoint. She focused on the hardships *she* had endured, the sacrifices *she* had made.

It is natural to see every life situation through our own lens. However, by doing so, we overlook the perspective of the other person (which is what happened with Bulbul's mother). We fail to step into the shoes of the other person. In the process, we end up making them feel unheard.

Having gone through the three mistakes made by Bulbul's mother, it's easy to find fault and point out what she did wrong. However, consciously or unconsciously, we all make similar mistakes in our conversations. We rarely listen with the intention of understanding the other person; instead, we listen to reply, to rapidly offer advice, to swiftly 'fix' their problem. We're either talking or thinking about what to say next.

Back when I was starting out on my journey, if I met someone in our community at a Satvic gathering and they talked about their health problems, I would jump in right away with advice. If I had gone through something similar, I'd tell them about it and quickly explain how I fixed it. Because I felt that I knew so much. I felt I could help them. Often, I was more focused on sharing what *I* knew, rather than truly understanding *their* problems.

This approach, though well intentioned, I realized, wasn't really helping them. Later in my life, I learnt about a practice that made me see this tendency of mine. It led me to completely change how I communicate. We will cover this practice in more detail later in this chapter. But the main idea here is that it's easy to see the mistakes Bulbul's mother made, yet many of us have a tendency to do this ourselves, in different relationships in our lives.

The Crazy Optician Example

Let's take an example to clarify this concept better. Imagine you've been experiencing issues with your eyes and decide to go to an eye specialist (optician) for help. After hearing your complaint, he removes his glasses and hands them to you.

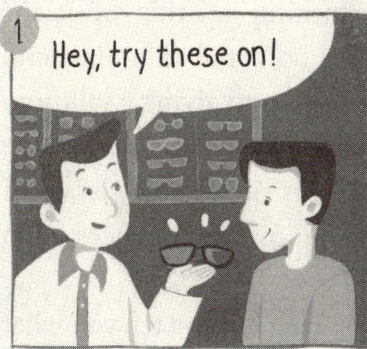

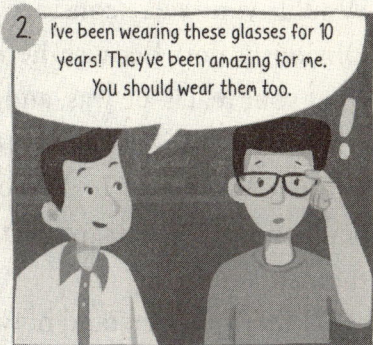

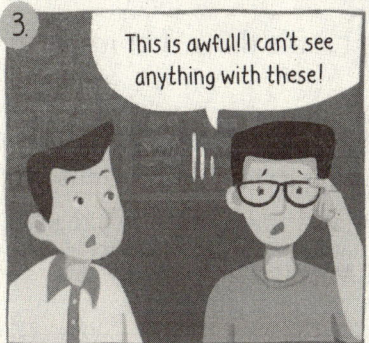

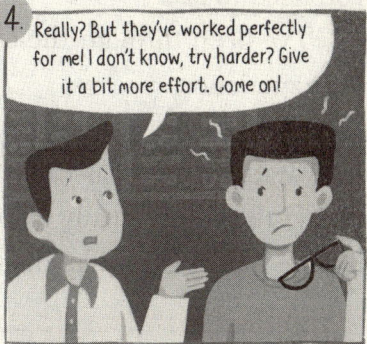

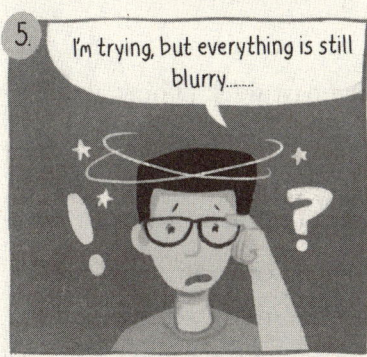

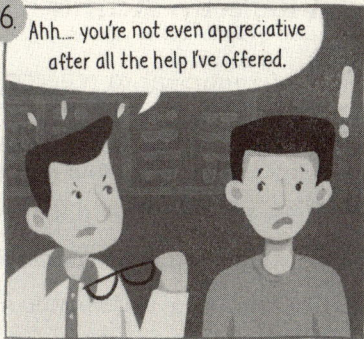

Would you ever consider returning to this optician? Obviously not! Because he never bothered to understand what your real issue was, and jumped into giving a solution.

This scenario is not just true for the optician or for the mother. We all do it. We often distribute our 'glasses of perception' to others, projecting our own experiences on to their situations.

'I totally understand how you feel. Let me tell you what you need to do.'

'I've been through the exact same thing. Let me share my experience.'

Each time we hastily offer someone *our* world view, *our* paradigm, *our* glasses for seeing the world, without first taking the time to truly understand *them*, we don't realize, but we become just like that crazy optician!

A Reflective Activity

Take a moment to reflect on the past week. Think about the various interactions you've had. It might be a personal conversation with your partner, children, parents or a close friend in which emotions were involved.

Once a few recent conversations come to mind, read the following statements. Pause for thirty seconds after each one and think:

- How often did you provide advice without first genuinely understanding the other person?

- How frequently did you find yourself cutting off the other person mid-conversation?
- Who are the people in your life with whom you find yourself doing this most often?

As these sentences sink in, you may find certain names or faces coming to mind, possibly highlighting a pattern in your interactions. This realization is the first step. But the question still remains: How can we break out of these patterns? How can we evolve into better listeners and more empathetic individuals? Let us learn as we proceed.

This marks the turning point in our chapter. We want to introduce you to a powerful tool drawn from Stephen Covey's book, *The 7 Habits of Highly Effective People*. This is a practice, a tool, a golden rule that we've embraced for many years now, and have witnessed its magical effects in transforming relationships first-hand.

The Golden Rule: Seek First to Understand before Being Understood

How does this work? The answer is simple: Before you seek to be understood by the other person, take time to fully and deeply understand *them*. Before sharing *your* perspective in a conversation, take the time to deeply and completely understand *their* perspective.

In order to do this, you must step out of your own shoes and gracefully **slide into the other person's shoes** for that moment. In other words, you must momentarily shed your own outlook and step into theirs. In that moment, you see the world how *they* see the world, not how *you* see the world.

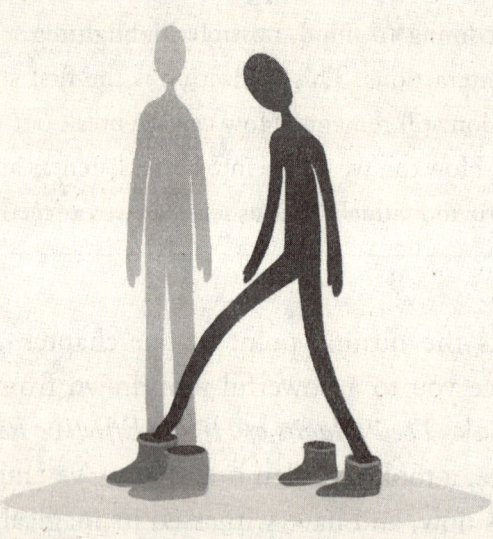

The question arises: 'But on practical grounds, how do you really do this? Do you just sit there listening to the other person, nodding your head and shaking your head, saying yes to everything?'

No. Not at all. There is a method to follow when seeking first to understand, and while it might seem unfamiliar or even a bit challenging initially, it is actually quite simple.

The Method: How to Seek First to Understand

Step 1: Listen with Undivided Attention

This means that when the other person speaks, your focus is unwaveringly on their words. No interrupting, no daydreaming, no checking your phone, no glancing at the clock—just looking into their eyes while they share.

But also, it's more than that. True understanding happens when you not only listen with your ears and eyes, but you also **listen with your heart.** You listen not just to their words, but also to what's behind those words. You listen not just to what they're saying, but also to what they're feeling. You basically enter their world and experience the world through *their* lens.

Step 2: Repeat What They Say in Your Own Words

For instance, Bulbul says, 'I don't like school any more. I'm sick of it.' If her mum were to repeat what Bulbul said in her own words, she could say, 'Bulbul, it sounds like you're really frustrated with school, and it's making you upset and angry.'

Repeating what the other person said, in your own words, serves a dual purpose:

- First (and perhaps more importantly), knowing that you have to restate what they're saying in your own manner naturally compels **you to listen more deeply.**

It enhances your own understanding of what the other person is saying.

- Second, when you reflect their words back to them, it makes **them feel truly understood**, often leading them to open up with you even further.

In summary, the two-step process to follow when seeking first to understand is (1) to listen with undivided attention, and (2) to repeat what they say in your own words.

Now that you've gained insights into what to do, it's equally important to be aware of what not to do in this process.

What Not to Do When Seeking First to Understand

✗ Don't Jump to Give Advice

Resist the urge to quickly offer advice or provide counsel—'you know, you should have done this' or 'you should do that'. Listen with the intention to understand, not with the intention to reply.

✗ Don't Compare

Avoid comparing their situation to your own or someone else's. Saying, 'I went through the same thing' and then launching into your own story or experience is considered comparing.

> ### ✗ Don't Assess the Situation through Your Own Lens
>
> Don't assess their situation while you're standing in your own shoes. Instead, leave your shoes behind and temporarily step into their shoes, their frame of reference, their life. See the situation as *they* see it, not how you see it.

There's one more crucial point to remember: This practice won't work unless it stems from a **genuine desire** to understand the other person. If your intention isn't sincere, if you're not truly interested in understanding the other person, we wouldn't recommend attempting it. In fact, doing so could create a false sense of openness and vulnerability that might backfire when the other person realizes that you weren't actually invested in understanding them. This can leave them feeling hurt and let down. So, be sincere in your attempt to understand; it's the foundation of this practice.

Now that you know the process, let us see how Bulbul's conversation with her mother might have unfolded if she had been aware of these principles.

Bulbul and Her Mother: A Transformed Connection

Bulbul: I . . . I just hate school, Mum. I'm just so tired of it.

Mother: What's wrong, beta? Is something troubling you?

Bulbul: *(frustrated, raising her voice slightly)* It's just . . . school doesn't make any sense to me. It's not helping me in any way.

Mother: Hmm . . . So my daughter is feeling stressed about going to school.

(Notice, here the mother isn't passing judgement on whether Bulbul's thoughts are correct or not. Instead, she's merely listening and repeating what Bulbul said, in her own words.)

Bulbul: This calculus and algebra I'm learning—I don't think any of this is actually going to help me in the real world . . . I . . . just want to quit . . . I want to quit school and do something better with my life, Mum.

Mother: Hmm . . . So you feel that you're wasting your time . . . you're not learning what *really* interests you . . .

(Again, notice how the mother is simply repeating Bulbul's words without offering guidance, interrupting or making comparisons.)

Bulbul: Yeah . . . sort of. Mum, remember I told you about being an artist? Like Dali, like Picasso? I just don't think these subjects in school are going to help me in any way! This is why I just don't want to go to school.

Mother: Mm-hmm . . . *(As she nods her head, showing that she's fully engaged and focused on her daughter's words.)*

Bulbul: I feel really passionate about art. I want to train to become an artist . . . *(pauses)* Not a mathematician. I really feel like I'm just wasting my time away . . .

Mother: Hmm. So, you're feeling really drawn to art, and you're worried that focusing on subjects like maths is taking you away from what you truly love and want to pursue.

Bulbul: Yeah, exactly. *(after a pause)* But you know, Mum, as I'm saying this, I also feel there's another side to all this. What if . . . what if there's a point to all this maths and algebra that I'm just not seeing?

Mother: It's okay to question, beta.

Bulbul: Yeah, I guess. I mean, I do understand that having a basic education is important for me. Like, if I don't complete school, how can I even think about getting into art college?

Mother: So you know that education matters. But you're confused. Confused between what you truly want and what's needed for your dreams.

Bulbul: That's exactly it, Mum. It's just so . . . *(sighs)* stressful, you know?

Mother: I understand, beta. It's difficult, for sure.

Bulbul: *(opening up)* And, Mum, there's something else I've been wanting to share . . . Remember the other day in school when I got the lowest score in my maths class? I only got 40 out of 100. I had studied hard for it, Mum. I actually prepared for it. But now, I'm worried I might actually fail this year. Honestly, I'm thinking it might be better to quit than to fail.

Mother: Hmm. It's really hard to give your all and still feel like you're failing. And sometimes, quitting can seem like the simpler way out. *(Notice how the mother has been careful not to jump in with advice or judgements. She's still simply echoing Bulbul's feelings back to her.)*

Bulbul: Yeah, Mum . . . I just feel . . . so lost! What do you think I should do?

~

Did you observe the remarkable impact that genuine understanding can make? Could you sense the change in Bulbul as her mother allowed her to fully express herself? By truly understanding Bulbul's feelings, her mother brought them together on the same side of the table, looking at the problem together, instead of being on opposite sides. When Bulbul realized that her mother understood her feelings, she even felt comfortable asking for advice.

Since Bulbul has asked for advice, now the mother can definitely offer guidance, and share what she considers will be best for her daughter. The difference, this time, will be that Bulbul will be receptive.

However, it's important for the mother to still be sensitive while doing so. If the advice gives rise to any unease or hesitancy for Bulbul, the mother should switch back to a listening and understanding mode. Thus, by **seeking first to understand, before being understood,** the mother builds a solid relationship with her daughter, built on trust, understanding and openness.

Theodore Roosevelt once said, '**Nobody cares how much you know until they know how much you care.**' This is a powerful statement. If you aim to have an impact on someone, you must first become a person they can rely on and have faith in.

> 'Instead of putting others in their place,
> put yourself in their place.'
>
> —Amish proverb

Four Things That Happen When You First Seek to Understand

1. You Help Them Empty Their Vessel

Let's imagine someone comes to talk to you about something that's sensitive to them. It's as if they come holding a vessel. This vessel carries their feelings, thoughts and emotions. When they start speaking, the load of their vessel slowly begins to lessen. But, what do you think will happen if you interrupt them and quickly offer your advice? Will they have enough space in their vessel to accommodate your suggestions? No, because a vessel that is already full cannot take more.

On the other hand, when you fully listen to them, when you allow them to share everything on their mind, you essentially allow them to completely empty out their vessel. Only when their vessel is emptied can they truly consider or welcome any new ideas, advice or perspectives from you.

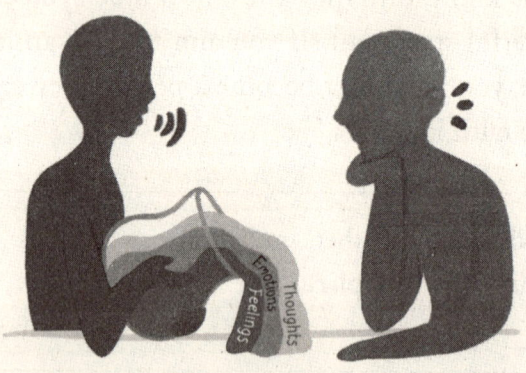

2. **They Open Up Quickly**

People tend to open up rapidly when they sense a genuine desire to understand them from the other person. This is true whether it's with a partner, child, parent, friend or colleague. If they believe you'll accept them unconditionally despite what they reveal—rather than criticizing, advising or ridiculing—they are more likely to express their feelings (notice how Bulbul opened up about her maths score when she sensed her mother's intent to understand, not judge?).

And when they do open up, it initiates a soul-to-soul connection. Gradually, like a rose letting go of its petals one by one, they reveal layer after layer of themselves. Eventually, they feel safe enough to reveal their innermost petals—their most delicate, innermost and tender feelings. Remember, your sensitivity to their emotions and sincere intent to understand is extremely important in this process.

3. **Sometimes, Advice Isn't Even Needed**
   Often, when the person opens up, they end up finding their own solutions. They untangle their own issues, and the answers are automatically revealed to them in the process. In such situations, allow the person to speak and share until the solutions become clear to them.

   At other times, they may actually require an outside perspective and guidance. If it is so, it's important to offer it only after you have fully understood their situation and when it is genuinely sought by them.

4. **You Greatly Strengthen Your Relationship with Them**
   In today's world, deeply understanding someone is a huge way of showing your respect towards them. In fact, one of the most meaningful gifts you can give is the **gift of authentic listening**—not merely to their words, but also to their underlying feelings. By doing

this, you make huge investments in your relationship with them.

> 'One of the most sincere forms of respect is actually listening to what another has to say.'
>
> —Bryant H. McGill

Deep listening isn't a new-age trend. It's actually a timeless, ancient practice—one that's been around since time immemorial. In fact, we can see Lord Krishna himself practising it in the beginning of an epic war scene.

Lord Krishna's Example

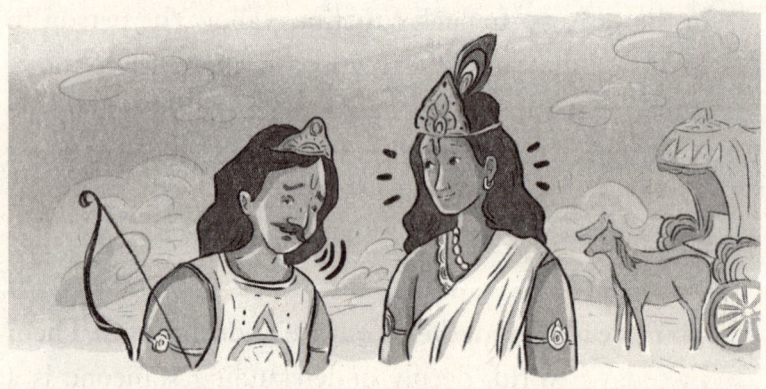

The Bhagavad Gita, an ancient Hindu text that forms a part of the Mahabharata, describes a scene set on a battlefield. The battle is between two branches of the same family. Arjuna is a prince on one side of the family. He's also one of the lead warriors in the fight. Lord Krishna is his charioteer (the one who drives and controls Arjuna's horse chariot).

Right before the war is about to start, Arjuna goes to see who he will be fighting against. This is when he sees his relatives, brothers, uncles, grandfathers, nephews and teachers all standing on the other side. Arjuna is considered the greatest warrior, but the thought of killing so many people from his own family leaves him overwhelmed with emotion. It fills him with so much sorrow that his body starts shaking, and his bow slips from his hand. He tells Krishna about his deep reluctance to fight.

As Arjuna pours out his reasons for not wanting to fight to Krishna, he passes through various states of confusion, frustration, depression and grief, finally reaching the depths of his distress. Yet, there's something very interesting we can observe here from Krishna's actions. Throughout all this, Krishna remains totally silent, paying full attention to Arjuna. From verses 28 to 47 (chapter 1) of the Bhagavad Gita, Krishna does not speak once. Krishna knows the solutions to all of Arjuna's confusion, yet for twenty verses, He simply listens, giving him the space to say all that he wants, without interrupting.

Finally, in chapter 2, Arjuna says, 'Now I am confused about my duty and have lost all composure because of weakness. In this condition, I am asking You to tell me clearly what is best for me. Now I am Your disciple and surrender unto You. Please instruct me.'

Finally, when Arjuna has completely emptied out his vessel, and he explicitly asks Krishna for help and guidance, that's when Krishna starts sharing his wisdom with him.

Therefore, through his actions, Krishna exemplifies the importance of giving someone the space to fully 'empty their vessel', before they are prepared to absorb or accept new perspectives or advice.

Teachings from the Buddha and the Bible

It's not just the Gita. In Buddhist philosophy, the practice of seeking to understand before being understood is termed 'compassionate listening'. Thích Nhất Hạnh, a late Buddhist monk, often referred to as the 'Father of Mindfulness', wrote a book titled *The Heart of Buddha's Teachings*. In this book, he wrote, 'Deep listening is the foundation of right speech. If we cannot listen mindfully, we cannot practice right speech. No matter what we say, it will not be mindful because we will be speaking only our own ideas and not in response to the other person.'

In the Holy Bible, in 'Proverbs' Chapter 18, verse 13, it is said, 'The one who gives an answer before he listens—this is foolishness and disgrace for him.'

It's fascinating how so many ancient texts demonstrate the immense power of deep listening and understanding. Either through their teachings or by actually demonstrating it in action.

Real-Life Stories from Our Community

Though rooted in ancient philosophy, this practice is not just a philosophical concept to read about, sit back and appreciate. It's also extremely practical in real life. For many years, we've been sharing it with thousands of people across the world through our online twenty-one day programme. The posts that our participants send to our community group after the session on understanding often leave us surprised. We would like to share some with you.

Sunita Yadav   •••
18 February

My husband and I were very happy. We went out, chilled and participated in all the social activities. But, for the last two months, I noticed a change; he started mentioning that he was experiencing pain in various body parts every day. I was scared and took him to the hospital to see if he had any health issues. We spent almost Rs 3 lakhs on all his health check-ups to see if there was any issue internally.

Thankfully, by God's grace, all his reports were normal. Everything was fine, but he still repeatedly complained that he felt pain and unease within his body. But I wasn't ready to listen to what he was saying. I used to ignore his words. He was internally depressed, but he would hide all his emotions so that I would be happy.

In today's session, I learnt to seek first to understand. So I sat with my husband at 10 am, I spoke to him and listened to everything he shared, including all his concerns about depression. He cried for about an hour. Soon, his internal pain began to fade away. I actually experienced the power of true understanding. Thank you, Satvic Movement. Through this principle, I got my husband back, physically as well as mentally. I will never forget you guys for as long as I live.

Prakash Chandra   •••
9 November

Today in the morning, my seven year-old son started crying, saying he didn't want to go to school. My usual response would have been to tell him that there's no reason to bunk school, reminding him he's well, doesn't have a fever or cold, and that he'll just end up watching TV all day at home, and blah blah blah.

But today, I TRIED TO UNDERSTAND why he didn't want to go to school. I didn't reason it out with him. I just listened.

In between the crying, he mentioned that some boy in his class is bullying him, and that's why he doesn't want to go. I had never really heard him before. Today, I did, and then I tightly hugged him after that.

Then, together with my wife, we calmed him down and told him that we don't run away from situations, we fight them. When mumma-dadda are near, he doesn't need to fear.

Obviously, we still need to take action against the boy who's bullying him. But I really felt at ease that my son could freely express himself when I tried to understand him.

One thing I've learnt through this process is 'Connection Before Correction'. It has beautifully changed and nourished all my relationships. Thank you, Satvic team.

Juhi Patel
24 April

•••

Yesterday morning, my househelp didn't come. Normally, when she missed a day and returned, I would start by saying that she's made it a habit to be absent without any reason. But today, when she came, I didn't say anything. She silently started her work, almost as if she was expecting some scolding or blaming words, as usual. Soon, she couldn't hold back anymore, and this was the conversation that followed:

Malti (my househelp): Aunty, I know I didn't come yesterday and that's why you're upset with me... You're not even talking to me...

Myself: No Malti, there is nothing like that.

Malti: Aunty, I didn't come because of my son. When he was walking to his school yesterday, someone on a bike hit him. My son got injured... I had to rush him to the hospital. That's why I couldn't come to work.

Myself: Oh! He was hit by a bike? (repeating her words) Malti, how is your son now?

Malti: He's okay now, Aunty. But I need to go back to the hospital in two days for his dressing change.

Myself: Malti, the day you have to take him to the hospital, please take that day off. And here's 100 rupees for the hospital expenses. And don't worry, this won't get cut from your salary; this is extra.

Instead of arguing and giving the threat of leaving the job as usual, this time Malti burst into tears and bent down to touch my feet. Not only this, but she also said, 'Aunty, you please don't do the housework yourself. As soon as I return from the hospital, I'll come and I'll do all the washing and cleaning work.' This time, I burst into tears, truly understanding the depth of the mantra, 'Seek first to understand, before being understood.'

Addressing Some Common Questions

Now that you've learnt nearly everything you need to know about the practice, here are some frequently asked questions and answers, to provide you with absolute clarity about its application.

1. **You said every time they say something, I have to repeat what they said in their own words. Does this mean I have to keep agreeing with everything they say? What about my feelings though?**

   No. The concept of seeking first to understand before being understood does not mean that you should agree with everything the other person says. It's not about suppressing your feelings or opinions. Instead, it's about genuinely comprehending their perspective before you share yours.

   After they complete their sharing, if you choose to share your perspective, it's perfectly fine even if you disagree with them. The key is that you're not rushing into agreement or disagreement. You're choosing to thoughtfully respond at the right time. And guess what? By doing so, the other person will also be more likely to understand your view (even if it is the opposite of theirs) because you've fully heard them out and allowed them to empty their vessel first.

2. **I applied this habit recently. I was at the office, and one of the employees came to me. She said, 'I want**

one day of leave, sir.' I remembered this principle and I repeated back what she said in her own words, 'Oh, so you want one day leave.' Then she said, 'Yes, sir, it's my sister's wedding.' I again repeated, 'Oh, it's your sister's wedding.' This went on for a few minutes, and in the end, the employee got very frustrated. What did I do wrong?

It's important to remember that not every situation requires you to repeat the other person's words. This step is most effective in situations wherein genuine emotions are involved, and the matter of discussion is sensitive for the other person. For instance, for straightforward matters like a simple leave request, you don't need to repeat what they say. But if the same employee comes to you and shares that she's feeling disconnected from her work, that's when using the step of repeating what they said back to them can be most impactful.

3. **Wouldn't this process take a lot of time? When I have the perfect advice for the other person, why do I have to wait to let them first vent and explain, when I already know what I want to say? A five-minute conversation will end up taking twenty or thirty minutes if I practise this method.**

    Well, yes, it's true that this practice takes time. In fact, you should only use it when you have the time. If you're in a rush, it might not even be suitable. However, while it may take a few extra minutes in the short term, it actually saves a lot of time in the long term.

Let's say your partner approaches you with an issue that is bothering them. You might give quick advice and wrap up the conversation in five or ten minutes. But what might end up happening is that your partner might not feel truly understood. They might even feel hurt, even if they don't show it. They might bottle up their feelings within themselves, leading to a bigger conflict down the line, which you will need to spend much more time trying to resolve.

So, yes, it takes more time upfront, but it saves time in the long run.

Concluding Thoughts about the Practice

Listening to someone with your whole heart, without interrupting them, is one of the loudest forms of kindness and the most precious gift you can give someone.

With this, we come to the end of habit five, 'Nourish Relationships'. By following the two principles outlined in this habit—letting go of unresolved issues and seeking first to understand before being understood—you'll greatly nourish your relationships, experiencing more joy, freedom and health.

Our request is that you don't let these concepts just be pages in a book. Implement them in your day-to-day living. You will see how these seemingly small changes will blossom your relationships in ways you couldn't have imagined. After all, the real luxuries of life are not the branded clothes we wear, the high-tech gadgets we use, the high-end cars we drive or the lavish house we live in. The real luxuries in life are the relationships we nurture, the memories we share with our loved ones, the laughter that fills our homes and the warmth of companionship that sustains us.

The next habit will explore a vital aspect of our lives that consumes a significant chunk of our day—our work! Prepare to embark on a journey where you'll encounter a fish attempting to climb a tree, soar through the skies from London to Delhi and meet Parth who loved his sandwiches with cheese, all the while uncovering one of the most thought-provoking habits in this book.

Habit 6

Live with a Purpose
Worth Jumping Out of Bed For

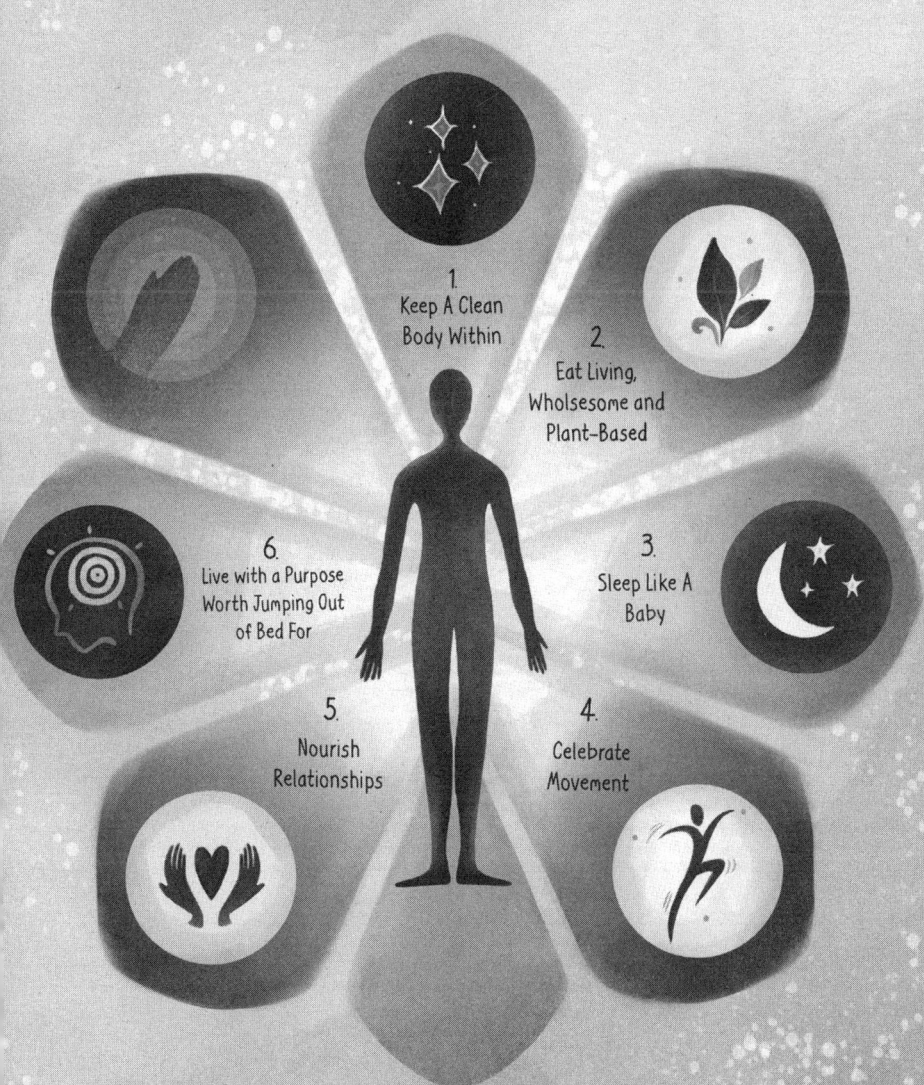

1.
Keep A Clean
Body Within

2.
Eat Living,
Wholsesome and
Plant-Based

3.
Sleep Like A
Baby

4.
Celebrate
Movement

5.
Nourish
Relationships

6.
Live with a Purpose
Worth Jumping Out
of Bed For

12

Your Purpose Is Waiting for You

Imagine yourself as a car. Picture your four wheels, representing the first four habits from this book.

Wheel 1: Keep a clean body within
Wheel 2: Eat living, wholesome and plant-based
Wheel 3: Celebrate movement
Wheel 4: Sleep like a baby

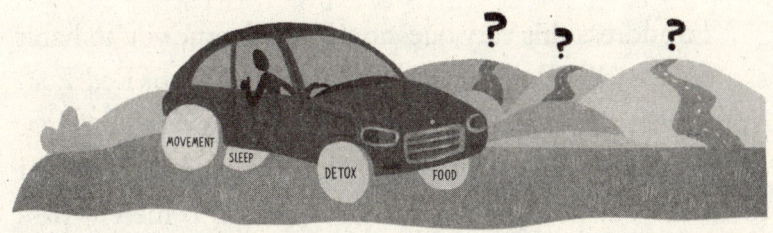

By following the first four habits, you've pumped air into all four wheels. Now the car is prepared, refurbished and ready to navigate even the roughest roads of life.

In the fifth habit, you learnt all about relationships. This means you've also prepared the driver inside the car to have better relationships with other drivers, reducing the chance of accidents on the road.

Now, the car is set. The driver is ready.

Yet, there's one major thing still missing.

What is it?

Well, it's the path!

What's the path which you want to take this car towards?

You can have the best-quality car, fitted with the most powerful engine, with its tyres fully inflated. But, if you don't know which direction to steer it in, if you don't know where to take it, what good is this highly efficient car?

In other words, what good is a healthy body if you don't know what to do with it? If you don't know what its purpose is? What is the value of excellent physical health if it isn't aligned with a meaningful path or purpose?

To address this very question, we welcome you to habit six: 'Live with a Purpose Worth Jumping Out of Bed For'. What does this mean? When you wake up every morning, you should have something to look forward to. If you want to reach your peak health, it's not enough to merely 'pass your days' or 'get through life'. You should have something that excites you—and that, dear reader, is what happens when we live in sync with our 'purpose'.

'Purpose' may seem like a heavy, grand word that's often thrown around lightly. But in simple terms, your purpose is nothing but your reason for waking up every morning, your inner calling, your reason for being.

Wherever you are, whoever you are, irrespective of your age, and irrespective of your profession, you have come with a special purpose on this Earth.

Here's what you can expect by the end of this chapter:

- First, you will learn about the fundamental connection between your health and your purpose.
- Then, you will learn six ways to check whether or not you're living in alignment with your purpose.
- Last, you will learn about the two crucial elements that come together to create your purpose.

Before we start, we want to clarify that it's unlikely you'll find your purpose by the end of this habit. That's not even the intention. Finding your purpose is not something you can do in a day or overnight. Our goal is to simply introduce you to this powerful concept, which many are unaware of, and help you take the first step towards it.

As you read, there is a chance that many answers will come to you automatically, like pieces of a puzzle seamlessly fitting together. Or, the process might be more gradual, requiring weeks or even months of reflection. This is because as we're progressing through this book, we're moving from the gross to the subtle. The first few habits addressed your gross, physical health. They were relatively straightforward to understand and practise. But now, we're learning about concepts that address subtler aspects of our health, which need more time for reflection and contemplation.

So our request to you is that as you read this chapter, don't rush into finding any answers. Allow your journey to unfold at its natural pace. Habit six is the one that requires the most time to actually implement in daily life.

Now, with our foundation all set, let's move to our first topic.

Purpose: How Is It Even Connected to Our Health?

The answer to this unfolds through a fascinating real-life story.

In the early years of starting Satvic Movement, Harshvardhan and I met a doctor who practised natural healing in the south of India. He ran a health centre in Pudukkottai, Tamil Nadu, which served as a sanctuary where people from across the nation could come and regain their health. At seventy-five years of age and with a wealth of experience and knowledge, he was affectionately called 'Guruji' by his students. One story that Guruji shared had a lasting impact on us.

Once, a middle-aged woman named Seema visited Guruji. She was suffering from multiple chronic lifestyle diseases. Upon meeting her, Guruji suggested that she should come and stay at the centre for at least a month, confident that she would see an improvement in her health within that time frame. Convinced, Seema left her home and family, came, and fully immersed herself in the regimen prescribed there: nutrient-rich meals, regular sleep, morning yoga, detox juices, consistent exercise and enlightening lectures. As the days turned into weeks, Seema's dedication to the programme remained unwavering.

However, fast forward to the end of the month, and despite her properly following everything, Seema barely saw any improvement in her condition. She was confused. She even felt disappointed. She went to Guruji with her dilemma, and said, 'I've done everything I was told. I followed all your advice. And yet, here I stand, with nothing changed in my body. Why isn't it working?'

Guruji listened to Seema intently. He then carefully reviewed her routine and soon realized that she had actually been quite meticulous in following it, leaving him equally puzzled as to why she saw no improvement in her health. Then, after a long and thoughtful pause, he asked her an unexpected question: 'Seema, let's say all your health problems disappear today. What would you do differently in your life? How would your life change?'

Taken aback, Seema struggled to find words. She searched for an answer. After a moment of silence, she said, in a soft, almost inaudible voice, 'Nothing. My life wouldn't really change. My son and daughter are both married. They are living their own lives. And my husband is absorbed in his work. I will just go back home and continue as before, finding ways to pass my days, trying to fill my time.'

This response was a revelation for Guruji. In that moment, he realized that what Seema was missing was not a change in diet, or more healing therapies. What she was missing was a purpose. She was missing a reason to look forward to each new day.

Guruji then asked her to close her eyes and said, 'Seema *beti*, think back to your childhood. Think about those moments when you felt the happiest, the most carefree.'

As Seema breathed deeply, some memories started to surface. Guruji continued, 'Picture those activities that captured your full attention, the ones you lost yourself in for hours. What were you doing?' He allowed a pause, giving Seema time to immerse herself in these reflections.

Then, slowly, he guided her further, 'Now, reflect on the skills that came to you naturally, the talents that set you apart even as a child. What were you known for? What did you love to do without anyone having to ask?'

In this serene state, Seema began to connect with parts of herself long forgotten. After a long pause, Seema opened her eyes. Her face seemed to light up as she said, 'Guruji, many happy memories crossed my mind, but one thing that kept reappearing was my love for art. I used to paint a lot as a young girl. It was my source of joy. Ever since I've gotten married, I haven't picked up the paintbrush.'

Hearing this, Guruji looked her in the eye and said, 'Seema, your time here is done. Now go home. Continue to follow the health principles you've learnt here, but more importantly, pick up that paintbrush again.'

Following Guruji's advice, Seema returned to her home.

Fast forward to a year later, Seema and Guruji crossed paths again. With keen interest, Guruji asked, 'How have you been, Seema? Have you seen any improvement in your health problems?'

Seema's reply caught him off guard. 'Health problems? What health problems, Guruji?'

Confused, Guruji reminded her, 'You came to our health centre in Pudukkottai wanting help for various health issues. Remember?'

With a radiant smile, Seema responded, 'Ah, of course I remember. But shortly after I returned home, my health started to improve dramatically.'

Intrigued, Guruji asked, 'Really? How did you manage that?'

'As you advised, Guruji, I picked up my paintbrush and I haven't looked back. You know, I even had exhibitions at an art gallery! Over the past year, I've sold many paintings.'

Guruji noticed something astonishing about Seema at that moment—she looked more alive, more vibrant and more energetic than he had ever seen her before.

The moral of this story, as Guruji explained to us, is the undeniable connection between a sense of purpose and our health. When Seema went back home, she started living a life that made her excited for each new day. Believe it or not, this sense of purpose is what helped her the most in getting better. It played the most important role in her recovery.

This, dear reader, isn't just an isolated case unique to Guruji's wisdom; it's backed by cultures around the world which are known for their longevity and well-being. In fact, some of the longest living people in the world have already uncovered this secret! Come, let's see how.

Ikigai: The Longevity Secret from Okinawa

Remember the Blue Zones we mentioned earlier in this book? These are unique regions around the world where people not only live exceptionally long lives but also have the lowest incidence of chronic lifestyle diseases.

If you ever go to these places, you'll find that there are a lot of people here who are living past the age of 100. They are often called 'centenarians'. And no, these aren't frail, weak, bedridden people; they're fit people who are living fulfilling lives. Although their largely plant-based diet is a well-studied factor that contributes to their longevity, researchers have discovered that there's another surprising element that's just as important. It's not about food. It's not about exercise. It's something more intangible.

It is their 'ikigai'. This is particularly common among those living in Okinawa, a Blue Zone near Japan. For them, 'ikigai' isn't just a buzzword—it's a fundamental life principle—**a deeply ingrained sense of purpose or mission in their lives**. Having an ikigai is considered to be one of the most powerful factors responsible for their long and healthy life.

In the documentary *Live to 100: Secrets of the Blue Zones*, a doctor in Okinawa shares his experience of doing regular visits for people who are over 100 years old. After checking on their physical and mental condition, guess what's the next question he always asks his patients? It's this—'What's your ikigai?' The doctor even says that if these older people lose their ikigai, they might die.

Another interesting finding in Okinawa was that the word 'retirement' doesn't even exist in their vocabulary. People there continue to work into their sixties, seventies, eighties, and even nineties. It's not merely about staying active; they actually remain part of the working world. They might be only tending their gardens to bring home fresh produce or running a stall at the local market just for the morning hours. But what's important is that, even in the later stages of their lives, they are involved in work that gives their life a meaning. This keeps their minds engaged, providing them with a reason to get up every morning, and imbuing them with a constant sense of purpose, right up to their final days.

Now, you don't have to travel to Okinawa in Japan or to the other Blue Zones to witness the power of having a purpose. You can also see it in your own family or social circle. Do you know anyone who retired at the age of sixty or sixty-five? Have you noticed how their life changes if they don't have something meaningful to do after they quit working?

I saw this happening with my own grandfather. As long as he was engaged in some kind of a routine, as long as he had something to look forward to in his day, somewhere to go every morning (whether it was going to his workspace, going to the market to buy fresh groceries for the house, going to his place of worship, or to meet his group of close friends at the park nearby), he remained healthy, happy and active. I always saw him smiling. But one by one, as he stopped these routines, the enthusiasm that he once held for life began to disappear. As a result, his physical health also started to deteriorate.

So the crux of everything you've read so far is simple: Without having a purpose or something to look forward to, it is challenging to be in your peak health. Whether we're in our eighties or in our twenties, whether we're old or young, we all need a purpose in life.

In fact, a study published by the *American Journal of Health Promotion* in 2022, which took data from approximately 13,000 participants, asked them to complete a questionnaire to determine their subjective sense of 'purpose in life'. The study concluded that those with the highest sense of purpose had:

- A 46 per cent reduced risk of mortality
- A 13 per cent reduction in the risk of sleep problems
- A 43 per cent lower risk of depression
- Lower loneliness ratings
- And higher levels of optimism

Now, having read about Seema and Guruji, and having learnt about the people in Okinawa, there's a chance that you might be wondering, 'What's *my* purpose? Am I even living it?' Well, to help you assess exactly this, here's a short quiz.

Six Ways to Check if You're Living Your Purpose

Review the following six questions, each with an option A and an option B. Tick the one that most closely aligns with your current situation. While answering, keep in mind the last thirty days of your life. And remember, honesty is key for an accurate result.

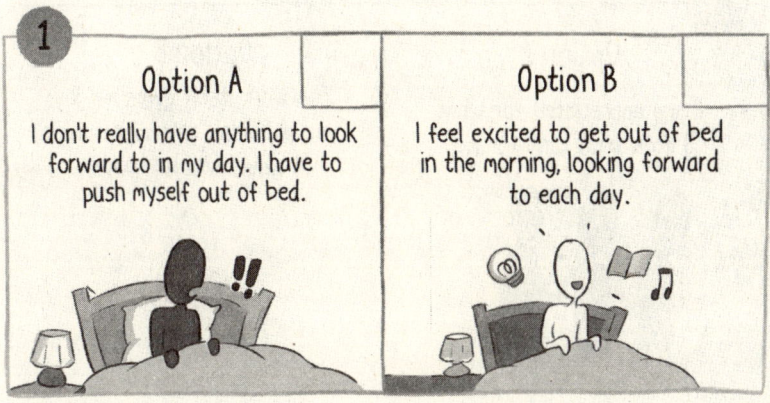

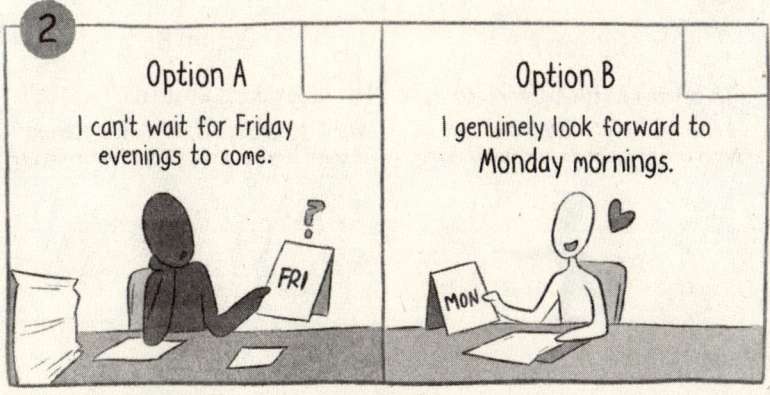

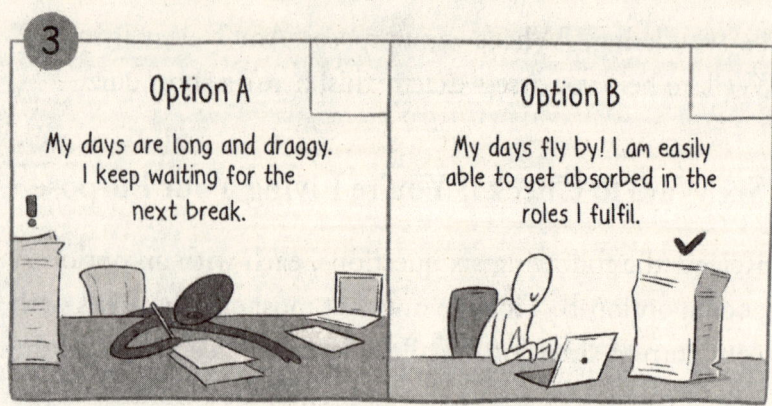

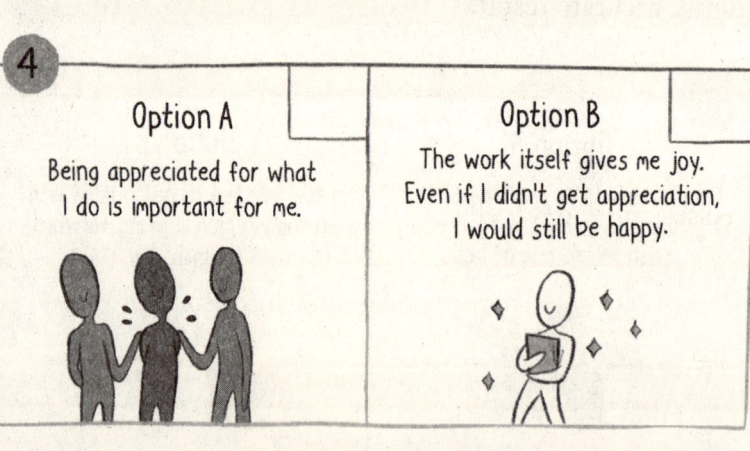

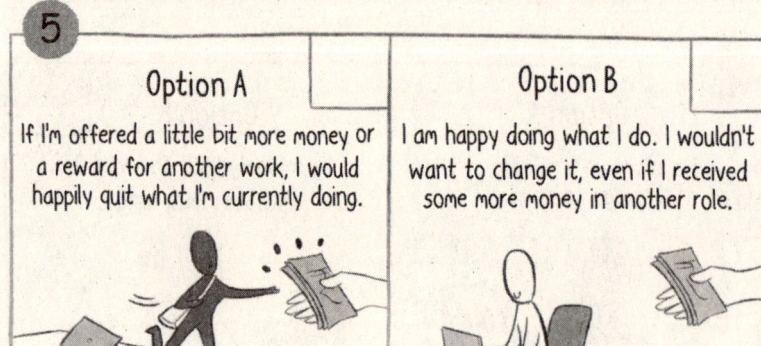

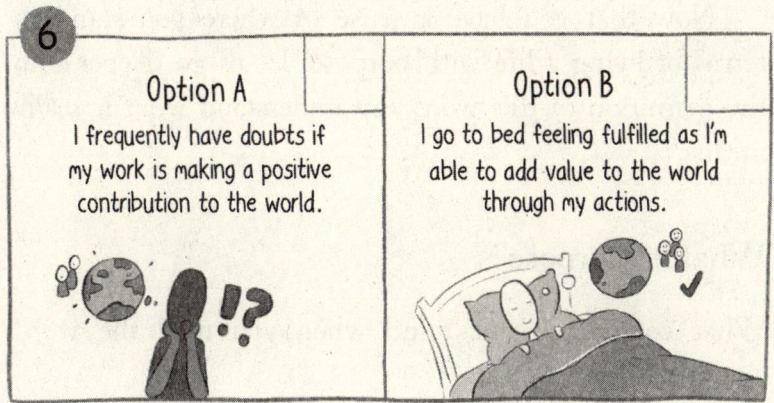

6

Option A

I frequently have doubts if my work is making a positive contribution to the world.

Option B

I go to bed feeling fulfilled as I'm able to add value to the world through my actions.

Make sure you have ticked the options that best fit your current life situation.

Assessing the Results:

Now, count how many ticks you have for option A and option B.

- If you find that the majority of your answers are As, it's a sign that your life is not yet aligned with your purpose. This is an opportunity for introspection and growth.
- On the other hand, if you have more Bs, it's a sign that you're on a path that is aligned with your purpose!

Remember, it's natural to have a mix of As and Bs, as life is not always so black and white. Use these six questions simply as a guide to help you think and introspect.

Now that you have a sense of where you stand in terms of living a life with purpose, let us go deeper into the definition of this word and understand what it really means.

What Is 'Purpose'?

What comes to your mind when you read the word 'purpose'?

Does it bring to mind certain goals? Or ambitions? Or perhaps talents? Or, do you feel that there's something more to it?

Well, it's difficult to define the word 'purpose' in one single English word, but 'inner calling' comes close.

In this book, when we say 'purpose', we see it as a combination of two key elements. It's at their intersection, at their confluence point, where your purpose lies.

The first key element is your innate strengths (your intrinsic talents and abilities). And the second key element is service to others (which involves dedicating one's time and efforts for the betterment of others), for the greater good. When you use your innate strengths to uplift the lives of others, that becomes your purpose.

In other words, when you employ your inherent talents and abilities—those skills that come naturally to you—in ways that meaningfully contribute to and improve the lives of others, you are living your purpose.

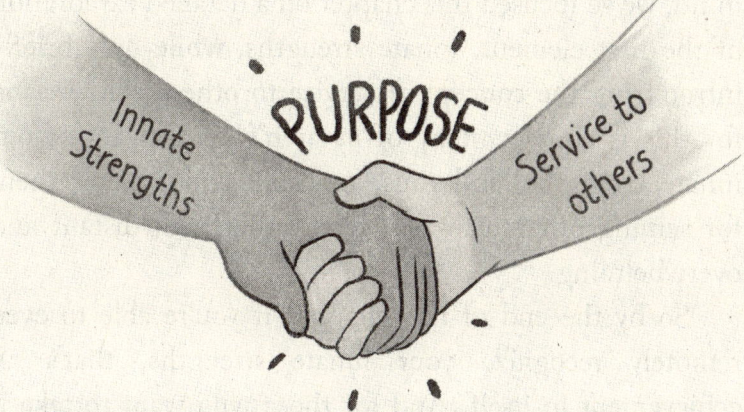

> **Note:**
>
> When analysing the 'purpose' of our life, it can have varying levels. For the context of this book, we have primarily focused on its relevance to our worldly duties. While there is so much more that could be explored about this topic from a spiritual perspective, we will leave this for our spiritual teachers to guide us.

Now, we understand that this idea of purpose, as inspiring as it is, may feel very idealistic. You might wonder, 'How can I think about service when I don't even know what my innate strengths are?'

Though using your strengths to serve others is ideal, our intention in this book is to help convert lofty, idealistic, high-level concepts into practical realities. With this in mind, we've focused this chapter on a detailed exploration of the first element, innate strengths, while only briefly introducing the concept of service to others. The reason for this is simple: many of us aren't even aware of our innate strengths, and thus, to think about using them for serving others can feel very far-fetched, distant and overwhelming.

So by the end of this chapter, if you're able to even remotely recognize your innate strengths, that's an achievement in itself. And for those who want to take it one step further, who want to use those strengths to serve others, we will touch upon how to do that as well.

So, What Are Innate Strengths?

These are your intrinsic strengths and abilities. They are those natural qualities and skills that are a part of your character, almost as if they are hardwired into your being. Think of them as your 'birth gifts'—the particular talents that you were born with.

Because of these birth gifts, or innate strengths, the potential within an individual is tremendous, even infinite. We really have no idea what we are capable of.

Remember, innate strengths are not skills you've acquired along the way. They're the abilities you were born with. Imagine you came into the world carrying a suitcase full of gifts. They're a part of who you are.

Take learning to play a musical instrument as an example. Two people may have the same teacher and practise the same amount, but one might master it quickly while the other struggles. That ease in learning is a sign of an innate strength in music.

Now, the real challenge is that many of us don't put these innate strengths to good use. We keep these birth gifts safely in a corner—unwrapped, gathering dust—waiting for a day sometime in the future when we'll open these, when we have time. But often, that time never comes. And thus, many of us go through years, decades and sometimes even our entire lives without ever unpacking these birth gifts that we were blessed with, without tapping into our true potential.

Let's take the example of a person who's naturally good at writing, but their job requires them to crunch numbers at a computer all day. Their work isn't allowing them to tap into their true strengths. Similarly, think of someone who is incredibly empathetic and great at connecting with people, yet they have a job that requires them to work alone most of the time. They're not using their innate gifts either. And what about a person who has exceptional leadership skills? If they're stuck in a role where they can't make decisions or inspire others, they're also not leveraging their innate strengths.

When we do work that doesn't match our innate strengths, it's like trying to swim against a strong current—it's hard and exhausting. Even simple work feels difficult and leaves us feeling frustrated and stressed because it doesn't fit our skills. At the end of the day, we don't feel fulfilled.

Reflection Activity

Before we move on, let's pause for a minute to reflect. Look back at the last week of your life and consider these two questions:

- What did you spend the majority of your day doing?
- Was this activity something you're naturally good at? Does it align with your innate strengths?

Now that you know what 'innate strength' means, here's a short story that beautifully shows what happens when we spend time on things that are not our innate strengths.

The Fish that Tried to Climb a Tree

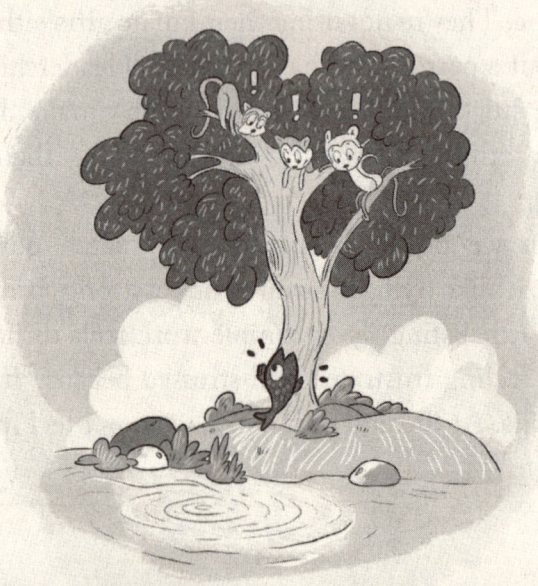

Once upon a time, in the heart of a lush green forest, there was a crystal clear pond. There were delicate water lilies floating on its surface, and various fish darting through its waters. Among these fish living in the pond, one was named Nemo.

One sunny day, she unexpectedly found herself out of the water, at the foot of a tall tree. As she looked up, she saw six baby monkeys joyfully swinging and leaping from branch to branch, their laughter echoing through the forest. Nemo was enthralled! Her heart swelled with desire. 'I want to do that too!' she thought.

She started trying to mimic the monkeys. She flopped and wriggled, attempting to climb the trunk of the tree, but each attempt only led to failure. The harder she tried, the farther she fell on the ground. And why wouldn't she? After all, she was a fish, not a monkey.

Feeling utterly defeated, Nemo whispered to herself, 'I can't do this. I'm just not good enough.' She lay on the ground, her tiny heart heavy with feelings of rejection, defeat and helplessness.

Just then, a wise sage passed by. He noticed little Nemo lying on the ground. Recognizing her struggle, he gently scooped her into his hands and returned her to the pond, her true home. Instantly revitalized, away went Nemo, flapping her fins, gliding effortlessly through the water, finally in her element once again, where she truly belonged.

The Lesson

The story of Nemo carries a deep lesson. Nemo was a fish, meant to swim, not to climb a tree. Yet, she judged herself based on a skill that was never in her true nature. This left her feeling inadequate and rejected, like she wasn't good enough.

Have you ever experienced something similar in your own life? Have you ever felt that you're like a fish trying to climb a tree? Like maybe you're not in your own 'pond'? Like you're doing something which is not your true nature? This could be for any reason—social expectations, family pressures, financial needs.

Well, you're not alone. Many of us find ourselves trapped in roles or responsibilities that don't quite fit our true nature. But, what we don't realize is that when we spend the majority of our day, month or year doing work that doesn't align with our innate strengths, it is as absurd as a fish trying to climb a tree!

In the long run, such a mismatch takes us a step away from experiencing peak health. Because we don't feel fully content, satisfied or happy from within. We pass years, even decades, with an unshakable feeling of incompleteness, as if we're square pegs living in a round-hole world.

> 'Everyone is a genius. But if you judge a fish by its ability to climb a tree, it will live its whole life believing that it is stupid.'
> —Commonly attributed to Albert Einstein

How This Applies to Our Personal Lives

Satvic Movement is a fast-growing movement, with thousands of people attending our online workshops every month. Managing such a large organization involves complex technical work. This is something that Harshvardhan takes care of. His strength in the domain of technology is simply extraordinary. He has reports and spreadsheets open in front of him all day long. He manages all things tech, oversees software development and manages the financial aspects of the movement. If I look at the same spreadsheet, I may probably get a headache, but for him, it's effortless, even joyful. Numbers, data, analytics and technology are his 'pond', his natural habitat. I've seen that even during the most hectic days, he remains invigorated because he's operating within his zone of innate strengths.

In contrast, when it comes to design, writing, scripting for videos and other creative work, those tasks fall into my domain because they come naturally to me. I could spend hours doing creative design work without getting tired. If Harshvardhan were to tackle these tasks, he would actually go crazy. That's because creative thinking and design are part of my birth gifts, just as technology and numbers are his.

We are fortunate to have identified our own 'ponds'. It took us a long time to find them—it was a journey. But now, instead of trying to improve our weaknesses, we focus on continuously building upon our natural strengths. That's not to say everything is perfect; there are times when we have to operate outside of our ponds. However, about 80 per cent of our work aligns with our natural abilities, making it deeply fulfilling.

> 'We each have unique abilities, strengths, personalities and capacities inbuilt within our body and mind. When we identify and engage these, we embrace our *sva-dharma*—occupational duties that we are "wired" for in this life.'
> —S.B. Keshava Swami,
> in his book *Gita 3*

When we align with our innate strengths, not only do we find fulfilment doing it, but there's one other very interesting thing that happens. We feel as though we're being 'pushed forward' on our path. Let's understand this further using an analogy.

What Air Travel Teaches Us about Innate Strengths

Do you know how long it takes for an airplane to go from New Delhi to London? It takes about ten hours. And do you know how long it takes for the same plane to come back from London to New Delhi? Well, you'd be surprised. It takes only eight and a half hours.

The plane, the distance, the engine and even the pilot are all the same. So, why such a big difference in travel time? The answer lies in the direction of the wind.

Throughout most of the year, winds blow predominantly in a westerly direction—meaning from London towards Delhi. When the plane travels from Delhi to London, it faces a headwind, a wind blowing in the opposite direction to the one the plane is travelling in. Despite the aircraft's best speed, it's in a constant struggle against these opposing winds, making the trip longer.

However, on the return trip from London to Delhi, the aircraft enjoys the benefit of a tailwind—a wind blowing in the same direction as its course. This tailwind pushes the aircraft forward, enabling it to complete the journey in less time, thus saving almost two precious hours.

In the same way, when we operate outside of our innate strengths, we have to deal with a headwind that slows our progress and saps our energy. We're in a constant struggle because we're trying to fly against the wind. But when we work in alignment with our innate strengths, we're pushed forward, not just through our own capabilities, but by a force that's greater than ourselves—a tailwind that makes our lives easier and seamless. Thus, the experience feels less like a struggle and more like a flow. Not only are we more efficient, but we also work with a greater sense of confidence and happiness. There are still obstacles that come in the way. We still have to put in our best effort. But it comes from a space of joy.

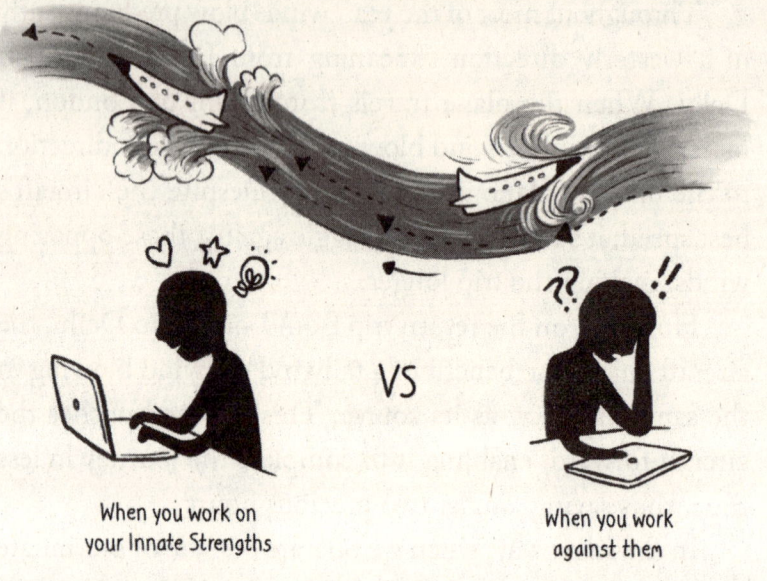

When you work on
your Innate Strengths

VS

When you work
against them

Reflection Activity to Help You Discover Your Innate Strengths

If you're still wondering what your innate strengths might be, here's an interesting activity to help you find clarity. It poses eight thought-provoking questions.

Here's what you have to do: read each question, think about it and then, you may jot down your responses in the space provided.

Note: While examples are provided for each question, consider them simply as starting points. Allow your imagination to expand beyond these examples.

1. What are those tasks that you can do effortlessly? What are those activities that come naturally to you? (Examples: writing, public speaking, playing an instrument, arranging data on a sheet, repairing cars)

2. What gets you in the state of flow? What are those activities that make you lose track of time, and even forget to eat and drink when you do them? (Examples: cooking, programming, playing a certain sport)

3. What are the things that your friends and family usually seek your help with? (Examples: helping with tech problems, relationship advice, fashion guidance, financial planning)

4. What extra tasks have you taken on at work or in your life just because you love doing them? (Examples: designing flyers, mentoring people, organizing events)

5. Think back to your childhood. What kinds of activities were you naturally inclined towards? (Examples: drawing pictures, building models/Lego structures, writing poems or stories, dancing, performing plays or skits)

6. Which class did you enjoy the most back in your school days? (Examples: science, arts, language, computers, environmental education, mathematics, business)

7. Which topics do you love learning about? What do you geek out about? (Examples: sustainability, yoga, culinary arts, spirituality, technology)

8. Imagine 1 crore rupees have just been deposited into your bank account. All of your life's needs, as well as your family's needs, are taken care of—now and in the future. You can't save this money or put it in a bank account; you have to use it. How would you use this money? (No examples for this one!)

Find the Common Threads

Once you're done answering the questions, take some time to review your responses. Look for any common threads or overlapping patterns among them. Then, underline or highlight those common threads which you find.

For instance, you might find a recurring theme of activities such as drawing, designing flyers and a love for art-related subjects. This indicates an innate strength in artistic creativity and visual expression. Another example: You may find recurring themes involving mentoring others, offering relationship advice and choosing subjects like psychology or spiritual learning. This points towards an innate strength in empathy, counselling and guiding others.

Now please take a few moments to review your answers. Once you've done this, you may write these common thread areas (which you've underlined) in the box below:

The common threads you've identified are likely your innate strengths. Don't be surprised if you find three to four of them—that's common and natural.

> Though self-reflection is a great way to find out what your birth gifts are, another way is to draw upon the advice of any mentors, coaches or spiritual guides you may have in your life. They may have the ability to see beyond what you can see yourself, and tell you what your innate strengths are.

Once you've found what your innate strengths are, you may discover that what you're spending 80 per cent of your day doing is already aligned with them. If so, celebrate the alignment! That's wonderful.

Or, you may discover that what you're doing in life right now is completely unrelated to your innate strengths. If that's so, don't worry. Continue reading, and further in this chapter, you will learn how you can start your journey towards this alignment, from exactly where you are now.

The Second Element: Service to Others

Earlier in this chapter, we discussed how your purpose is a combination of two key elements. We've covered the first one (innate strengths) at length, but what about the second element (service to others)? Come, let's learn.

What Does 'Service to Others' Mean?

In its simplest form, service means dedicating one's time and effort for the betterment of others, for the greater good. How can we assess if our actions genuinely count as service? A good rule of thumb is to ask, 'How many lives am I positively affecting with my actions?'

To understand this, let's look at the three levels at which we can operate our lives:

First Level: Self-Centric Work

If your work is motivated solely by personal gain, thinking only about how you will benefit from it, what you will gain out of it, you are at the level of self-centric work. Here, you always think, 'What's in it for me?' This is operating at the most basic layer.

Second Level: Family-Centric Work

If your actions serve to benefit not just you, but also your immediate family or loved ones, that becomes family-centric work. You're in the mindset of, 'As long as my family is happy and they are taken care of, I'm happy.' By doing so, you're broadening your scope of service, but it's still very far from the pinnacle.

Third Level: Community and Beyond

This level transcends your own self and your family. Here, you use your life not just to add value to your near and dear ones, but you think beyond that. You use your being as an instrument in the service of people, humanity at large, animals, Mother Nature or God. Thus, when you serve others, with a heart full of compassion and without selfish motives, that is considered *seva*. When you're in this mindset, you think, 'I have already been given so much. I have been so blessed. How can I now contribute in meaningful ways to the world?'

How Can We Combine Our Innate Strengths and Service?

This really depends on your innate strengths, your capacity, available resources and the needs of your community. There's no one-size-fits-all approach, but to provide some inspiration, here is an example.

Let's say there is a woman whose innate strength is cooking, and she decides to set up a small kitchen. If she operates at the 'self-centric work' level, her primary thought would be, 'How can I gain the maximum money through this work?' In pursuit of this goal, she will do anything to make the food sell more—whether it involves using lower-quality ingredients or using chemical additives, simply for taste, even when she knows that they are not the best for her customers' health.

On the other hand, if she approaches her cooking as a form of service, her mindset shifts. She may still charge for her meals and make a profit, but now, her foremost thought becomes, 'How can I best serve others through this food?' With this perspective, she could decide to prepare food that uplifts the health of people, and thus, make wholesome, nutritious, plant-based, Satvic food, benefiting both human health and our animal friends.

This shift in intention from *taking* to *giving* can transform the same innate strength—cooking and serving food—into a meaningful purpose that contributes positively to the community.

Service is not only expressed in specific tasks but also in your intention in each and every moment. For example, if someone is a medical professional, therapist or caregiver, the next time they walk into their clinic, instead of thinking, 'What can I *take* from my patient? How can I benefit from them?', they could enter with the thought, 'How can I *give* them the best possible care? My primary intention is always to uplift *their* life, not to fill my own pockets.'

These examples are just a starting point to spark your imagination. Now you can think about how you could use your innate strengths in service of others, in your own unique way.

Why Is 'Service to Others' an Important Element of Purpose?

When we focus solely on our innate strengths, that certainly brings us joy, proficiency and a sense of satisfaction. We excel in what we're naturally good at and enjoy the process. However, this satisfaction might not be long-lasting. Over time, we may get bored with that work. We might start to question, 'Why am I doing this? What's the use of it?'

But when we channel these same innate strengths towards the betterment of others, to uplift them, help them, serve them, we experience a deeper, more lasting fulfilment. This fulfilment nourishes us even in the long term. That's one reason why it's the blend of innate strengths and contribution to others that really makes your purpose. Because we don't feel satisfied just by earning and accumulating more for ourselves; we feel true joy and bliss in giving and serving others.

Just as living, whole, plant-based foods nourish our body, similarly, service opens the heart and nourishes our soul. The Holy Bible beautifully puts it across: 'Each of you should use whatever gift you have received to serve others, as faithful stewards of God's grace in its various forms' (New Testament, 1 Peter 4:10).

In fact, all our religious teachings teach us to move beyond the small world of 'I, me and mine', and instead explore how we can sacrifice, serve and bring happiness to others. When we selflessly serve others, our own happiness arises automatically. To the degree we live in the concept of 'I', we experience illness. When we shift our paradigm to 'we', we experience wellness.

But How Do We Begin?
How to Make All this Practical?

Now that you've understood both the elements that come together to form your 'purpose', and have an idea as to what your innate strengths could be, you might be wondering, 'But where do I start?' Questions about money, family expectations and social pressure might be flooding your mind. 'Is this even practical?' you may ask.

Well, as we shared with you in the beginning of this chapter, habit six ('Live with a Purpose Worth Jumping Out of Bed For') takes the most time to fully incorporate into your life. Because it's not just difficult to identify your purpose, but it's also challenging to wholeheartedly live it. Even when we know what we're hardwired for, various things distract us from the path of our inner calling—expectation of others, financial needs, desire for appreciation, etc.

So, here's what we suggest:

- You **don't have to make drastic changes** right away. There's no need to quit your job or drop everything you're doing. It's important that you don't do anything that leaves you financially unstable.
- Instead, start small. If you've pinpointed something as your strength, **spend just thirty minutes each day focusing on it**, along with your current work/job. Whether it's yoga, entrepreneurship, teaching, finance,

music, technology, making food or whatever else that you feel you're good at and also enjoy doing, give it half an hour of your day.

- Depending on what that innate strength is, you could actually **practise it** in those thirty minutes. Or, you could **educate yourself** more about it. In other words, move towards mastering that skill. This could be in any way—by reading books about it, by taking courses on it, etc. The best time to do this is in the early-morning hours. That's when you have the greatest focus and the highest chance of entering the state of flow, as we learnt in habit three.

- As you keep practising and learning more about your subject matter, **you'll notice doors starting to open.** Over time, you will find opportunities to align your birth gift with your profession. You may even find opportunities that allow you to truly serve others through your gift. When that happens, you may choose to switch roles or continue with your current one while pursuing your birth gift part-time. Both are valid choices.

Personally, after many years of running Satvic Movement and sharing this health knowledge with others, I realized that I had a birth gift left unwrapped in my suitcase. This gift was for singing *kirtan* (devotional songs) and playing the harmonium. Since I had left it unopened for so long, it had begun to gather dust. But once I realized it was there, I didn't want to ignore it. So, I started small. Amid my busy, hectic days, I found thirty minutes every morning to learn kirtan. For me, early mornings worked best for focusing on this. I began by learning from online videos and practised daily. I tried not to break the chain (as we learnt in habit four, 'Celebrate Movement'). Eventually, I felt confident enough to start playing in front of crowds at our Satvic gatherings and events. When I opened this birth gift, I was able to add value not only to my own life, but also to the lives of others who listened to the kirtan. Initially, I thought I had become too old to sharpen this skill. However, I soon realized that we are never too old to unwrap our birth gifts, or to dream a new dream.

The bottom line is: start with practising your innate strengths for just thirty minutes every day and trust that doors will open.

Concluding Thoughts about This Practice

We would like to close this chapter with a final story. This is about a man named Parth, who is an IT engineer in his mid-thirties, living in Mumbai. One day, as he's eating lunch in his office cafeteria, he opens his lunch box to find a cheese sandwich. 'Ah, not again! I don't want another cheese sandwich,' he complains. His colleagues, sitting with him, glance over and continue eating, largely unaffected.

Days pass, and the scene repeats. Parth keeps complaining about his monotonous cheese sandwiches. One day, one of his colleagues speaks up, 'Parth, if you're not happy with the cheese sandwiches, request your wife to prepare something different.' Parth looks at his colleague and responds, 'Wife? I'm not even married. I made this sandwich myself this morning!'

Dear reader, this story is a perfect metaphor for what many of us are doing in life. We complain about circumstances we've created ourselves, about a life we've built for ourselves.

Who should stop making the cheese sandwiches?

Parth.

And who will benefit from that decision?

Parth.

If you find yourself saying, 'I'm stuck here; I don't want to do this', if you spend your whole month just wishing for a better life, then you're just like Parth with his cheese sandwiches. If you're unhappy, make a change. Remember, you are choosing the life you live. Nobody else.

As we end this chapter, our message for you is simply this: You have been given brilliant birth gifts that may be lying unopened. Society might make you think you have no gifts, no strengths or that you should set them aside. That's not true. You have a special place where you can flourish. Don't spend your whole life leaving your unique gifts wrapped up, unused. Open them and share them with the world. Use them to serve others. And remember, as Guruji taught us, as the Okinawans taught us, as little Nemo and the sage taught us, **the secret to peak health isn't just in staying alive; it's about finding a reason to live for!**

In the next chapter, we'll move to the last and final of the seven habits of the Satvic Revolution. The story of the prince that is coming up is perhaps our favourite in this whole book!

Habit 7

Live in the Mode of Surrender

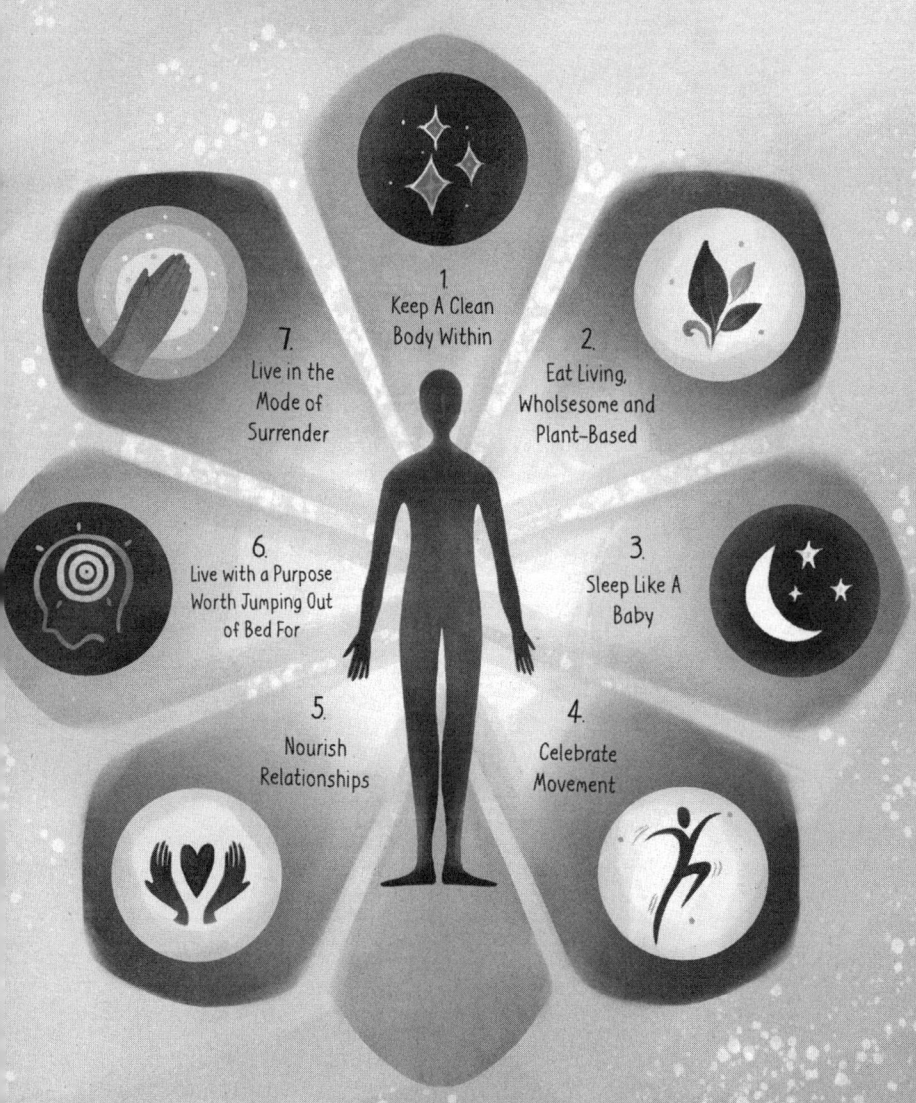

1. Keep A Clean Body Within

2. Eat Living, Wholsesome and Plant-Based

3. Sleep Like A Baby

4. Celebrate Movement

5. Nourish Relationships

6. Live with a Purpose Worth Jumping Out of Bed For

7. Live in the Mode of Surrender

13

How to Stay
Calm during Any Chaos

It was 1 April 2023. As a raindrop splashed on to my wrist while Harshvardhan and I stood on stage, I knew we were entering one of the most challenging moments of our lives.

We were at the Satvic fest, hosted in New Delhi. Up until then, this was the largest physical gathering we had ever had at Satvic Movement. Our team had poured their heart and soul into planning this event over the past three months. The line-up was vibrant and diverse, with some talks, yoga sessions, an exquisite Satvic dinner and a musical performance led by our team. The venue was an expansive, gorgeous garden surrounded by lush trees and covered in beautifully arranged decorations.

More than 500 people had come together for this Satvic fest, many having flown from distant cities to be part of it. For the majority of them, it was their first time attending a physical gathering we had organized. To say that expectations were high would be an understatement.

Sitting on an outdoor stage decorated with white jasmine and bright orange marigold flowers, Harshvardhan and I were hosting a question-and-answer session with the attendees. The atmosphere felt electric. The crowd was engaged, hanging on to every word.

It was about an hour into the event when the unexpected happened: I felt a raindrop land on my wrist. My heart sank. April rains in New Delhi are as rare as they are unpredictable. I knew we weren't prepared for the rain.

Before we knew it, we were hastily guiding the crowd under a canopy of trees. But it wasn't enough; the heavens opened, and the rain became heavy. Soon our beautifully dressed guests were drenched. Our carefully laid out food began to get wet, and our once-beautiful venue turned into a ground of mud puddles. Some people who had travelled miles to join us were seen making their way to the exit. We could sense the frustration in the air. To make matters worse, the large speakers we'd set up for the musical evening got wet in the rain and stopped working.

Thankfully, the venue had one indoor hall, but it was not designed to accommodate 500 people. We managed to squeeze everyone inside, wet and packed tightly together.

As the two of us stood at the front, alongside our team, 500 pairs of eyes looked at us, each probably wondering why we weren't prepared for the rain. But only we knew that there was no way we could have covered the entire outdoor venue. Even our team members looked at each other, worried. We didn't have a plan B.

When you've invested months of hard work into something, seeing it washed away (quite literally!) is not an easy feeling to deal with. My heart began to beat a bit faster. I felt nervous and helpless. I didn't know what to do.

Just as a tear was about to fall from my eye, a powerful thought surged through my mind, holding the tear back. The thought was clear and resonant: 'There is a Divine force at play. Trust it.' I looked at Harshvardhan, and somehow, I knew that the same realization had occurred to him.

Holding on to this thought, I felt the nervous tension in my body begin to slowly dissolve, replaced by a surprising sense of calm and clarity. Somewhere deep within, a strong sense of understanding had emerged: although things weren't happening as per our original plan, they were happening as per a larger, grander plan. This allowed us to not be overly affected by what was going on. It allowed us to think clearly and ask ourselves, 'What's the best we can do right now?'

With everyone packed in the hall, we asked them to sit down and made them comfortable. Together with our team members, we decided to lead a short meditation. As we did so, gradually, the tension in the room seemed to melt away; everyone became calm.

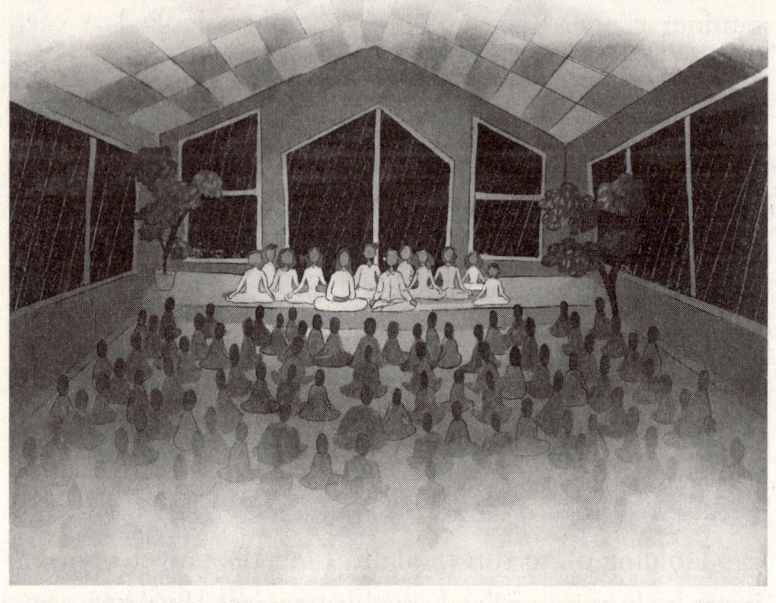

Soon after, the rain slowed down. We talked to the chefs and told them to start serving dinner right away. Sure, we had lots of puddles created by the rain in the entire venue, but we somehow managed.

Ultimately, we even held the musical performance which was led by our team, although it was not on the large outdoor stage we'd originally planned, but in the indoor space. Looking back, we think it was actually better—more cozy and intimate. In the end, the event didn't turn out how we had envisioned it, but it didn't matter. Everyone left the fest with a smile on their face and warmth in their heart.

The situation was such that it would have been very easy for us to become anxious, lose our composure, and make poor decisions. Had that happened, everyone would likely have left in the middle of the event, frustrated. However, the simple thought that whatever was happening was for the ultimate best allowed us to approach the moment with a sense of surrender, yet still do our best. In accepting things as they were, we found the ability to make the right decisions.

This mindset was shared not just by the two of us, but by the entire Satvic team. We believe it was this simple thought that saved the event. This attitude of surrender has helped us not once, not twice, but countless times throughout the journey of Satvic Movement. Whether dealing with negative criticism, technical glitches in our large online workshops or unexpected departures from the team, this mindset has helped us maintain our calm amid any chaos.

Now, here's a question for you: How often do you find yourself in situations that are totally out of your hands? When you want something, but the total opposite ends up happening?

For instance, you're reading this book and you're inspired to make changes in your life. You hoped your whole family would be supportive, but things don't go according to plan, and they simply don't understand your choices.

Or imagine this: You're in a relationship with someone you really care about, and you've planned to spend the rest of your life with them. But one fine day, they tell you that they want to end the relationship, and it's genuinely because of no fault of yours.

Lastly, imagine this: you've been working for years in a company, steadily climbing the corporate ladder, only to discover that a younger, less experienced colleague has been promoted over you.

In situations where things don't go as planned, how do you usually feel? Do you feel that 'life has been unfair to me', or think that 'I don't deserve this', or even wonder, 'Why is this happening to me?'

Whether we like it or not, all of our lives are full of challenges. One moment you're excitedly planning a trip to a wedding, and the next, travel restrictions have you grounded. You think you've found your soulmate, only for them to say, 'We need to talk.' Life is a roller coaster of ups and downs, but each time we hit a low point, many of us find ourselves severely stressed, worried, frustrated and sometimes even depressed, completely bowled over by life.

But here's an important distinction: We can't always prevent these stressors from coming our way. **But, we do have a choice in how we react to them**. This choice—whether to let these stressors affect us or not—is entirely within our control. We could either choose to sail through them gracefully and come out stronger, or we could struggle and fall further behind.

Would you like to develop a power within you that allows you to stay unshaken even when stressful situations arise? A resilience that keeps you centred, be it during a financial setback, an unpleasant work situation or a relationship issue? This might seem like an idealistic, far-fetched reality right now. But, if you found yourself nodding 'yes' to those questions, then this seventh habit is precisely for you. It's the final key of the Satvic revolution.

Introducing habit seven: Live in the Mode of Surrender.

In this habit, you will learn two mindset shifts that will help you remain calm even during the most difficult times of your life.

So sit tight, get comfortable and let's begin!

What Does 'Surrender' Really Mean?

'Surrender' may seem like a heavy nine-letter word, but in essence, it means accepting things as they are. In other words, it's about having the ability to see a higher plan in life's situations.

This might sound a bit abstract, so let's simplify it. When we can remind ourselves that everything happening in our lives is ultimately for the best and that there is a higher plan for us, even if we can't see it at the moment, that's when we are living in the mode of surrender.

Don't Get Caught Up with the Terms

When we rise in the morning and go out, we feel delighted to see everything around. The sun shines, the wind blows, clouds bring rain, crops grow, grains flourish, fruits ripen, flowers bloom and seasons change—we are all just witnesses to these events. We know that we are not the ones making these things happen. Just as there is a scientist behind the invention of a complex computer, similarly, we recognize that there is some Supreme Power that orchestrates these natural phenomena.

Different cultures and religions refer to this Supreme Power by various names. Some call it Krishna, others, Rama, Waheguru, Allah, Jesus, Shiva, or simply God. Some prefer terms like Higher Consciousness or the Universe, and many use names that aren't even mentioned here.

Please remember, the specific name is not what holds importance here. For the sake of clarity and consistency, we will use the term 'God' in this chapter, but feel free to interpret it in a way that aligns with your own faith or belief system. Should you become caught up by the terminology, or firmly hold on to either belief or disbelief, you may miss out on one of the most beautiful habits discussed in this book, and we certainly wouldn't want that to happen. So, dear reader, we humbly request that you don't get caught up in semantics, but take the essence of the learnings.

The First Mindset Shift to Remain Calm amid Any Chaos:

Trust the Divine Plan

Most of us have created a plan or a road map for ourselves, of how we would like our lives to unfold. This plan might look something like this:

'I will work hard and get into the college of my dreams.'

'Soon after, I'll get that high-paying job.'

'Then, I'll get a raise and buy a new car.'

'Eventually, I'll get married.'

'In due time, I will go on that much-needed vacation.'

'Then, I'll settle into a beautiful new home.'

'And somewhere down the line, I will definitely have a couple of kids running around.'

Your plan might look entirely different; however, the point is, we've all created this imaginary ladder of success. For now, let's call it our 'self-created plan'.

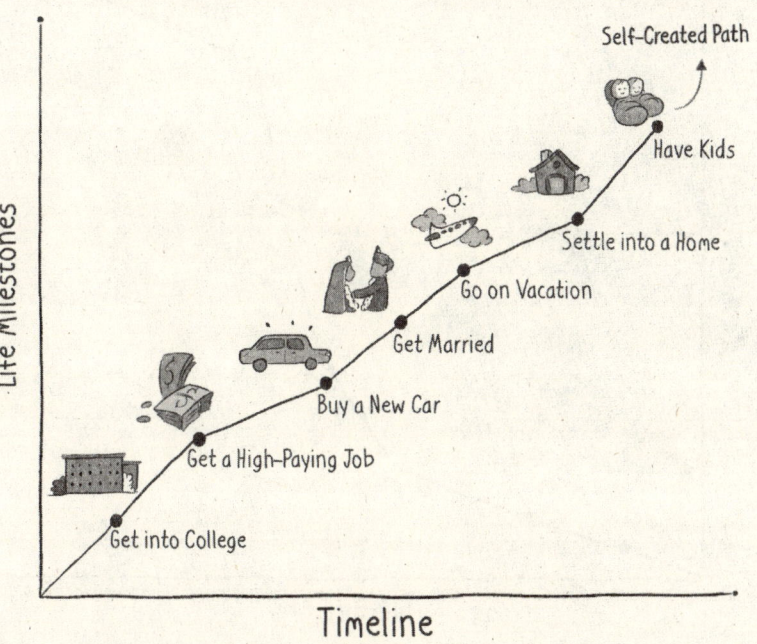

But, the question to ask is: Does life always follow this self-created plan? Does reality always align with what we hope and expect? Well, sometimes it does, but often it doesn't. This means that even though we create a plan for ourselves, our lives don't always adhere to it, and that's where the 'Divine plan' comes into play.

You can think of the 'Divine plan' as God's plan for us. In other words, it refers to the path that a higher power, God, the Universe or whichever Divine force you believe governs existence, has laid out for us. This Divine plan is shaped by our own past actions, or past karmas. This plan is the actual course that our life runs in accordance to.

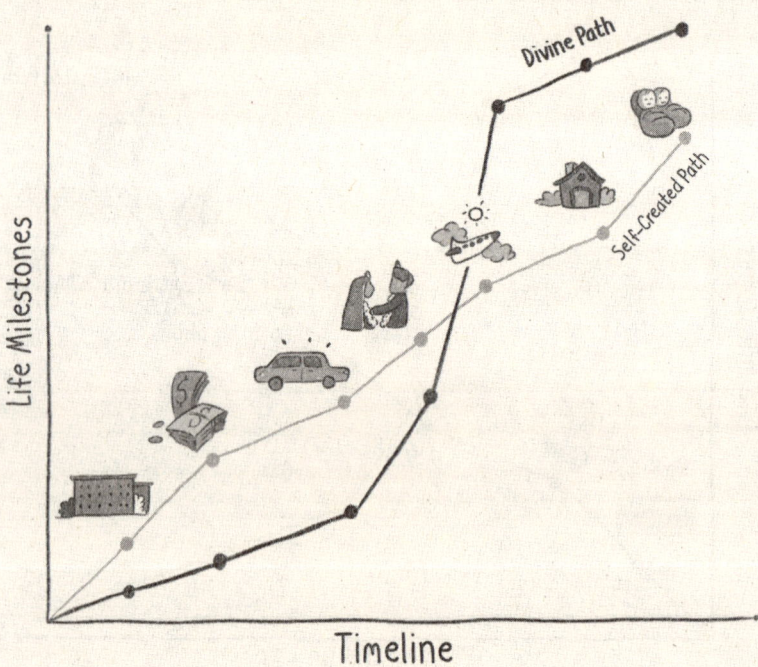

When the two plans (our self-created plan and the Divine plan) closely align, we feel satisfied, because things are going exactly as we had hoped. We feel content because we're getting everything we desired.

What happens when the Divine plan surpasses your own plans? When you receive more than you anticipated? Say you applied for a certain job but got an offer from a more lucrative one. Say you share your work online, only to find it's going viral and bringing you unexpected fame. Say you invest in some real estate and the value of your investment skyrockets. Or say you book a standard room for a vacation, but upon arrival, you find that you've been upgraded to a luxury suite at no extra cost. In all such instances, when God's plan is even better than your own self-created plan, you feel ecstatic. You celebrate with joy and thoroughly enjoy yourself.

And what about other times when this Divine plan falls below the self-created plan? When life doesn't go as planned? Say you work hard and expect a promotion, but it's given to someone else. Say you make a good investment but it results in a financial loss. Say you've been wanting a child but aren't able to bear one. Or say you hoped for a daughter but get a son. In all such situations, when the higher plan appears less generous than your own, you feel frustrated, disappointed, worried or even angry. If your aspirations were particularly important to you, you might even feel depressed. Such emotional responses, particularly when intense or prolonged, ultimately deteriorate your physical and mental well-being.

Now, in those difficult moments, if you remember and hold on to just one simple thought, it can make all the difference. The thought is this: 'There's a higher force guiding my journey, one that understands what's best for

me, even when I can't see it.' When you're able to realize
that your life events may not always be following your self-
created path but are instead governed by a greater path,
then you automatically find the strength to remain calm,
composed and joyful, even amid chaos.

For some of you, the concept of a higher force guiding
our paths might seem vague and elusive. Logically, it
may not even make sense. The concepts that we are now
discussing are not as black and white and may not be easy
to suddenly accept. However, this has been one of the
most powerful realizations in both of our journeys. It has
enabled us to remain resilient and avoid a lot of needless
stress when things haven't gone as per our plan. In this
story of the Clarke family, we hope to bring more clarity to
this concept, making it more tangible and relatable.

The Incredible Story of the Clarke Family

The Clarke family resided in England during the early
1900s, living a life of financial hardship. They had many
dreams and aspirations, but their topmost desire was to
go on a cruise holiday to the United States. The daughter
spoke endlessly about it with her friends, and their son
would often daydream about the trip. For years, Mr Clarke
scrimped and saved, penny by penny, to afford this holiday
for his family.

Then one evening, during dinner, Mr Clarke surprised
his family. He revealed tickets for their dream voyage which
was just a few months away. Mrs Clarke was so elated that

she baked a cake to mark the occasion, and the kids were jumping on the sofas and shouting with joy. That night, the kids even slept with the tickets tucked under their pillows, dreaming about all the fun they would have in America.

The next day, as their son was coming home from school, he was eagerly waiting to hold the ticket to the United States in his hands again. Wanting to get home quickly, he decided to take a shortcut. As he was jumping over a fence, something unexpected happened—a stray dog chased him and bit his leg, leaving the small boy crying in pain. He was taken to the hospital where he was administered an injection to protect against infection.

Fast forward to a few weeks later. Mr Clarke returned home from work a little later than usual. He looked visibly distressed.

Mrs Clarke asked him, 'What happened, my dear? Was everything all right at work today?' Mr Clarke explained that he had called their booking agent, and during their conversation, he happened to mention that their son had been bitten by a dog and had been given injections. As soon as he mentioned this, the agent informed Mr Clarke that they would have to cancel their tickets immediately, as the travel rules did not allow anyone who had recently been bitten by an animal to travel on the ship, as it posed a danger to other passengers.

Upon hearing this, Mrs Clarke burst into tears. All their dreams and aspirations had been ruined. She then delicately informed the children, taking care to not make her son feel guilty for the trip's cancellation.

As the son heard the news, he broke down. This had been his only dream for so many years. He had told all his friends about the trip and had been looking forward to it every passing day. The kids clung to their cancelled tickets, looking at them as if they were some kind of lost treasure. The parents tried to lift the children's spirits, reassuring them that they would go in a couple of years. But for now, with their dreams shattered, the kids remained quiet, with no smiles on their faces. The atmosphere in the house remained gloomy for the next many months, and the joy that once filled their home seemed to have evaporated.

Some time later, Mr Clarke rushed back home, panting and breathing heavily. He kept ringing the doorbell until Mrs Clarke opened the door. Mr Clarke yelled for the kids to come down to the drawing room immediately. 'Kids! Kids! Come, come now!' Mrs Clarke was so nervous, her heart was beating fast. She asked her husband what had happened. Mr Clarke continued to breathe heavily, his whole body in shock. It seemed as though a strange sense of fear had overtaken him. As the kids came down, Mr Clarke rushed to them and hugged them tighter than ever before. He broke down in tears. Mrs Clarke didn't know what was happening. She had never seen her husband behave like this before. She tried to understand what was troubling him, thinking, 'Why is my husband behaving like this? Why is he so anxious and tense?'

Then she noticed that Mr Clarke was holding something in his hands—it was a newspaper. She took the newspaper from him, and the headline read, 'The Titanic Has Sunk!'

Mrs Clarke's eyes became moist as she saw her husband cry and kiss their kids. 'We were meant to be on board, honey,' cried Mrs Clarke. 'Today, we wouldn't be together if we had boarded that ship.' The atmosphere in the home shifted from sadness to a sombre sense of relief. It dawned on them that all this time, when they so desperately yearned for something they couldn't attain, a higher plan had been quietly unfolding.

The Lesson

The Clarke family's story serves as a reminder that life doesn't always go as we want. They had painstakingly saved up for a trip to America—what we would call their 'self-created plan'. When their plans were cancelled, they were disheartened and devastated. It wasn't until much later that they realized how the seemingly unfortunate incident of their son being bitten by a dog actually saved them.

In our own lives, we, too, encounter situations that initially appear unfavourable from the outside. However, this story reminds us that what appears to be a setback, may actually be a blessing. It reminds us to stay equanimous and refrain from rushing to judgements when something bad happens in our lives. It reminds us to navigate through life's ups and downs with Grace, because there is always a higher plan in place.

So in all those moments in your life, when you find yourself frustrated, disappointed or upset, here's a gentle reminder to give yourself:

When things don't unfold as I wish, there's no reason to brood over it. Know that the Divine plan is much more thought through than my self-created plan, even if I cannot see it right now. Let me not look up to God as a victim and ask, 'Why is this happening to me?' Instead, let me look up as a seeker and ask, 'What could my learning from this situation be?'

This shift of mindset is easier said than done. But if you start embracing it, in even the smallest challenges you face, you'll be able to handle them gracefully and won't be tossed up and down by the waves of life. Gradually, you'll find yourself feeling more peaceful from within, understanding that life is unfolding exactly as it should, orchestrated by a wisdom far greater than your own.

Time for Some Reflection

Step 1: Take a few moments to look back at your life and identify three instances when things didn't go your way. It could be not securing admission to your dream college, not landing a job at your desired firm, a project you really wanted not coming your way, or even a heartbreaking break-up with someone you cared deeply for. Essentially, think about situations where you found yourself asking, 'Why is this happening to me?'—times when you felt rejected, dejected and unhappy. Jot down these three situations in the space below.

1.

2.

3.

Step 2: Now that you've written down those instances, it's time to reflect on them. Can you see any potential good that could have come from these situations? Maybe they helped you to grow, taught you invaluable life lessons or strengthened your emotional resilience. Write down your reflections, whether positive or not, in the space below.

1.

2.

3.

Looking back, were you able to recognize how some of the hardest situations in your life may have happened for your ultimate good? If yes, it's a testament to your ability to find meaning even in adversity. However, if your answer is no, that's fine too. Sometimes, it's difficult or even impossible to see anything good that could have ever come out of a situation. But the reality is, whether we realize it or not, each event in our life is unfolding for a reason. And some day, when we look back, the dots will all connect.

> 'You can't connect the dots looking forward; you can only connect them looking backward. So you have to trust that the dots will somehow connect in your future.'
> —Steve Jobs

Surrender the Outcome, Not the Effort

The first mindset shift we explored to remain calm amid chaos was to 'Trust the Divine Plan'. But as you read this, you may have wondered, 'If life is already laid out for me by this higher plan, why should I put in any effort? Why not just sit back, relax and let destiny take its course?' In fact, when I heard about this idea for the first time, I thought, 'Won't this turn me into a lazy person, who just waits for things to happen?'

But, here's the thing: Surrender doesn't mean surrendering your actions, your efforts or your responsibilities. It simply means **surrendering, or letting** go of your attachment to the results, to the outcomes, to the rewards.

This may sound like very high-level philosophy, but it's actually really simple! Let us explain using an example. Imagine you're taking care of a garden. You can water the plants, remove the weeds, fertilize the soil, etc. Those are your actions, your efforts. But whether the plants actually bloom and produce fruit—that's the outcome. While your efforts might increase the chances of a good yield, there's no guarantee. The weather, pests or other factors which are not in your control also play a role.

Living in the mode of surrender simply means taking care of your garden with your best, perfect actions, but not becoming attached to the fruits that may or may not come.

Essentially, living in the mode of surrender involves two steps:

1. Doing your actions, your duties, with utmost perfection.
2. Leaving the result, or the outcome of your actions, in the hands of God.

If you don't perform your actions to the best of your abilities, that's not surrender. That's laziness. Surrendering involves doing your very best, doing everything within your control, and yet, accepting whatever outcome you get as a result.

This mindset isn't something you can practise only occasionally or just when things go wrong. Rather, it's one that you can embrace even in the smallest aspects of everyday life, be it in your relationships, your exams, your job or even your health.

Wisdom from the Bhagavad Gita

Chapter 2, verse 47 states: 'You have a right to perform your prescribed duty, but you are not entitled to the fruits of action. Never consider yourself to be the cause of the results of your activities, and never be attached to not doing your duty.'

Wisdom from the Yoga Sutras

Many centuries ago, when Sage Patanjali wrote the Yoga Sutras, the foundational texts of yoga philosophy, he outlined five *Niyama*s (duties directed towards ourselves). The last and final Niyama he shared was something called 'Isvara Pranidhana'.

The term 'Isvara Pranidhana' is made up of two words.

- 'Isvara' translates to 'Supreme Being', 'God' or 'the Higher Power'.
- 'Pranidhana' means 'to surrender' or 'to devote'.

Essentially, Isvara Pranidhana is the practice of fully surrendering oneself to God or the Higher Power. It refers to having complete faith in the guiding and protective power of the Absolute Reality, living with a deep sense of being guided and cared for by something greater.

The Second Mindset Shift to Remain Calm amid Any Chaos:

Don't Impose Your Plan on the Higher Plan

Often, the world teaches us to approach God with a long shopping list.

A house by the sea

The latest new TV

A rich, good-looking partner

A car that's faster

A raise in my pay

A luxurious holiday

A lot of us treat prayers like a wish list: 'Help my daughter get married' or 'Get me that promotion', or 'Please let my favourite sports team win!' or 'Please get my in-laws' visit cancelled'.

In doing so, we do something without realizing—we end up imposing our limited plan on a greater plan, one that is far beyond our understanding.

Do you know who else tried to impose his will on the Divine plan? The prince. We want to share his story with you to illustrate this second mindset shift. We find that stories are the best way to learn and remember, and this is our favourite one. So let's dive into the tale of the prince and his wants.

The Story of the Prince and His Wants

Once upon a time, there was a kingdom, and all its residents were extraordinarily happy. They enjoyed good health and abundant wealth. The king and his family cherished their kingdom deeply. However, there was only one issue: the king was unable to find a suitable girl for his son, who was the prince.

The prince was approaching the end of his ideal marriageable age, and the king had left no stone unturned. He had reached out to all the neighbouring kingdoms, inquiring about their eligible princesses, and he had even scoured his own kingdom for a suitable partner for his son. But despite his efforts, nothing seemed to work out.

One day, about to lose all hope, the king summoned the prince into his chamber and said, 'We've tried everything, my son. Nothing is working. Now, only God can help us. Why don't you pray to Him?'

Taking his father's advice to heart, the prince embarked on a quest to find God. During this journey, he faced many difficulties. He went through scorching heat, torrential rains and biting winter. He travelled across fields, mountains, lakes and many tough terrains. Despite injuring himself along the way, he finally reached the gate of God.

After waiting for a few days, he finally had the opportunity to meet God. As soon as he entered, the prince bowed in reverence, saying, 'God, we owe everything to you. Our kingdom is prosperous, my family is wonderful and our people are the best anyone could ask for.'

Intrigued, God asked, 'That's wonderful, son. What brings you here?'

'There is just one problem. I am unable to find a wife. I'm not able to get married,' said the prince.

'Is that it?' God chuckled. 'Well, don't worry. This will be taken care of.'

Before the prince left, God inquired, 'Is there anything else you want? You've come a long way.'

'No, I have everything else I could ever wish for,' the prince replied. 'Just a wife and I'll be the happiest person alive.'

'Very well, consider it done,' said God.

As the prince approached his kingdom, he found it already buzzing with celebrations. There was a festival going on throughout the kingdom. His father had found a beautiful bride for him, and the people were overjoyed. The prince and his new bride married soon after, and the kingdom erupted in delight.

As the prince and princess spent more time together after their marriage, they came to realize that they were unable to bear a child. As the news spread, the kingdom fell into a state of despair. Concerned for the future of the kingdom, the king called for doctors from far and wide. The locals tried every home remedy they knew of. But despite these efforts, nothing seemed to work. A sense of despair filled the air, enveloping the kingdom in a mood of sadness.

This time, the princess approached the prince and said, 'Remember how you went to seek God's help when you

404   The Satvic Revolution

were struggling to find a wife, and how that led you to me? Why don't you go back to Him? I'm certain He will help us once again.'

Intrigued by the idea, the prince agreed that it was worth a try. Setting out once more, he went through the same difficult terrain again. He sustained injuries along the way, and managed to finally reach God.

As he bowed in reverence, God greeted him, saying, 'Ah, it's you again. You were here before.'

The prince replied, 'With your grace and mercy, we have everything we could wish for. Our kingdom is prosperous, our family is healthy, our people are happy and now, I also have the most wonderful wife.'

God then asked, 'So why have you returned? Is everything okay?'

The prince responded, 'There's just one thing missing: we are unable to bear a child. If you could grant us just this one blessing, the future of our kingdom will be secure.'

God replied, 'Is that all? How many children would you like?'

The prince said, 'Just one child would be enough to fill our lives with joy.'

God nodded and said, 'Consider it done. No problem.'

As the prince prepared to return to his kingdom, God posed another question: 'Is there anything else you desire? You've come a long way.'

The prince shook his head and said, 'No, God, by your mercy everything is already wonderful. Just a child and I'll be the happiest person alive.'

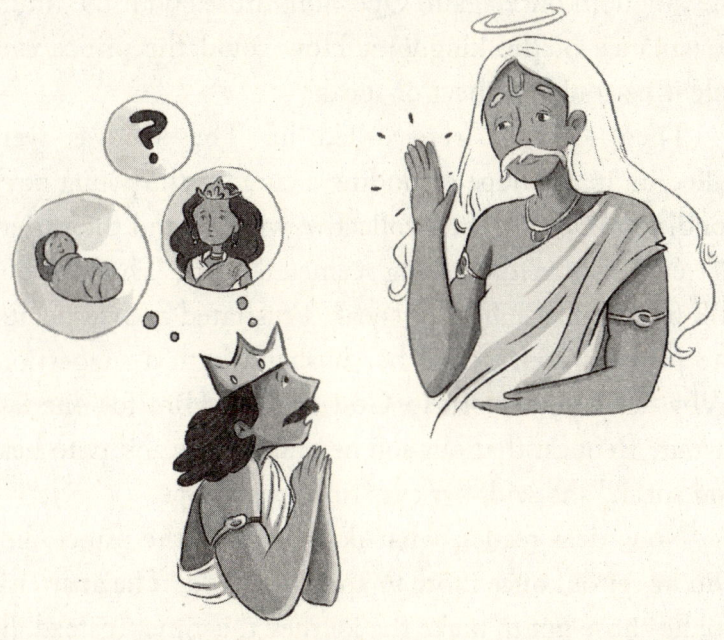

The prince returned to his kingdom to find that joyous news had already filled the air: his wife was pregnant. The entire kingdom erupted in jubilant celebrations; donations were made, feasts were prepared and grand parties were thrown. Everyone was ecstatic. Soon enough, a beautiful, chubby and cheerful baby boy was born, embodying everything the couple could have wished for. The celebrations in the kingdom continued for many weeks.

Fast forward to a year later, and the prince and princess were playing with their child, when they discovered a serious issue: their baby boy was unable to hear or speak. As word of the young heir's condition spread throughout the kingdom, a cloud of sorrow and worry spread across the kingdom once again. Questions arose about the future governance of the kingdom: How could the prince ever rule if he could not hear or speak?

Then, doctors were called in. The Vaidyas were called in, in the hope of finding a cure for the young boy's condition. Despite their collective wisdom and the variety of treatments tried, nothing seemed to work. The baby boy still wasn't able to hear or speak. Frustrated and desperate, the princess approached her husband with a suggestion. 'Why don't you return to God and ask Him for one last favour? Request that our son be granted the ability to hear and speak,' she said, her eyes filled with hope.

Now, dear reader, what do you think the prince did? Did he set out once more to approach God? The answer is no; he chose not to make the journey this time. Instead, he looked at his wife and said, 'I'm certain that if I go back to God with this request, He will grant our child the ability to hear and speak. However, I fear that afterwards, our son might speak such utter nonsense that I'll find myself praying for him to be silent.'

The Lesson

Each time the prince asked for something, he genuinely believed that getting it would make him the happiest person on the planet. But after some time, he found himself wanting something else. He failed to realize that his wishes, though earnest, might not necessarily make him happy in the long run.

This prince lives in all of us. We may not have a kingdom, but we've got wishes—lots of them. We keep praying to God, thinking, 'This is it. If I get this, it'll make me the happiest person alive.' We go to different temples, gurdwaras and mosques, begging for different things each time. Some of us even enter into transactional relationships with God, promising donations if our wishes come true. However, there are two problems with this approach:

1. **We have unlimited desires**
   As soon as we get what we originally desired, we forget about it. Then, we want something else. We have a new desire. As soon as we get that, it's gone. We again have a new set of desires, leaving us perpetually unsatisfied and continuing to ask for more and more.

2. **We often don't know what is genuinely best for us**
   We're short-sighted. We have a very limited view. Yet, throughout our lives, we impose our will and demands on God through our prayers. He might even grant our prayers, but they may not be what's best for us.

So, the lesson I take away from this story is simple: Don't make your prayers a wish list. Stop asking God to fulfil every fleeting desire. Trust that He knows what's best for us. If we could see the wonderful plan He has in store, we'd realize it's better than anything we could ask for. And in recognizing that, we'd feel content, with no need to keep asking for more things. This is what it truly means to live in a state of surrender.

Rather than imposing our own plans and desires of what we think should happen, let's turn our focus to expressing our gratitude. Instead of asking God, 'Can I please have this?' we can say, 'Thank you, God. You have given me so much.' **When we become grateful instead of wishful, we experience a deep sense of satisfaction and love for the life we have.**

To sum up these thoughts, there's a beautiful quote from the book *The Journey Home* by Radhanath Swami that encapsulates what we've discussed so far.

> 'It is better to pray to God for the strength to overcome the temptations, difficulties, and doubts in order to do His will, rather than for Him to do our will.'
>
> —Radhanath Swami, *The Journey Home*

In other words, when we pray, let's ask for the strength to follow the Divine plan that God has designed for us, rather than insisting that God follows our own crayon-drawn plan, that we have made for ourselves. This shift in perspective can make all the difference in how we view and interact with the world around us.

To Sum Up This Chapter

We've learnt two key mindset shifts to embrace, in order to stay calm amid chaos: 1) Trust the Divine Plan, and 2) Don't Impose Your Plan on God's Plan.

Concluding Note

To conclude, I'd like to share one last story from my childhood that had a profound impact on me. My mum and dad have always been extremely hard-working. Growing up, I saw them dedicatedly running their business, which specialized in producing modular kitchens. A couple of years earlier, they had taken a big step by establishing their own factory to manufacture these kitchens. The factory was quite large, situated in the outskirts of Delhi, equipped with top-quality machinery.

Given their busy schedules, it was usual for my parents to return home late in the evening. But this was not a problem because growing up, I lived in a joint family with twenty people living in one home. However, there was one evening that I'll never forget. It was around 8 p.m., and they still hadn't returned home. I kept calling my mum, but she didn't answer.

As the minutes ticked by, I was getting ready to sleep in my aunt's room when my mum finally picked up the call.

I asked her, almost furious, 'What happened, Mumma? Why are you coming home so late? When will you be back?'

To that, my mum didn't respond.

'Mum! Where are you?' I said. Then, I heard her weeping. My mum was crying.

'Our factory caught fire, beta,' she said.

It turned out that the newly established factory, which housed their dreams and hard work, had caught fire due to a short circuit. This enormous facility had been reduced to ashes, and all my parents could do was stand there, helpless, and watch their factory go up in smoke. Fortunately, the fire hadn't resulted in any casualties. I was young at that time and probably didn't grasp the financial loss this situation entailed. Shortly after sharing what had happened with me, my mum hung up the phone.

I attempted to sleep, but I found it impossible to do so knowing that my mum was in tears. After a few hours, I tried calling my dad. When he answered, I couldn't hold back my concern, 'What happened, Papa?'

His response left me utterly astonished. He calmly informed me that he had gone out with mum for dinner. I couldn't believe my ears, 'But, Papa, the factory has burnt to ashes, and you've gone out for dinner?' He reassured me not to worry, and that he and Mum would return home late at night, urging me to get some sleep.

As I listened to him speak, there was something peculiar about his tone. He didn't seem to have even a tinge of worry in his voice.

I was confused. How come my father was not worried? Did I miss something? By this time, exhaustion finally overcame me, and I drifted off to sleep, my mind still swirling with questions.

The next morning, I hurried to their room, wanting to know what had happened. When I arrived, my fears were confirmed: the factory had indeed suffered a devastating fire, and everything was reduced to ashes.

But what surprised me was that my father still didn't seem upset. Unable to contain my curiosity and concern any longer, I asked him, 'Papa, can I ask you something? If the factory has burnt down to ashes, why aren't you upset?'

He replied with a calm tone, 'Who said the factory has burnt down to ashes?'

I was confused and said, 'Mumma told me that the factory was burnt down!'

To which he replied, 'Beta, who said the factory has burnt down to ashes? All our mistakes have burnt down to ashes. We'll start anew from tomorrow.'

That single sentence changed something profound inside me. Witnessing such strength in my father's eyes taught me more than any lesson from school ever could. Usually, a situation like that could leave someone depressed for months to come, but I couldn't see a tinge of sadness in him.

Even when seemingly unpleasant things happen, having the ability to see the good, to let go of what we can't control, and to believe that even the worst situations are part of a bigger plan, all without wishing they hadn't happened—that takes a special kind of strength. I saw that strength in my father, and ever since, I've tried to live my life with that attitude of surrender, especially for things I have no control over. I guess what happened at the Satvic fest was just a small reflection of this value that I learnt from him.

Imagine if we could practise this value in every situation in our lives—whether we're stuck in a long traffic jam and running late for work, or dealing with the disappointment of a project we've worked hard on being rejected by our boss. Whether we end up missing a flight for an important event, or face a rejection from someone we dearly love. If we could handle everything, from the smallest to the steepest lows of our life, with grace, courage and an attitude of surrender, we could free ourselves from so much existing and future stress, and thus live a life of bliss, joy and peak health.

As we conclude this chapter, we've not only completed the seventh habit, but all the seven habits of the Satvic Revolution. If you're reading these words right now, you deserve a pat on your back. Wherever you are, give yourself a pat on the back! Now, what remains is the final chapter of this book. In this last chapter, we'll bring everything together and sum up the journey so far, sharing our four concluding messages with you, and a poem that's very close to our hearts.

14

Conclusion—This Is Where It Begins

One sunny day, in the heart of a bustling kingdom, a famous sculptor made his way to the royal court of a wise and wealthy king. The king's court was absolutely spectacular, with sunlight streaming through its large stained glass windows, intricate patterns drawn on its shiny marble floors, and sweet melodies by classical musicians playing all day long.

As the sculptor entered the king's court, he brought with him three beautifully sculpted statues. Each of the three statues was of a human figure, about 6 feet in height, made using smooth, high-quality clay. What was remarkable was that the statues looked exactly the same. They were also incredibly detailed, demonstrating the sculptor's mastery at his craft.

The king, captivated by their beauty, expressed, 'These are truly magnificent! How much do they cost?'

The sculptor, with a hint of pride, responded, 'Your Majesty, the first statue is priced at five hundred. The second is valued at fifty thousand, and the third, at 5 lakhs.'

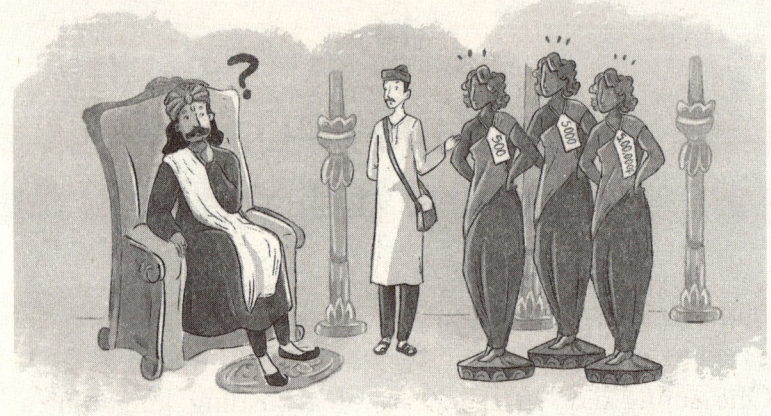

Upon hearing the sculptor's response, the king was taken aback. When the king inquired about why there was such a massive price difference, the sculptor refused to share the reason. This left everyone in the court—from the ministers to the courtiers—equally puzzled. 'Why such different prices when all three statues are exactly the same?' the king wondered aloud.

Then, the king summoned one of his ministers to come and investigate the reason behind the huge price difference among the three statues. As the minister approached, he examined each statue meticulously from every conceivable angle. He assessed their colour, their material, the flow of their curves and the precision of their edges. Despite his inspection, he found no difference at all. From the shape of their noses, the curve of their lips, the outline of their ears, the style of their hair, and even the drape of their clothing—all three statues appeared identical. This left the king more baffled than ever.

Then, the king called minister after minister to inspect the three statues. But all the ministers who came were equally bewildered. Now, the king was getting frustrated.

Finally, the king called his favourite and most talented minister, Rama, who was known for his wisdom and insight. The king presented Rama with the same challenge. Understanding the complexity of the task, Rama requested some time for a thorough examination. The king agreed.

Then, Rama carried out a detailed inspection of the three statues. He scrutinized every aspect, hoping to uncover even the slightest variance that might justify their varying worth. But after a few hours, he found himself standing in the same position as the other ministers before him—utterly confused, unable to discern any difference at all.

Finally, after some time, an idea struck him. Rama rushed off and came back with three red marbles. Everyone in the court—the ministers, the king and even the sculptor—watched intently, intrigued by what Rama might be attempting.

With the court's full attention, Rama proceeded with his experiment. He took the first marble and placed it into the ear of the first statue. To his astonishment, the marble rolled out of that same statue's other ear. This outcome sparked a murmur of surprise from everyone in the court.

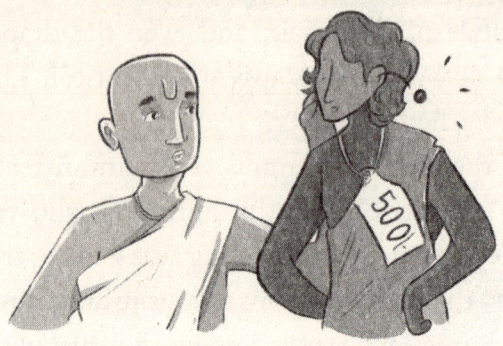

Encouraged by this discovery, Rama then took the second marble and inserted it into the ear of the second statue. This time, the marble emerged from that statue's mouth. This peculiar outcome deepened the mystery, leading to puzzled looks and whispers from the audience.

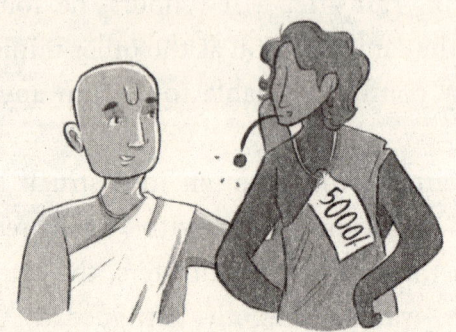

Finally, Rama placed the third marble into the ear of the third statue. Unlike before, this time, the marble never came out. It just vanished inside, making a sound as though it had rolled deep within that statue. It was as if it had been swallowed, leaving no trace of its passage.

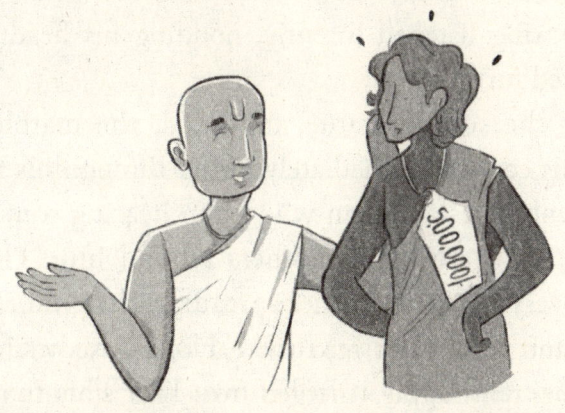

Rama was elated. He had found his answer. He turned to the king, with a tone of victory in his voice, and announced, while pointing to the third statue, 'This, my Lord, is the most precious of the three!'

The sculptor, who had created the three statues, bowed down to Rama, congratulated him and said, 'Yes, he is correct!'

However, the king, though impressed by Rama's confidence, was still confused. He wanted an explanation. 'Tell us, Rama, how have you come to this conclusion?' the king asked.

Then, Rama explained, 'My Lord, when I placed the marble in the first statue's ear, it rolled out of his other ear. This symbolizes a person who hears but lets everything he hears pass out through the other ear. It represents someone who listens but does not retain what is heard. Such a trait is not valuable. That is why this statue has the lowest worth.'

The king listened intently, nodding his head. Rama elaborated further.

'For the second statue, my Lord, the marble went inside his ear and immediately exited through his mouth. This symbolizes a person who upon hearing something, is quick to share it with others around him. He talks about everything he learns, spreading that information to friends and acquaintances. However, he fails to internalize and apply it in his own life. This too is not a commendable quality. Therefore, this statue is also considered of lesser value.'

The king's eyes widened in realization as Rama concluded his explanation. 'But when I placed the marble in the third statue's ear, it vanished, my Lord. This statue symbolizes a person who truly digests what he hears. He fully absorbs the information, internalizes it and makes it a part of his being. This is the mark of the superior individual who not only listens, but actually applies the knowledge. Without a doubt, this kind of person represents the highest form of wisdom, and thus, his statue has the highest worth.'

The king, deeply impressed by Rama, approached him with open arms and hugged him. He also purchased all three statues from the sculptor. The ministers, witnessing this moment, joined in the celebration. The atmosphere became charged with a sense of achievement and appreciation for the lesson that had unfolded in the royal court.

The Lesson for Us

This story carries an important lesson for each of us. Throughout this book, you've gained immense knowledge, and now, you have a choice—which type of statue do you want to be like?

In the context of this book, the first statue represents those who consume all the information but retain very little. The knowledge simply slips away, from one ear to the other, without having a lasting impact.

The second statue represents a person who reads everything attentively, even discusses it with others, but when it comes to applying that knowledge in real life, they fall short. Their learning doesn't translate into meaningful change.

Then there's the third type of person. They not only read but they also ensure that the knowledge permeates their being and guides their actions. These individuals hold the highest value because they turn learnings into actual change and thus, experience real-world results.

People often say that knowledge is power, but the truth is, **knowledge by itself is not enough**. The real power comes from applying that knowledge effectively. The story shows us that the goal of learning isn't just to accumulate information, but to bring about personal transformation.

The aim of this final chapter is to help you with that. In this chapter, we will summarize everything you've learnt so far. We will weave together the varied threads of wisdom you've picked up along the way into a realistic plan which you can actually follow in your day-to-day life, setting you on the path to real success!

Here's how you can expect this chapter to unfold:

- First, we'll engage in a practical activity that provides you with a clear road map for applying the seven habits to your life.
- Next, we will share our four closing messages with you. These messages will address the most common traps people encounter when they adopt these seven habits, and guide you on how to avoid them.
- Last, as a token of our gratitude to you for making it this far, we would like to unveil the larger vision behind the Satvic Revolution, showing you how this book is just the beginning of something much, much bigger.

So sit tight and get comfortable as we embark on the final chapter of our splendid journey together.

The Final Activity—Bringing It All Together

On the pages that follow, you'll find a list of all the principles we've covered for each of the seven habits. Next to each principle, you'll see two columns: one labelled 'I Can Start Now', and another labelled 'Not Ready for this

Yet'. All you need to do is read each action step and mark the column that fits best for you. If you're ready to start a habit right away, tick the first column. If you're not convinced or prepared to begin, then mark it in the second column for now.

When deciding what goes in each column, don't just think about today or this week. Think about the next month. Can you stick with the habit for thirty days? If yes, go ahead and mark it as something you can start immediately.

Remember: the goal here isn't perfection—it's creating a list that's practical. Be honest about what you can realistically start right now. Even if you only identify three or four immediate steps, that's great! It's far better to succeed at a few changes than to fail with an overly ambitious list that you end up quitting two weeks later.

Ready? Let's get started.

	I Can Start Now	Not Ready For This Yet
Habit 1: Keep a Clean Body Within		
Eat Your Dinner by 7 p.m. **Why:** In a world where our bodies are bombarded with toxins, internal cleanliness is key to health. By eating an early dinner, we allow our inner healer, our praanshakti, adequate time to cleanse the body and remove the toxins from within. **How:** Aim to eat dinner by 7 p.m. On days when this is not possible, the next best option is to eat a light dinner, avoiding an excess of grains and pulses.		

	I Can Start Now	Not Ready For This Yet
A bonus suggestion: **Start Your Morning with a Glass of Cleansing Juice** **Why:** Drinking a cleansing juice in the morning on an empty stomach aids the praanshakti in its cleansing work. **How:** Ash gourd juice is an excellent option for a cleansing drink. Just have a glass of it on an empty stomach every morning, and wait for at least one to one and a half hours before eating anything. If you can't find ash gourd juice, then any green juice, fresh coconut water or celery juice are excellent alternatives.		
Habit 2: Eat Living, Wholesome and Plant-Based		
No Dead Food (Eat Living) **Why:** Processed foods (such as chips, store-bought biscuits, breakfast cereals, namkeen, instant noodles, factory-made sauces, etc.) lack the vital life energy that our body needs. These foods are laced with food colours, preservatives and artificial flavours. They are designed to have a long shelf life, but ironically, they actually shorten our life. **How:** Before purchasing any food item, check which list it falls under (red, yellow or green). Additionally, make dead foods invisible in your environment. Out of sight, out of mind. Also remember to replace, not remove.		

	I Can Start Now	Not Ready For This Yet
No Refined Food (Eat Wholesome) **Why:** Nature provides foods as whole entities, each element playing an important role in its nourishment and digestion. The moment we remove one part—like the bran in grains—we're left with a refined food that has lost its nutritional value. **How:** Replace white sugar with unrefined/minimally refined options like dates or jaggery. Opt for whole grains and millets over refined grains.		
No Animal-Based Foods (Eat Plant-Based) **Why:** Eating meat affects our health on multiple fronts—physically, mentally and spiritually. Furthermore, in the case of dairy, the stress hormones from the cow are transferred to her milk. Additionally, three quarters of the world's population today struggles to digest the lactose found in milk. **How:** Embrace a plant-based lifestyle by quitting or at least reducing meat, fish and eggs. Switch from commercial animal milk to plant-based alternatives like home-made coconut or almond mylk.		

	I Can Start Now	Not Ready For This Yet
Habit 3: Sleep Like a Baby		
Disconnect from Technology One Hour before Sleep **Why:** Deep sleep is our body and mind's highest healing and recharging time. The prime sleep hours are known to be from 10 p.m. to 2 a.m. Using gadgets just before sleep disrupts melatonin production and overloads our mind with content, disrupting our natural sleep rhythm. **How:** Create a wind-down routine. To do this, disconnect from technology at least one hour before sleep and switch from high-stimulation activities to low-stimulation activities (such as reading, engaging in a recreational hobby, etc.).		
Wake Up in the Golden Hours (5 a.m.) **Why:** Waking up at 5 a.m. gifts us three extra hours every morning that we can dedicate to our personal growth. It's like opening a window to our creative genius thoughts and getting access to a flow state. **How:** Establish a solid reason for waking up early. Many find that reason in their '3M morning routine', focusing on movement, meditation and mastery. In addition, remember that in order to wake up early, we simply have to focus on sleeping early.		

	I Can Start Now	Not Ready For This Yet
Habit 4: Celebrate Movement		
Move Every day—Don't Miss Twice in a Row **Why:** When you move your body through various physical activities, you supply your cells with more oxygen, give your whole body a detox, boost your digestive system, and even uplift your mood. A body in motion stays alive. A body without motion decomposes. **How:** The key to consistency is to find a form of movement that feels like a celebration rather than an obligation. Don't break the chain. If unexpected events come up, don't miss twice in a row. Also, to ensure consistency, find an accountability partner.		
Habit 5: Nourish Relationships		
Let Go of Unresolved Relationships **Why:** Just as a constantly running AC in an unused room drains electricity, unresolved relationships—even those from a decade ago—continue to drain your life energy, or praanshakti. **How:** Communicate with the people you have strained relationships with, using the techniques outlined in the chapter.		

	I Can Start Now	Not Ready For This Yet
Seek First to Understand before Being Understood **Why:** When we don't truly listen to others, or only offer shallow forms of listening, we leave them feeling unheard, isolated and misunderstood. Mastering the art of seeking first to understand is underrated but an extremely powerful way to improve our relationships and our overall emotional well-being. **How:** Put aside the desire to offer advice, interrupt, compare or judge while the other person is speaking. Provide them with your undivided attention. Only after ensuring you've fully understood their perspective should you share your own thoughts.		
Habit 6: Live with a Purpose Worth Jumping Out of Bed For		
Identify Your Innate Strengths and Use Them to Serve Others **Why:** Studies from the Blue Zones show that a common trait among people who live extraordinarily long lives is that they have a deeply ingrained sense of purpose or mission in their lives. This sense of purpose, of having something exciting to look forward to each day, not only engages our mind but also adds a spark to our life, ultimately contributing to our health and longevity. **How:** Start by identifying your innate strengths—your unique birth gifts that you're naturally good at. Then, find ways to use these strengths to serve others. As a practical first step, devote just thirty minutes a day to practise and hone your innate strengths.		

	I Can Start Now	Not Ready For This Yet
Habit 7: Live in the Mode of Surrender		
Trust the Divine Plan		
Why: Living in a mode of surrender allows us to navigate the ups and downs of our life with a sense of ease, without getting stressed or depressed. It allows us to remain unshaken and calm even during chaos.		
How: Trust the Divine plan. Have faith in the journey that has been laid out for you. It's likely a better plan than anything you could conceive. Rather than imposing your own plans and desires on what you think should happen, turn your focus to expressing gratitude for what you've already received.		

Please ensure that you've taken the time to carefully read through each action step, assigning it to one of the two columns.

Even if you've committed to just two or three action steps from the previous table, that's a great start. It's far more effective to select a few goals that you can fully apply to your life—turning them into concrete actions (much like the third statue)—than to ambitiously choose many goals, only to find out a few months down the line that you're overwhelmed and all your learnings are slipping away (like the first statue).

There's power in starting small, and from there, you can build up to slowly incorporating more and more steps. Eventually, as you continue on this path, you'll discover that:

THE FIRST STEP IS NEVER JUST A FIRST STEP.

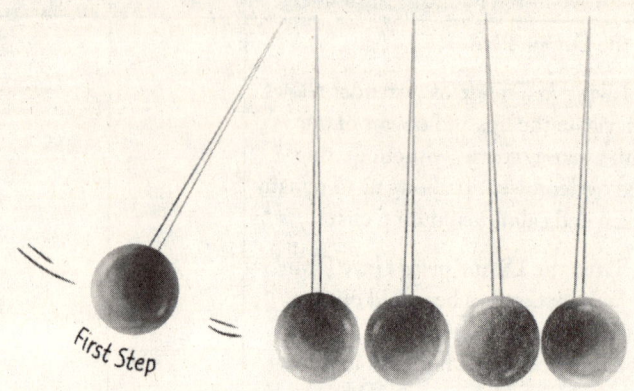

As you start living even one habit, it will naturally create a ripple effect, leading to the formation of new, positive habits, often without you even realizing it. So, focus on what you can do, not on what you can't, and start making changes from there.

Now, having completed the reflection activity, we want to share something important with you.

The knowledge that we have shared in this book is the same knowledge that we have been sharing with people from all corners of the world for many years. Yet, in our journey of guiding countless individuals, we've come to understand that not everyone experiences the same level of transformation. Some, despite possessing the knowledge and wisdom, fall into certain traps.

In the next section of this chapter, we want to share ways to avoid these common traps through our four concluding messages. Our aim is to help you steer clear of these traps right from the beginning, so there are no pitfalls stopping you from reaching and maintaining your peak health.

Our Four Concluding Messages for Your Journey

Message 1: Stay Connected to This Knowledge

As you embark on this journey, there will be many obstacles on your path. Whether you get stuck with those obstacles or seamlessly overcome them will depend on one thing: how connected you are with this knowledge. It's only when we stay in touch with this knowledge, that we garner the strength to not be swayed from our path. This is because the influence of our external world is so strong that over time, it's easy to let these habits slip from memory and gradually fade away.

So how do you stay connected to the knowledge? Well, here are a few ways we would like to suggest:

1. Join Satvic Movement's Twenty-One-Day Online Health Workshop. We start a new batch of this programme frequently. It covers the same seven habits but allows you to get a deeper understanding of each one. Participating in this programme will help you immensely in solidifying concepts that you've already learnt. Also, if you find it difficult to adapt to the habits alone, this programme will help you to connect with a community of like-minded people in your area.

2. If you'd like to delve deeper into any of these seven habits, we have dedicated online workshops for each one at Satvic Movement.

- For Habit 1 (Keep a Clean Body Within), we have the Three-Day Juice Fast.
- For Habit 2 (Eat Living, Wholesome and Plant-Based), we have the Seven-Day Satvic Food Workshop.
- For Habit 3 (Sleep Like a Baby), we have the Twenty-One-Day Early Waking Workshop.
- For Habit 4 (Celebrate Movement), we have the Twenty-One-Day Yoga Workshop.

If you want to learn how to reverse chronic lifestyle diseases naturally, we have the Seven-Day Healing Workshop.

To know more about these programmes, you can visit our website: www.satvicmovement.org

3. We've also compiled a list of some excellent books and documentaries on the same topics that we've discussed in this book. You can read or watch these to deepen your understanding. To access this resource list, simply scan the QR code below or visit satvicmovement.org/book/resources. We keep updating this list with the newest educational material.

Message 2: Be Disciplined But Also Know When to Be Flexible

We have witnessed many people falling into the trap of extremism. Once, we received a message from Sandeep, who was experiencing a lot of stress after learning and implementing the habits. When we asked him why, he explained that the stress stemmed from his struggle to strictly follow the habits he had learnt.

For instance, on a special occasion, his mother insisted that he should join some relatives for dinner at 8 p.m., but he declined because he was determined to stick to his 7 p.m. dinner schedule. This made his mother a little upset. On another occasion, his grandmother offered him a barfi which was a part of *prasad*, but he spat it out when he realized it contained refined sugar and dairy products. This made his grandmother upset. Then, one night, his younger sister called him, expressing that she wasn't feeling her best and needed someone to talk to, but he declined because he had committed to not using gadgets after 8 p.m. Now even his sister was upset.

Like Sandeep, we have spoken to quite a few people who rigidly adhere to rules and norms, often at the cost of flexibility, adaptability, and their social and emotional connections. They become hardliners. Extremists. And this tendency is particularly common in the early stages of one's journey.

Maybe you can relate to this, maybe you can't, but it's a trap you definitely don't want to fall into. Why? Because extremism is not sustainable. You won't be able to live these habits for long if you become an extremist. These habits are meant to liberate you and bring you happiness, not to bind you and make you miserable.

By becoming an extremist, you create stress for yourself but even worse, you might end up creating stress for others around you. You constantly worry about maintaining an exceedingly high level of control, viewing these habits as a strict set of rules. This creates distance in your relationships with loved ones, because they may feel they come second to your rules, reducing the quality and depth of your relationships.

How can you avoid becoming an extremist? Well, be disciplined, but also know when to be flexible. There will be moments when you must be flexible, particularly when dealing with the genuine emotions of your family members and loved ones.

For instance, take the case of Sandeep, whose grandmother had lovingly prepared barfi as part of a prasad offering. In this situation, Sandeep could easily maintain his discipline while also considering his grandmother's feelings. He could have actively been involved in the prasad-making process and created something that aligned with his food choices. Or, if that wasn't feasible, he could have graciously accepted a small portion of the barfi, knowing well that at that moment, he is deciding to prioritize his grandma's sentiments above his own discipline, knowing well that he is making an exception and this won't become the norm. When he does this, he should do it out of love, out of a genuine desire to bring happiness to his grandmother, and not out of force or pity.

What really helps in practising this is to be clear about what your **negotiables** and **non-negotiables** are. Out of everything that you have put in your first column (habits you have decided to follow), there may be a few things which you feel sure and determined about. Those are your non-negotiables; you don't compromise on them, no matter what happens.

However, there may be other things you want to follow but know you can't adhere to 100 per cent of the time. Those are your negotiables. For example, it could be eating dinner by 7 p.m., or it could be putting down your digital devices by 8 p.m.

You need to communicate your non-negotiable list to others around you.

So, for example, Harshvardhan and I are committed to not consuming animal products; it's on our non-negotiable list. We won't negotiate on this habit, no matter what happens. If we visit a friend's or family member's home, we call them in advance and request that they prepare food without dairy products for us. On the other hand, there are many values and habits on our negotiable list, like eating by 7 p.m., or celebrating movement each day. We do our level best to follow them, but if situations arise where we can't, we don't create a fuss or become too rigid.

Knowing your negotiables and non-negotiables helps you avoid becoming an extremist. You'll know when to be disciplined but also when to be flexible.

Message 3: Don't Look Down on Others Who Are Following Different Habits

As you live these new habits, you may notice a tendency to judge others who aren't following the same path. For instance, you might see someone consuming processed foods and think, 'Ah, they're so uninformed. They don't even know how much this is harming their body.' Or when you witness someone dominating a conversation without listening to the other person, you might think, 'They don't even understand the basics of communication.' Perhaps when you see someone waking up at 9 a.m., the thought might arise, 'Look at them, wasting their life away.'

Each time you catch yourself having such thoughts, remember that this is your ego speaking. This tendency to look down on others is a subtle one, but it's deeply damaging. While you may never express these judgements openly, internally you may begin to view others as 'wrong'. In doing so, your ego inflates, creating an illusion that you are superior to others. Falling into this trap completely defeats the purpose of living these habits.

So how do you avoid becoming a snob who looks down on others? Remember that everyone is on their own unique journey. By passing judgement, even if it's only in your mind, you're disrespecting their journey. Even if we mentally judge our family as wrong without voicing these thoughts, we are still sending negative energy their way. They can sense this, and in return, they may send negative energy back to us. This cycle of mutual negativity makes it impossible to follow the seven habits in harmony.

The right attitude to have is this:

'I am doing what's best for me based on what I know, and others are doing what's best for them based on what they know. I may not agree with them but I accept them wholeheartedly for who they are.'

When you carry this attitude in your heart, you'll find it much easier to live these habits cheerfully.

Remember: the essence of Satvic living is love. You may follow the healthiest diet, the most disciplined routine and have the most noble purpose, but if you criticize, compare, complain or compete with others, even if it's only in your mind, then you lose the very essence of this way of life, which is to carry love in your heart at all times. Never allow this to happen. Always remember: the greatest of all qualities, the greatest of all virtues is love.

Message 4: If You Want to Change Someone, Be a Lighthouse Yourself

Many of you often ask us, 'How do I bring my partner on board?'; 'How can I guide my children on the right path?'; 'My parents just don't listen—they are too moulded in their habits—how do I possibly change them?'

This can be one of the hardest things to do. In fact, it's what I struggled with the most when I first started this lifestyle. When I came back from attending the first four-day camp with my teacher, I wanted to throw out the packets of processed food and sugar from my house. I wanted to turn our whole kitchen upside down. But when my mum saw me doing all this, she thought I'd gone crazy—following some temporary fad which I'd soon forgo. This created a slight distance between us, because I really wanted everyone in my family to follow these principles, even when they didn't want to.

It wasn't until much later that I learnt the powerful mantra: 'Be a lighthouse, not a critic.'

You see, there's a huge difference between a lighthouse and a critic.

A lighthouse stands tall on the edge of the ocean, casting light in all directions. This light serves as a guide to the ships, enabling them to navigate safely to shore. The lighthouse does not go around looking for people or ships to provide its light to. Its sole purpose is to be a source of light itself, and due to its nature, it effortlessly illuminates the path for others.

This is very different from being a critic, who focuses on constantly telling other people what's right and what's wrong, pinpointing faults and passing judgements.

If you want to live these habits with love and harmony, be a lighthouse. Because when it comes to influencing others, criticism or enforcement rarely works. Instead, it pushes people away. They feel like you're 'policing' them. If you want your family, your partner, your kids or anybody else to also live these habits with you, don't force them to. Don't impose yourself on them. Instead, accept their choices, even if they differ significantly from yours. Meanwhile, live

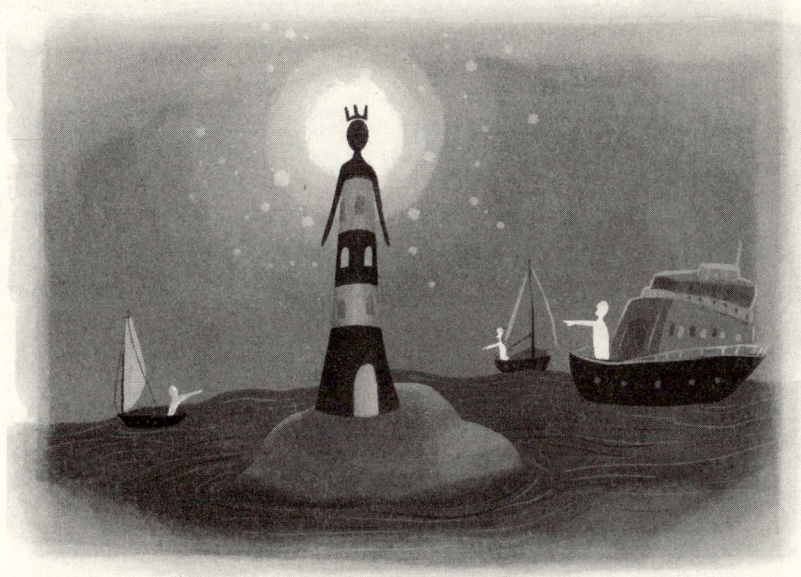

the change yourself. Incorporate this knowledge into your daily life first. As they witness your transformation and start to see the benefits you are enjoying, they may come themselves and ask you why you're making these lifestyle changes.

So, if you want to sustain this change, remember to:

Be a lighthouse, not a critic.

Be a role model, not a judge.

Inspire, don't enforce.

So those were our four concluding messages for you. To summarize:

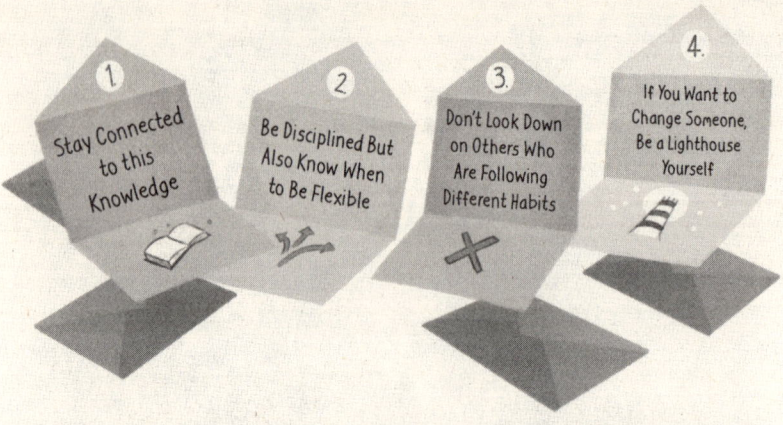

As we come to the end of the final chapter, we can now say that we have successfully shared with you all the tools in this book.

Remember, the habits you've learnt are more powerful than you think. Don't take them for granted. While much can be said about health, and there are a thousand different paths to wellness, what you've learnt in this book are the key elements—the 20 per cent that will yield 80 per cent of the results.

As we approach the final pages, Harshvardhan and I want to express our deepest gratitude to you. While writing this book, we often questioned whether we were sharing too much, whether anyone would read these words until the very end. Yet here you are, having journeyed with us from the first chapter to these last pages. We bow in respect to your commitment and thank you from the depths of our hearts for walking with us on this profound journey.

Before we part ways, there's one last thing we must share. The habits you've learnt—yes, they will undoubtedly improve your life. But they are more than personal routines; **they are catalysts for change in this world**. They are catalysts to create a revolution. A Satvic Revolution.

With every choice you make, with every decision you take, with every purchase you make, you are voting. You are voting for a world. When you live these habits with joy, you are voting for a Satvic world.

What is this Satvic world? What are we talking about? Since you've stayed till the very end, you need to know. This vision is what we at Satvic Movement are working towards—a vision etched in our hearts, a mission that ignites our purpose, a blueprint of a new world that pulses through our veins. This book and everything you've learnt, is just a small part of this vision.

What is this Satvic world we speak of? What is this vision? Allow us to share.

The Vision

Imagine a world where health is the norm, not an exception,
As people live in sync with Mother Nature's perfection.

Where every individual realizes the power of the healer
      sitting inside,
Giving it a chance to heal, repair, fix and constantly guide.

Where illnesses and diseases are rare,
And doctor visits are reserved only for urgent care.

Imagine a world adorned with Satvic centres in every city,
Where people can come and connect with their like-
     minded community.

Within each centre resides a cafe, serving Satvic food
     that heals,
And tiffin services delivering living, wholesome and
     plant-based meals.

The weekly farmers' market here provides the freshest
     veggies and fruits,
Connecting people to their farmers, and thus back to
     their roots.

The big open *yogashala*s here provide abundant
     opportunity and space,
For each one to celebrate the movement their heart
     can embrace.

There are also workshop halls where wisdom is
     constantly flowing,
With hundreds of Satvic educators, people are
     continuously growing.

Imagine a world where processed food loses its allure,
As people are no longer interested in food that's impure.

A world where fast-food giants bow to the demand for a
    healthier menu,
And even McDonald's and Burger King are considering a
    total renew.

Fries are forgotten, as demand for unhealthy food drops,
And as you stroll down streets, you see more fresh juice
    than liquor shops.

A world where cigarettes have become a thing of the past,
And dying from cancer and heart disease is no longer in
    anybody's forecast.

Imagine a world where empathy and respect you can
    abundantly find,
A world which is compassionate to every kind.

A world where we humans no longer view ourselves as
    superior to our animal friends,
As for all species, there is love and care that transcends.

A world where animals are no longer hurt or killed,
Not for their food, not for their skin, not for their milk.

Imagine a world where the same compassion extends to
    Mother Earth,
Where even large corporations start understanding a
    green planet's worth.

Big businesses say no to using plastic, which chokes our
    oceans deep,
And yes to sustainable practices, thus making a huge leap.

Imagine a world where the educational systems for our
    children extend beyond calculus, algebra, geography
    and athletics,
And also teach the importance of true health and value-
    based ethics.

Imagine a world where stress and depression have hit an
    all-time low,
Free from lust and greed, each person's face has a special
    glow.

Where selfless giving and service is the norm,
Where goodness, joy, love and health thrives in every form.

This is not a dream, neither a vision, nor a whim that will
    succumb,
But a blueprint of a Satvic world, and its making has
    already begun.

Remember, our dear reader, every choice you make creates
    this reality,
Every small action you take ripples out in ways you may
    not even see.

When you live with intent, each habit you've learnt,
You pave the path to not only your own peak health,
But also to a Satvic world, in turn.

With that, we close this last chapter of our book.

Sending you boundless love,
Subah, Harsh
and the entire Satvic Team

Acknowledgements

We feel humbled and grateful to share this timeless wisdom with you. However, we truly feel this book is not ours alone. While the two of us have put it together, it is the collective effort of many special people who have contributed immensely to bring it to life.

First and foremost, we'd like to thank both of our mothers, who are embodiments of selfless service. They have built the foundation of everything we ever do, being the strongest pillars of our lives. They tolerated us being on the computer all day long when we could've been doing things they may have preferred.

Next, I'd like to thank my father. He was the one who pushed me to start Satvic Movement in the first place. He gave me the most precious gift in my life: belief. He was the first one to ever believe in me. He saw my potential and worth when I couldn't see it in myself. A lot of the core values I carry in my life have emanated from him.

We'd also like to thank our two elder sisters, Vartika and Prachita, and our younger brother Ishat—for loving us unconditionally and for being such beacons of inspiration, joy and wisdom in our lives.

We extend our heartfelt thanks to all the masters, teachers and gurus who have shaped us. It would fill many pages if we name each one. In particular, we want to mention Acharya Mohan Guptaji. I met him first when I was only seventeen years old. He taught me how I could heal my body by changing simple habits. He gave me hope when all hope was lost. He introduced me to the healer within me.

We also pay homage to the teachers we couldn't meet: Acharya Lakshman Sharmaji and Sheshadari Swaminathanji. They wrote timeless books on health and healing which we spent many years reading and studying.

We thank Shivender Nagarji—a teacher who has been selflessly sharing the wisdom of the Gita. A lighthouse himself, he's been illuminating the path for many along their spiritual journey, including ours.

We thank Brian and Anna Marie, who run the Hippocrates Health Institute, a place where a lot of our learnings were born.

To the teachers we've mentioned here and to all the other extraordinary teachers who have enriched our lives, we bow in reverence.

Also, a big thank you to Lovyaa Garg, for bringing these seven habits to life through her beautiful illustrations, for being so warm and patient, and for creating and recreating many illustrations.

Thank you to our researcher Jordan Smith, for being so meticulous in verifying every fact, claim and the research presented in this book, ensuring its accuracy and integrity, and for being such a joy to work with.

We would like to thank our two doctors— Dr Anand Gopalakrishnan and Dr Shailendra Chaubey— for reviewing the chapters, giving us their feedback and ensuring that every concept shared is in alignment with medical science.

Thank you to two special spiritual guides: Radheshyam Das Prabhu and Sesa Prabhu, for their thoughtful, in-depth review of the last two habits, ensuring that they are in alignment with scriptural wisdom.

Our hearts swell with gratitude when we think of all the Satvic team members whose collective efforts have made this book a reality. To name a few, we thank Mun, for organizing the feedback calls with the community. Christina, for her honest and critical feedback. Radhika, for constantly reminding us to not rush the process and give it the time it deserves. Anandi and Lipika, for being ready to do any kind of research work, no matter how tight the deadline. Himadri, for having the courage to tell us the limitations of the philosophy and then painstakingly finding ways to fix each one. A big thank you to all other Satvic team members who allowed us to take a step back from our daily work and immerse ourselves in the writing process.

Our sincere gratitude to the hundreds of early readers of this book from the Satvic community. Thank you for taking the time to sit through the two-hour reading sessions every Sunday morning, and then patiently filling out the long feedback forms with your honest and raw thoughts, telling us what real-life problems you face while living these habits. There were times when we would read your feedback and say to each other, 'Oh my, what a powerful community!' Your feedback made such massive contributions to this book, and it wouldn't have been what it is without you.

Also a big thank you to the whole team at Penguin Random House India. Writing a book was a distant dream for us till a few years ago. But you made it come alive! Thank you to our editor Deepthi, not only for being so patient with us as we continuously pushed deadlines, but also for giving us the opportunity to write this book in the first place.

Lastly, we thank Mother Nature, our loving, eternal mother, and God, our Divine, life-giving father, for choosing us as instruments to spread this message, for blessing us with all the people in our lives who we've listed above, and for providing us with the wisdom and strength to take this timeless knowledge forward.

References

In this section, we have included a detailed list of scientific research studies and references for each chapter in the book. With the assistance of a dedicated researcher, we have tried our best to provide as much useful information as possible regarding the sources of the material. We trust that readers, especially those seeking to delve deeper into the research, will find this compilation beneficial.

Introduction

'Real health comes when your physical, mental and spiritual health are all well-nourished and thriving.' Hawks, Steven. 2004. 'Spiritual Wellness, Holistic Health, and the Practice of Health Education'. *American Journal of Health Education* 35(1): 11–18. https://doi.org/10.1080/19325037.2004.10603599

'. . . and even your spiritual health—allowing you to grow across all areas of your well-being.' Ng, S.M., Josephine K.Y. Yau, Cecilia L.W. Chan, Celia H.Y. Chan and David Y.F. Ho. 2005. 'The Measurement of Body-Mind-Spirit Well-Being'. *Social Work in Health Care* 41(1): 33–52. https://doi.org/10.1300/j010v41n01_03.

Chapter 1: The Twelve-Step Health Test

'Sanskrit shloka from a traditional Nature Cure text.' *Swadheen Swasthya Maha Vidya (1500 Shlok). NATURAL LIFESTYLE.* Natural Life Style Shloka 23–24.

'If you're not clearing your bowels every day, it means that the waste that was supposed to exit your body is staying and collecting inside.' Pan, Ruili, Linlin Wang, Xiaopeng Xu, Ying Chen, Haojue Wang, Gang Wang, Jianxin Zhao and Wei Chen. 2022. 'Crosstalk between the Gut Microbiome and Colonic Motility in Chronic Constipation: Potential Mechanisms and Microbiota Modulation'. *Nutrients* 14(18): 3704. https://doi.org/10.3390/nu14183704.

'By implementing the habits you're going to learn about in this book, your body will naturally come to its optimal weight.' Müller, Manfred. 2010. 'Is There Evidence for a Set Point that Regulates Human Body Weight?'. *F1000 Medicine Reports* 2 (August). https://doi.org/10.3410/m2-59.

'Your skin is like a mirror, showing the reflection of your body's internal state.' Genuis, Stephen J., Detlef Birkholz, Ilia Rodushkin and Sanjay Beesoon. 2010. 'Blood, Urine, and Sweat (BUS) Study: Monitoring and Elimination of Bioaccumulated Toxic Elements'. *Archives of Environmental Contamination and Toxicology* 61(2): 344–57. https://doi.org/10.1007/s00244-010-9611-5.

'Hunger of the mind is the kind that craves something spicy, salty or sweet every few hours.' Volkow, Nora D., Gene-Jack Wang and Ruben D. Baler. 2011. 'Reward, Dopamine and the Control of Food Intake: Implications for Obesity'. *Trends in Cognitive Sciences* 15(1): 37–46. https://doi.org/10.1016/j.tics.2010.11.001.

'A healthy person experiences real hunger at least once a day.' Klok, M.D., S. Jakobsdottir and M.L. Drent. 2007. 'The Role of Leptin and Ghrelin in the Regulation of Food Intake and Body Weight in Humans: A Review'. *Obesity Reviews: An Official Journal of the International Association for the Study of Obesity* 8(1): 21–34. https://doi.org/10.1111/j.1467-789X.2006.00270.x.

'It is during deep sleep when the maximum healing of the body takes place.' Eugene, Andy R. and Jolanta Masiak. 2015. 'The Neuroprotective Aspects of Sleep'. *PubMed* 3(1): 35–40.

'Chronic pain . . . [is] your body's way of whispering to you that something is just not right within.' Havelin, Joshua and Tamara King. 2018. 'Mechanisms Underlying Bone and Joint Pain'. *Current Osteoporosis Reports* 16(6): 763–71. https://doi.org/10.1007/s11914-018-0493-1.

'One aspect that impacts how joyful you feel is your relationship with others.' Maes, Michaël et al. 2018. 'Early Life Trauma Predicts Affective Phenomenology and the Effects Are Partly Mediated by Staging Coupled with Lowered Lipid-Associated Antioxidant Defences'. *BioRxiv* (Cold Spring Harbor Laboratory). https://doi.org/10.1101/397711.

'. . . elevates levels of stress hormones like cortisol in your body, which is linked with problems.' O'Connor, Daryl B., Julian F. Thayer and Kavita Vedhara. 2020. 'Stress and Health: A Review of Psychobiological Processes'. *Annual Review of Psychology* 72(1): 663–88. https://doi.org/10.1146/annurev-psych-062520-122331.

Chapter 2: The Surprising Ancient Practice for Inner Cleansing

'But if we ignore the symptoms for several years, these toxins, or this accumulated waste matter can also lead to chronic lifestyle diseases such as diabetes, thyroid imbalance, hypertension, etc.' Riccio, Paolo and Rocco Rossano. 2019. 'Undigested Food and Gut Microbiota May Cooperate in the Pathogenesis of Neuroinflammatory Diseases: A Matter of Barriers and a Proposal on the Origin of Organ Specificity'. *Nutrients* 11(11): 2714. https://doi.org/10.3390/nu11112714.

'In the Aṣṭāṅga Hṛdaya, one of the primary classical Ayurvedic texts, these "toxins" are referred to as "āma".' Vāgbhaṭa. 2017. Aṣṭāṅga Hṛdaya of Vāgbhaṭa.

'We, as a generation, need constant detoxification today more than ever before.' Jackson, Erin, Robin Shoemaker, Nika Larian and Lisa Cassis. 2017. 'Adipose Tissue as a Site of Toxin Accumulation'. *Comprehensive Physiology* 7 (4): 1085–1135. https://doi.org/10.1002/cphy.c160038.

'In the *Charaka Samhita*, one of the foundational Ayurvedic texts, this digestive fire is termed "*jatharagni*".' Charaka. Charaka-samhita: translated into English. Calcutta: Avinash Chandra Kaviratna, (18901914).

'Today, even research studies are reaffirming what our age-old traditions have always said.' Simon, Stacey L., Jennifer Blankenship, Emily N.C. Manoogian, Satchidananda Panda, Douglas G. Mashek and Lisa S. Chow. 2022. 'The Impact of a Self-Selected Time Restricted Eating Intervention on Eating Patterns, Sleep, and Late-Night Eating in Individuals with Obesity'. *Frontiers in Nutrition* 9 (October). https://doi.org/10.3389/fnut.2022.1007824.

'These rhythms, driven largely by our exposure to sunlight, suggest that our metabolism and digestive ability are more active during daylight hours.' Mihaylova, Maria M., Amandine Chaix, Mirela Delibegović, Jon J. Ramsey, Joseph Bass, Girish C. Melkani, Rajat Singh et al. 2023. 'When a Calorie Is Not Just a Calorie: Diet Quality and Timing as Mediators of Metabolism and Healthy Aging'. *Cell Metabolism* 35(7): 1114–31. https://doi.org/10.1016/j.cmet.2023.06.008.

'In a recent study published in 2022, scientists looked at data from nine rigorous clinical trials involving 485 adults.' Deota, Shaunak, et al. 2023. 'Diurnal Transcriptome Landscape of a Multi-Tissue Response to Time-Restricted Feeding in Mammals'. *Cell Metabolism* 35(1): 150–65. https://pubmed.ncbi.nlm.nih.gov/36599299/.

Clinical study on Ash Gourd: Gupta, Prerna, Sivanand Chikkala, and Priyanka Kundu. 2019. 'Ash Gourd and Its Applications in the Food, Pharmacological and Biomedical Industries'. *International Journal of Vegetable Science* 27(1): 44–53. https://www.researchgate.net/publication/337854043_Ash_gourd_and_its_applications_in_the_food_pharmacological_and_biomedical_industries.

Clinical study on Ash Gourd: Dingare, Shraddha, et al. 2023. 'Overview of Ash Gourd as a Nutraceutical Source'. *International Journal of Pharmacy and Pharmaceutical Research* 27(1): 214–21. https://ijppr.humanjournals.com/wp-content/uploads/2023/05/16.Tushar-Undegaonkar-Dipasha-Sugnani-Shraddha-Dingare.pdf.

Chapter 3: Truths That Packaged Food Companies Hope You Never Find Out

'Some anecdotal accounts showed that even after several weeks of being left on the counter, some fast-food burgers hardly changed in their appearance or composition.' Greenwald, Morgan. 2022. 'Woman Alarms TikTok Users with Video of 24-Year-Old McDonald's Meal: 'Never Eating Fast Food Again'. *In the Know.* 28 July 2022. https://www.intheknow.com/post/a-woman-kept-a-mcdonalds-meal-in-her-closet-for-24-years-and-it-looks-good-as-new/.

'Multiple studies have indicated these additives have carcinogenic properties (cancer-causing properties).' Kobylewski, Sarah and Michael F. Jacobson. 2012. 'Toxicology of Food Dyes'. *International Journal of Occupational and Environmental Health* 18(3): 220–46. https://doi.org/10.1179/1077352512Z.00000000034.

Detailed studies on the health implications of chemical additives:

Hiasa, Yoshio et al. 1988. 'The Promoting Effects of Food Dyes, Erythrosine (Red 3) and Rose Bengal B (Red 105), on Thyroid Tumors in Partially Thyroidectomized N-Bis(2-Hydroxypropyl)- Nitrosamine-Treated Rats'. *Japanese Journal of Cancer Research* 79(3): 314–19. https://doi.org/10.1111/j.1349-7006.1988.tb01593.x.

Sasaki, Yu F. et al. 2002. 'The Comet Assay with 8 Mouse Organs: Results with 39 Currently Used Food Additives'. *Mutation Research/Genetic Toxicology and Environmental Mutagenesis* 519(1-2): 103–19. https://doi.org/10.1016/s1383-5718(02)00128-6.

Vorhees, C.V., R.E. Butcher, R.L. Brunner, V. Wootten and T.J. Sobotka. 1983. 'Developmental Toxicity and Psychotoxicity of FD and c Red Dye No. 40 (Allura Red AC) in Rats'. *Toxicology* 28(3): 207–17. https://doi.org/10.1016/0300-483x(83)90118-x.

'It exposed the lengths to which food companies go.' Moss, Michael. 2021. *Hooked*. Random House.

'Packaged foods are engineered for addiction.' Fuhrman, Joel. 2018. 'The Hidden Dangers of Fast and Processed Food'. *American Journal of Lifestyle Medicine* 12(5): 375–81. https://doi. org/10.1177/1559827618766483.

'Motivation is overrated. Environment matters more.' Clear, James. 2018. *Atomic Habits: Tiny Changes, Remarkable Results: An Easy & Proven Way to Build Good Habits & Break Bad Ones.* New York: Avery, Penguin Publishing Group.

Chapter 4: The Two Most Sneaky Culprits in Your Kitchen

'94 per cent of the rats preferred sugar water over cocaine!' Lenoir, Magalie, Fuschia Serre, Lauriane Cantin and Serge H. Ahmed. 2007. 'Intense Sweetness Surpasses Cocaine Reward'. Edited by Bernhard Baune. *PLoS ONE* 2(8): e698. https://doi.org/10.1371/journal. pone.0000698.

'When we consume sugar, the amount of dopamine released in the brain increases, just like the response triggered when we take an addictive drug.' Ahmed, Serge H., Karine Guillem and Youna Vandaele. 2013. 'Sugar Addiction: Pushing the Drug–Sugar Analogy to the Limit'. *Current Opinion in Clinical Nutrition and Metabolic Care* 16(4): 434–39. https://doi.org/10.1097/mco.0b013e328361c8b8.

Bennett, Connie. 'The Rats Who Preferred Sugar over Cocaine'. 2010. HuffPost. 10 September 2010. https://www.huffpost.com/entry/the-rats-who-preferred-su_b_712254.

'. . . excess sugar in our diet is stored as fat in our body, causing excessive weight gain.' Te Morenga, L., S. Mallard and J. Mann. 2012. 'Dietary Sugars and Body Weight: Systematic Review and Meta-Analyses of

Randomised Controlled Trials and Cohort Studies'. *BMJ* 346 (January 2013): e7492–92. https://doi.org/10.1136/bmj.e7492.

'Short-term studies also link high sugar intake to elevated blood sugar levels, diabetes . . .' Gulati, Seema and Anoop Misra. 2014. 'Sugar Intake, Obesity, and Diabetes in India'. *Nutrients* 6(12): 5955–74. https://doi.org/10.3390/nu6125955.

'. . . high triglycerides, increased blood pressure and heart disease.' DiNicolantonio, James J., Sean C. Lucan and James H. O'Keefe. 2016. 'The Evidence for Saturated Fat and for Sugar Related to Coronary Heart Disease'. *Progress in Cardiovascular Diseases* 58(5): 464–72. https://doi.org/10.1016/j.pcad.2015.11.006.

'When you eliminate refined sugar from your diet, it's amazing how quickly your body responds.' Della Corte, Karen, Ines Perrar, Katharina Penczynski, Lukas Schwingshackl, Christian Herder and Anette Buyken. 2018. 'Effect of Dietary Sugar Intake on Biomarkers of Subclinical Inflammation: A Systematic Review and Meta-Analysis of Intervention Studies'. *Nutrients* 10(5): 606. https://doi.org/10.3390/nu10050606.

'Our digestive system has to work extra hard to push it out of our body, and often, it isn't fully eliminated, resulting in incomplete digestion and thus the creation of toxins inside.' Iversen, Kia Nøhr, Johan Dicksved, Camille Zoki, Rikard Fristedt, Erik A. Pelve, Maud Langton and Rikard Landberg. 2022. 'The Effects of High Fiber Rye, Compared to Refined Wheat, on Gut Microbiota Composition, Plasma Short Chain Fatty Acids, and Implications for Weight Loss and Metabolic Risk Factors (the RyeWeight Study)'. *Nutrients* 14(8): 1669. https://doi.org/10.3390/nu14081669.

'. . . those who consumed more refined grains ended up with more belly fat and weight gain.' McKeown, Nicola M., Lisa M. Troy, Paul F. Jacques, Udo Hoffmann, Christopher J. O'Donnell and Caroline S. Fox. 2010. 'Whole- and Refined-Grain Intakes Are Differentially Associated with Abdominal Visceral and Subcutaneous Adiposity in Healthy Adults: The Framingham Heart Study'. *American Journal of Clinical Nutrition* 92(5): 1165–71. https://doi.org/10.3945/ajcn.2009.29106.

'. . . the more refined grains these ladies had on their plates, the higher their risk of developing obesity.' Liu, Simin, Walter C. Willett, JoAnn E. Manson, Frank B. Hu, Bernard Rosner and Graham Colditz. 2003. 'Relation between Changes in Intakes of Dietary Fiber and Grain Products and Changes in Weight and Development of Obesity among Middle-Aged Women'. *American Journal of Clinical Nutrition* 78(5): 920–27. https://doi.org/10.1093/ajcn/78.5.920.

Chapter 5: Animals: To Eat or Not to Eat?

'Meats, especially red and processed meats, are high in saturated fats. Over time, their consumption can elevate cholesterol levels in our blood.' Sun, Le et al. 2022. 'Red Meat Consumption and Risk for Dyslipidaemia and Inflammation: A Systematic Review and Meta-Analysis'. *Frontiers in Cardiovascular Medicine* 9. https://doi.org/10.3389/fcvm.2022.996467.

'As these fatty deposits continue to build in the arteries over the years (much like a clogged pipe), it makes them narrower and narrower.' Al-Shaar, Laila et al. 2020. 'Red Meat Intake and Risk of Coronary Heart Disease among US Men: Prospective Cohort Study'. *BMJ 371* (December): m4141. https://doi.org/10.1136/bmj.m4141.

'In 2020 the *British Medical Journal* published a study concluding that men who consumed about one serving per day of either processed or unprocessed red meat had a greater risk (upto 28 per cent) of heart disease . . .' Ibid.

'They found that people who switched to a plant-based diet had a 10 per cent reduction in their LDL (bad cholesterol) levels, compared to their peers who continued eating a meat-based diet.' Koch, Caroline A., Emilie W. Kjeldsen and Ruth Frikke-Schmidt. 2023. 'Vegetarian or Vegan Diets and Blood Lipids: A Meta-Analysis of Randomized Trials'. *European Heart Journal:* 44(28). https://doi.org/10.1093/eurheartj/ehad211.

'The World Health Organization (WHO) has also listed processed meat as a Group 1 carcinogen.' World Health Organization. 26 October 2015. *Cancer: Carcinogenicity of the Consumption of Red Meat and Processed Meat*. https://www.who.int/news-room/questions-and-answers/item/cancer-carcinogenicity-of-the-consumption-of-red-meat-and-processed-meat.

'Blue Zones . . . primarily eat a 95 per cent plant-based diet.' Buettner, Dan and Sam Skemp. 2016. 'Blue Zones: Lessons from the World's Longest Lived'. *American Journal of Lifestyle Medicine* 10(5): 318–21. https://doi.org/10.1177/1559827616637066.

'In a study published in the *European Journal of Clinical Nutrition*, researchers conducted an eighteen-week experiment with 291 corporate employees.' Mishra, S., J. Xu, U. Agarwal, J. Gonzales, S. Levin and N.D. Barnard. 2013. 'A Multicenter Randomized Controlled Trial of a Plant-Based Nutrition Program to Reduce Body Weight and Cardiovascular Risk in the Corporate Setting: The GEICO Study'. *European Journal of Clinical Nutrition* 67(7): 718–24. https://doi.org/10.1038/ejcn.2013.92.

'For adults leading a moderately active or sedentary lifestyle, the protein needed is 0.83 grams per every kilogram of body weight.' Joint WHO/FAO/UNU Expert Consultation. 2007. 'Protein and Amino Acid Requirements in Human Nutrition'. *World Health Organization Technical Report Series*, 935: 1–265. https://iris.who.int/bitstream/handle/10665/43411/WHO_TRS_935_eng.pdf;jsessionid.

'He trained pigs to play a video game using a joystick.' Helft, Miguel. 1997. 'Pig Video Arcades Critique Life in the Pen'. *Wired*. 6 June 1997. https://www.wired.com/1997/06/pig-video-arcades-critique-life-in-the-pen/.

'From our current scientific understanding, plants cannot experience pain.' Mallatt, Jon, Michael R. Blatt, Andreas Draguhn, David G. Robinson and Lincoln Taiz. 2021. 'Debunking a Myth: Plant Consciousness'. *Protoplasma* 258(3): 459–76. https://doi.org/10.1007/s00709-020-01579-w.

'It's not just the person who does the killing, but also all those involved in the process—those who kill, transport, cook, serve or eat the meat.' Manu-Samhita (5.51–52). Manu's Code of Law: A Critical Edition and Translation of the Mānava-Dharmaśāstra.

Chapter 6: Moo-ving Facts about Milk

'Cow's milk is referred to as 'Amrit'—the elixir of life.' N.V.R. Krishnamacharya. *The Mahabharata:* Anu 65-46, Tirupati: Tirumala Tirupati Devasthanams, 1983.

'*Gashu Amrutam raksha mana,*' meaning 'cow milk is Amrit, it shields us from diseases.' Shakala Samhita *The Rigveda:* 1-71-9 New Delhi: Delhi Vedic Trust, 19901997.

'Milk is sweet, tasty, gives us calmness, and increases vitality within us.' Sutrasthan, *Charak Sutrasthana*, 27/217-218, Dr Brahmanand Tripathi, Chaukhamba Prakashan, Varanasi; 2001.

'Allah has given us a drink from the cattle—pure milk, which is a palatable drink for those who take it.' *The Qur'an*, Surah 16: verse 66.

'Even the Bible mentions milk about forty-eight times in the Old Testament alone, each time in high regard, as something to aspire for.' *The Holy Bible,*

'In fact, as per the findings of Animal Equality India, the calves are separated from their mothers within just a few hours after birth' India, Animal Equality. 'Cow Appreciation Day.' Animal Equality India, 12 July 2022, https://animalequality.in/blog/cow-appreciation-day/.

'To counter this, they are injected with an illegal drug called oxytocin'. 'Dairy's Dark Secrets Exposed'. Animal Equality India. May 25, 2023 https://animalequality.in/news/2023/01/10/animal-equality-investigates-dairy-farms-markets-and-slaughterhouses-exposing-abuse-to-buffaloes/.

'The vast majority of dairy cows are considered 'spent' and no longer useful to the industry by the time they reach around eight years of age.'

Damodaran, Harsh. 2019, January 6. 'Uttar Pradesh's animal farm: The cow count.' *Indian Express.* https://indianexpress.com/article/india/uttar-pradeshs-animal-farm-the-cow-count-yogi-adityanath-beef-ban-slaughterhouse-ban-5524944/.

'But did you know that India is also one of the largest exporters of beef in the world?' The Wire: The Wire News India, 'India Emerges as Second Largest Beef Exporter in the World' March 5, 2024. https://thewire.in/trade/who-are-the-biggest-exporters-of-beef-in-the-world#:~:text=Brazil%20was%20the%20biggest%20exporter,the%20United%20States%20and%20Australiared.com/1997/06/pig-video-arcades-critique-life-in-the-pen/.

'The dairy, meat and leather industry are interdependent. The dairy industry churns out a large number of unproductive animals for slaughter every day, which in turn helps the meat and leather trade thrive. In other words, the meat and leather industry is heavily dependent on the dairy industry for its supply.' Deadly Dairy." n.d. India Deadly Dairy. https://animalequality.in/india-deadly-dairy/.

'They discovered that cows in pain showed significantly higher levels of cortisol (a stress hormone) in their milk.' Gellrich, Katharina, Tanja Sigl, Heinrich H. D. Meyer, and Steffi Wiedemann. 2015. "Cortisol Levels in Skimmed Milk during the First 22 Weeks of Lactation and Response to Short-Term Metabolic Stress and Lameness in Dairy Cows." *Journal of Animal Science and Biotechnology* 6 (1). https://doi.org/10.1186/s40104-015-0035-y.

'Researchers discovered that when cows experience increased stress due to higher temperatures or higher humidity in the dairy farm, it showed in the composition of their milk in the form of increased cortisol levels.' Mohammad, Si Nae Cheon, Geun-woo Park, Eska Nugrahaeningtyas, Jung-Hwan Jeon, and Kyu Hyun Park. 2023. "Assessment of Stress Levels in Lactating Cattle: Analyzing Cortisol Residues in Commercial Milk Products in Relation to the Temperature-Humidity Index." *Animals* 13 (15): 2407–7. https://doi.org/10.3390/ani13152407.

'They discovered that a staggering 68 per cent of the global population suffers from lactose malabsorption." "To break down lactose, our digestive tracts need to produce something called 'lactase.' Lactase is basically an enzyme that is vital for breaking down lactose present in milk, allowing the body to absorb and use it . . .' Storhaug, Christian Løvold, Svein Kjetil Fosse, and Lars T Fadnes. 2017. "Country, Regional, and Global Estimates for Lactose Malabsorption in Adults: A Systematic Review and Meta-Analysis." *The Lancet Gastroenterology & Hepatology* 2 (10): 738–46. https://pubmed.ncbi.nlm.nih.gov/28690131/.

'Researchers found that consuming any amount of dairy each day increases the odds of having acne by 25 per cent. And drinking two or more than two glasses of milk per day increases the odds to 43 per cent.' Juhl, Christian, Helle Bergholdt, Iben Miller, Gregor Jemec, Jørgen Kanters, and Christina Ellervik. 2018. "Dairy Intake and Acne Vulgaris: A Systematic Review and Meta-Analysis of 78,529 Children, Adolescents, and Young Adults." *Nutrients* 10 (8): 1049. https://doi. org/10.3390/nu10081049.

Chapter 7: How to Sleep Smarter at Night to Achieve More in the Day

'As a result, it is during sleep that wounds heal, old skin cells are replaced with new ones, our immune system actively defends against external threats, and the body undergoes thorough healing.' Adam, K. and I. Oswald. 1984. 'Sleep Helps Healing'. *BMJ* 289 (6456): 1400–01. https://doi.org/10.1136/bmj.289.6456.1400.

'An article published in the journal *Sleep* performed a fascinating study on the impact of sleep on the immune system and its effectiveness in fighting off the common cold.' Prather, Aric A., Denise Janicki-Deverts, Martica H. Hall and Sheldon Cohen. 2015. 'Behaviorally Assessed Sleep and Susceptibility to the Common Cold'. *Sleep* 38(9): 1353–59. https://doi.org/10.5665/sleep.4968.

'The researchers discovered that our glymphatic system actually becomes ten times more active during sleep, than when we're awake.' Xie, L. et al. 2013. 'Sleep Drives Metabolite Clearance from the Adult Brain'. *Science* 342(6156): 373–77. https://doi.org/10.1126/science.1241224.

'This, in turn, can lead to various neurological disorders, starting from small problems such as fogginess in the brain and lack of focus in our work, to bigger disorders over time, such as Alzheimer's and dementia.' Reddy, Oliver Cameron and Ysbrand D. van der Werf. 2020. 'The Sleeping Brain: Harnessing the Power of the Glymphatic System through Lifestyle Choices'. *Brain Sciences* 10(11): 868. https://doi.org/10.3390/brainsci10110868.

'Why, according to a recent Nielsen survey conducted on over 5600 people across twenty-five cities, do 93 per cent of Indians suffer from sleep deprivation?' Punj, Deepshikha. 2013. 'Understanding sleep afresh'. *The New Indian Express.* https://www.newindianexpress.com/magazine/2013/Jul/28/understanding-sleep-afresh-501056.html#:~:text=In%20a%20recent%20study%20conducted%20by%20AC,in%20concentration%20due%20to%20sleep%20deprivation%20and

'Why is India the second most sleep-deprived country in the world?' Sharma, Kalpana. 2023. 'India is the second most sleep deprived country: What we can do to fix our sleep habits'. *The Times of India.* https://timesofindia.indiatimes.com/life-style/health-fitness/health-news/india-is-the-second-most-sleep-deprived-country-what-we-can-do-to-fix-our-sleep-habits/articleshow/98728738.cms

'When the blue light from gadgets hits our eyeballs, it's as if our brain receives an alternate message, "Hold off on the melatonin! It's still daylight out there, not time to sleep yet!".' West, Kathleen E. et al. 2011. 'Blue Light from Light-Emitting Diodes Elicits a Dose-Dependent Suppression of Melatonin in Humans'. *Journal of Applied Physiology* 110(3): 619–26. https://doi.org/10.1152/japplphysiol.01413.2009.

'We now consume as much data in a day as an average person in the fifteenth century would have absorbed in an entire lifetime!' Kwik, Jim. 2020. *Limitless.* Hay House Inc.

'This not only keeps our minds on high alert, preventing us from sinking into deep sleep, but also makes that negativity seep into our subconscious mind.' Levenson, Jessica C. et al. 2017. 'Social Media Use before Bed and Sleep Disturbance among Young Adults in the

United States: A Nationally Representative Study'. *Sleep* 40(9). https://doi.org/10.1093/sleep/zsx113.

'There is no possibility of one becoming a yogi, O Arjuna, if one eats too much, or eats too little, sleeps too much or does not sleep enough.' Dvaipayana Krishna, Bhagavad Gita.

Chapter 8: Three Unknown Secrets of Waking Up Early

'In our Vedic scriptures, this period of time is referred to as the Brahma Muhurta. 'Brahma' signifies the Creator, and 'Muhurta' translates to Time.' Agni Purāṇa, Chapter 155. | Aṣṭāṅgahṛdayasaṃhitā (Sūtrasthāna), Vāgbhaṭa. Verse 2.1.

'You Gain Access to Your Creative Genius Thoughts.' Bowles, Nicole P. et al. November 2022. 'The Circadian System Modulates the Cortisol Awakening Response in Humans'. *Frontiers in Neuroscience* 16. https://doi.org/10.3389/fnins.2022.995452.

'In an insightful study conducted by scientists at Aachen University, researchers conducted brain scans on fifty-nine people.' Rosenberg, Jessica, Ivan I. Maximov, Martina Reske, Farida Grinberg and N. Jon Shah. January 2014. '"Early to Bed, Early to Rise": Diffusion Tensor Imaging Identifies Chronotype-Specificity'. *NeuroImage* 84: 428–34. https://doi.org/10.1016/j.neuroimage.2013.07.086.

'One fascinating discovery made by psychologist Csikszentmihalyi in his research is that people are at their most productive when they are in a state of flow.' Csikszentmihalyi, M. and I.S. Csikszentmihalyi (Eds). (1992). *Optimal experience: Psychological Studies of Flow in Consciousness*. Cambridge University Press. https://psycnet.apa.org/record/1988-98551-000.

'In essence, the flow state multiples the impact of any action.' Goh, Grace, Shane Maloney, Peter Mark and Dominique Blache. 2019. 'Episodic Ultradian Events—Ultradian Rhythms'. *Biology* 8(1): 15. https://doi.org/10.3390/biology8010015.

'The Visitor Who Knocks on Our Window Every Morning.' Gupta, Mohan 2017. *Rogo Se Bachav*. India: Natural Life Style.

Chapter 9: Move, Breathe, Celebrate

'Research studies clearly show a direct correlation between a person's health and the level of oxygen in their bloodstream.' Mairbäurl, Heimo. 2013. 'Red Blood Cells in Sports: Effects of Exercise and Training on Oxygen Supply by Red Blood Cells'. *Frontiers in Physiology* 4: 332. https://doi.org/10.3389/fphys.2013.00332.

'The growth of cancer cells is initiated by a relative lack of oxygen, and how cancer cannot live in an oxygen-rich environment.' The Nobel Prize in Physiology or Medicine 1931. n.d. 'Otto Warburg Biographical'. https://www.nobelprize.org/prizes/medicine/1931/warburg/biographical/, accessed 1 March 2024.

'Through sweat, you're getting rid of toxins and waste products, creating a cleaner internal environment.' Kuan, Wen-Hui, Yi-Lang Chen and Chao-Lin Liu. 2022. 'Excretion of Ni, Pb, Cu, As, and Hg in Sweat under Two Sweating Conditions'. *International Journal of Environmental Research and Public Health* 19(7): 4323. https://doi.org/10.3390/ijerph19074323.

'Movement is a direct way to drastically improve digestion.' Monda, Vincenzo et al. 2017. 'Exercise Modifies the Gut Microbiota with Positive Health Effects'. *Oxidative Medicine and Cellular Longevity* 2017: 1–8. https://doi.org/10.1155/2017/3831972.

'A single workout makes your brain immediately release dopamine, adrenaline and serotonin.' Lin, Tzu-Wei and Yu-Min Kuo. 2013. 'Exercise Benefits Brain Function: The Monoamine Connection'. *Brain Sciences* 3(4): 39–53. https://doi.org/10.3390/brainsci3010039.

'They discovered that exercising for four or more days per week was linked not only to significant reductions in sadness among these students but it also resulted in a 23 per cent reduction in suicide attempts among bullied students!' Sibold, Jeremy, Erika Edwards, Dianna Murray-Close and James J. Hudziak. 2015. 'Physical Activity, Sadness, and Suicidality in Bullied US Adolescents'. *Journal of the American Academy of Child & Adolescent Psychiatry* 54(10): 808–15. https://doi.org/10.1016/j.jaac.2015.06.019.

Chapter 10: Switch Off That Running AC inside You

'According to a WHO study conducted in twenty-four countries, 70 per cent of people reported experiencing one or the other kind of emotional trauma in their lives.' Benjet, C. et al. 2016. 'The Epidemiology of Traumatic Event Exposure Worldwide: Results from the World Mental Health Survey Consortium'. *Psychological Medicine* 46(02): 327–43. https://doi.org/10.1017/s0033291715001981.

'Our emotions actually have the power to change the biology of our body.' Yaribeygi, Habib et al. 2017. 'The Impact of Stress on Body Function: A Review'. *EXCLI Journal* 16(1): 1057–72. https://doi.org/10.17179/excli2017-480.

'The study shows how greatly our emotional state influences our immunity to illness, as well as our overall physical state.' Rosenkranz, M.A. et al. 2003. 'Affective Style and in Vivo Immune Response: Neurobehavioral Mechanisms'. *Proceedings of the National Academy of Sciences* 100(19): 11148–52. https://doi.org/10.1073/pnas.1534743100.

'If you have an unresolved relationship in your life, you may be unknowingly paying the price for it without even realizing it. The price you're paying is not in terms of money but something even more precious—your praanshakti, your life energy, your health.' Felitti, Vincent J. et al. 1998. 'Relationship of Childhood Abuse and Household Dysfunction to Many of the Leading Causes of Death in Adults'. *American Journal of Preventive Medicine* 14(4): 245–58. https://doi.org/10.1016/s0749-3797(98)00017-8.

'To a great extent, this act of expression naturally enables us to let go of these emotional burdens.' Pennebaker, James W. 1997. 'Writing about Emotional Experiences as a Therapeutic Process'. *Psychological Science* 8(3): 162–66. https://doi.org/10.1111/j.1467-9280.1997.tb00403.x.

'I realized that when you release unresolved relationships, even with just one person, you start to experience a significant lightness and joy in your being.' Song, Yiying et al. 2014. 'Regulating Emotion to Improve Physical Health through the Amygdala'. *Social Cognitive and Affective Neuroscience* 10(4): 523–30. https://doi.org/10.1093/scan/nsu083.

Chapter 11: The Most Precious Gift You Can Ever Give Anyone

'The Golden Rule: Seek First to Understand before Being Understood'. Covey, Stephen R. (1989) 2020. *7 Habits of Highly Effective People.* Simon & Schuster Ltd.

'If they believe you'll accept them unconditionally despite what they reveal—rather than criticizing, advising or ridiculing…' Itzchakov, Guy, Netta Weinstein, Dvori Saluk and Moty Amar. June 2022. 'Connection Heals Wounds: Feeling Listened to Reduces Speakers' Loneliness Following a Social Rejection Disclosure'. *Personality and Social Psychology Bulletin* 49(8). https://doi.org/10.1177/01461672221100369.

'And when they do open up, it initiates a soul-to-soul connection.' They feel safe enough to reveal their innermost petals—their most delicate, innermost and tender feelings.' Kawamichi, Hiroaki et al. 2014. 'Perceiving Active Listening Activates the Reward System and Improves the Impression of Relevant Experiences'. *Social Neuroscience* 10(1): 16–26. https://doi.org/10.1080/17470919.2014.954732.

'People tend to open up rapidly when they sense a genuine desire to understand them from the other person.' Kluger, Avraham N. and Guy Itzchakov. 2022. 'The Power of Listening at Work'. *Annual Review of Organizational Psychology and Organizational Behavior* 9(1): 121–46. https://doi.org/10.1146/annurev-orgpsych-012420-091013.

'Lord Krishna's Example'. Dvaipayana Krishna, Bhagavad Gita, Chapters 1–2.

'Deep listening is the foundation of right speech.' Nhất Hạnh, Thích. 2015. *The Heart of the Buddha's Teaching: Transforming Suffering into Peace, Joy and Liberation: The Four Noble Truths, the Noble Eightfold Path, and Other Basic Buddhist Teachings.* New York: Harmony Books.

'The one who gives an answer before he listens—this is foolishness and disgrace for him.' *Holy Bible,* Proverbs, 18:13 (ESV).

Chapter 12: Your Purpose Is Waiting for You

'Researchers have discovered that there's another surprising element that's just as important. It's not about food. It's not about exercise. It's something more intangible.' Buettner, Dan and Sam Skemp. 2016. 'Blue Zones: Lessons from the World's Longest Lived'. *American Journal of Lifestyle Medicine* 10(5): 318–21. https://doi.org/10.1177/1559827616637066.

'A study published by the *American Journal of Health Promotion* in 2022, which took data from approximately 13,000 participants, asked them to complete a questionnaire to determine their subjective sense of 'purpose in life'.' Kim, Eric S. et al. 2021. 'Sense of Purpose in Life and Subsequent Physical, Behavioral, and Psychosocial Health: An Outcome-Wide Approach'. *American Journal of Health Promotion* 36(1). https://doi.org/10.1177/08901171211038545.

'Each of you should use whatever gift you have received to serve others, as faithful stewards of God's grace in its various forms.' *Holy Bible*, 1 Peter, 4:10 (NIV).

Chapter 13: How to Stay Calm during Any Chaos

'If we could handle everything, from the smallest to the steepest lows of our life, with grace, courage and an attitude of surrender, we could free ourselves from so much existing and future stress, and thus live a life of bliss, joy and peak health.' O'Connor, Daryl B., Julian F. Thayer and Kavita Vedhara. 2020. 'Stress and Health: A Review of Psychobiological Processes'. *Annual Review of Psychology* 72(1): 663–88. https://doi.org/10.1146/annurev-psych-062520-122331.

'It's the final key of the Satvic revolution.' Butler, Jodie and Joseph Ciarrochi. 2007. 'Psychological Acceptance and Quality of Life in the Elderly'. *Quality of Life Research* 16(4): 607–15. https://doi.org/10.1007/s11136-006-9149-1.

Scan QR code to access the
Penguin Random House India website